Pediatric Orthopedics
A Guide for the Primary Care Physician

CRITICAL ISSUES IN DEVELOPMENTAL AND BEHAVIORAL PEDIATRICS

SERIES EDITOR: MARVIN I. GOTTLIEB, M.D., Ph.D.
Hackensack Medical Center
Hackensack, New Jersey
and University of Medicine and Dentistry of New Jersey—
New Jersey Medical School
Newark, New Jersey

DEVELOPMENTAL-BEHAVIORAL DISORDERS· Selected Topics
Volumes 1–3
Edited by Marvin I. Gottlieb, M.D., Ph.D., and John E Williams, M D.

PEDIATRIC COMPLIANCE: A Guide for the Primary Care Physician
Edward R. Christophersen, Ph.D.

PEDIATRIC ORTHOPEDICS: A Guide for the Primary Care Physician
Richard J. Mier, M.D , and Thomas D. Brower, M.D.

PRACTITIONER'S GUIDE TO DEVELOPMENTAL AND
PSYCHOLOGICAL TESTING
Glen P. Aylward, Ph.D

A Continuation Order Plan is available for this series A continuation order will bring delivery of each new volume immediately upon publication Volumes are billed only upon actual shipment For further information please contact the publisher

Pediatric Orthopedics
A Guide for the Primary Care Physician

Richard J. Mier, M.D.
University of Kentucky, and
Shriners Hospital for Crippled Children
Lexington, Kentucky

Thomas D. Brower, M.D.
University of Kentucky
Lexington, Kentucky

With Contributions by
Brian T. Carney, M.D.
David B. Stevens, M.D.

Springer Science+Business Media, LLC

Library of Congress Cataloging in Publication Data

Mier, Richard J.
  Pediatric orthopedics: a guide for the primary care physician / Richard J. Mier
and Thomas D. Brower; with contributions by Brian T. Carney, David B. Stevens.
     p.   cm.—(Critical issues in developmental and behavioral pediatrics)
  Includes bibliographical references and index.
  ISBN 978-1-4613-6080-3   ISBN 978-1-4615-2534-9 (eBook)
  DOI 10.1007/978-1-4615-2534-9
  1. Pediatric orthopedics. I. Brower, Thomas D. II. Title. III. Series.
  [DNLM: 1. Orthopedics—in infancy & childhood. WS 270 M632p 1994]
RD732.3.C48M54 1994
617.3'0083—dc20
DNLM/DLC   94-34760
for Library of Congress   CIP

ISBN 978-1-4613-6080-3

©1994 Springer Science+Business Media New York
Originally published by Plenum Publishing Corporation in 1994
Softcover reprint of the hardcover 1st edition 1994

Plenum Medical Book Company is an imprint of Plenum Publishing Corporation

To Rita, Kate, and Lizzie

—RJM

To Hania Kalinowski Brower

—TDB

Preface

Musculoskeletal problems are common in pediatric primary care and we have always found them interesting and fun to deal with. The primary care physician, someone who knows the child and the family, is in an excellent position to provide the initial evaluation of the child with a musculoskeletal complaint. This is true more than ever today as pediatricians and family practitioners assume an expanded role. As government does its best to restrict the number of specialist orthopedists, generalists will need to do more.

Unfortunately, many residency programs in primary care specialties do not provide the education in pediatric orthopedics necessary to do a good job. This book is our attempt to provide a solution to this educational problem. We have written it for generalists taking care of children and for trainees in pediatric and family practice residencies. It is not, obviously, an attempt to duplicate excellent and encyclopedic texts available. Rather, we are here trying to provide a framework for the effective evaluation of childhood musculoskeletal problems in a practical and problem-based manner. We hope it is useful and would be happy to hear from readers who see ways in which we could make it better.

We would like to express our thanks to the many souls who have helped us in this endeavor, including Drs. Nathan Hasson, Katie Tripp, Vesna Kriss, Al Selke, Rob Fulbrigge, Peter Wong, Sheila Woods, Patricia Woo, Madeleine Rooney, Daniel Lovell, Robert Rennebom, Holly Cintas, David Stevens, Keith VandenBrink, Brian Carney, Jerry Anderson, Janet Walker, Kevin Nelson, and Bryan Hall. Thanks go also to Tammy Anderson for her illustrations, Jean Garvey for her photographs, Susan Wagers for her technical advice, Peggy Meyers and her staff, Michael Garvey, Katie Garvey, Claire Garvey, Emily Wachs, and Julio Gaspar. Finally, thanks to all of the hardworking staff at Plenum Publishing Corporation.

Richard J. Mier
Thomas D. Brower

Lexington, Kentucky

Contents

1

The Orthopedic Examination

1.1. INTRODUCTION

The effective evaluation of any child with musculoskeletal difficulties requires attention to the story the family has to tell and a thorough physical exam. The frequency of nonorganic or nonspecific causes for problems of this nature is high. Even when specific organic causes are present, their subtlety of manifestation is such that a "shotgun" or undirected approach to diagnosis is often frustrating and expensive and can even be dangerous.

A thorough history and physical exam is not only the best way to make the diagnosis but is also an excellent way to demonstrate to the family that you as their physician are taking their child's problems seriously when, as often happens, no apparent organic cause becomes evident. Under these circumstances, their trust in you becomes extremely important if it becomes necessary to counsel watchful nonaction.

It is often necessary to explain to families that physicians are at their best when excluding diagnoses (as in "I'm sure he doesn't have cancer, polio, or arthritis") but that we are frequently unable to explain exactly what the child *does* have. A compulsive history and physical exam with several simple laboratory exams will do more to establish the trust necessary for parents to accept your explanation that nothing serious is at hand

1

than all the sophisticated laboratory and radiological evaluations available at your local hospital. Such trust is essential since many musculoskeletal problems require a longitudinal approach to diagnosis, with the child returning for follow-up and more sophisticated diagnostics over time if the problem persists.

1.2. CHILDREN ARE DIFFERENT

Not only are children different from adults, they are different one from another. The toe-walking of 12-month-olds should not be expected in 24-month-olds. What is a normal serum phosphorus for a 2-year-old (4.5–6.5 mg/dl) is not normal for a 22-year-old (3.5–4.5 mg/dl). An appreciation of the constancy of change in childhood is not only necessary to tell normal from abnormal but it makes things interesting as well.

Hip disease, for example, brings to mind different sets of explanations when it occurs in a 2-year-old than in a 12-year-old. A reluctance to treat children as developing organisms is a major impediment to their care.

1.3. THE GENERAL PHYSICAL EXAMINATION

In this chapter the details of the orthopedic examination will be reviewed. Before we do so, however, several aspects of the general pediatric examination that relate to musculoskeletal pathology merit mention:

1. General appearance: is this an ill-appearing child who is pale and listless, febrile, or hypertensive?
2. Weight: any recent loss, decreased subcutaneous tissue? What is the weight percentile for age?
3. Height: short (rickets, skeletal dysplasia, thyroid dysfunction, chronic inflammation), or tall (Marfan's)? What is the height percentile for age?
4. HEENT: signs of iritis (conjunctival reaction, corneal clouding, cataract), mucous membrane ulceration (SLE), or lymphadenopathy (neoplasia, collagen vascular disease)?
5. Cardiovascular: murmur (valvular insufficiency, endocarditis), rub, myocardial dysfunction or failure?
6. Abdomen: organomegaly (collagen vascular disease), or mass (neuroblastoma)?
7. Skin: café-au-lait spots, neurofibromata, heliotrope (the purple eyelid rash of dermatomyositis), nailbed telangiectasia (dermatomyositis), erythema chronicum migrans (the "bull's-eye" rash of Lyme disease), erythema marginatum (of acute rheumatic fever), purpura, other rashes?
8. CNS: weakness related to myopathy or neuropathy [muscle strength is graded on a five-point scale (the MRC Scale): 5 = normal strength; 4 = somewhat decreased; 3 = weaker, but moves against gravity; 2 = moves, but not against gravity; 1 = no movement but contraction visible; 0 = no movement whatsoever], hyperreflexia, atrophy, tonal abnormalities, loss of vibratory or position sense (Charcot–Marie–Tooth)?

9. Genitalia: pubertal development (relevant to prognosis for scoliosis or for predictions regarding leg length discrepancies), genital lesions of Reiter syndrome or gonorrhea?

1.4. THE ORTHOPEDIC EXAMINATION

To do this you need to know how. And to know how, a quick brushup on terminology is essential. Orthopedic consultants love to dazzle with a little "valgus" here and a little "cavus" there. Arm yourself with the list below.

Abduction: the lateral movement of the arms or legs from the median plane of the body; the outward movement of the fingers from the axial line of the hand which runs along the third metacarpal.

Acromelia: One type of short limb in which the distal part of the limb is short.

Adduction: the movement of an extremity toward the median plane of the body; the opposite of abduction.

Amelia: complete failure of limb formation.

Apophysis: any secondary growth center from the main body of a bone which does not participate in a joint. Traction on immature apophyses causes a variety of painful conditions (Osgood–Schlatter disease among them).

Axial: referring (usually) to the axes of the extremities in the "anatomical position." Preaxial refers to the radial and postaxial to the ulnar side of the hand and forearm. Axial also refers to the major joints of the central skeleton, including those of the chest, spine, and pelvis. Spondylarthritides typically affect axial joints, as opposed to peripheral joints.

Calcaneus: referring to the heel bone; often used to describe a deformity such that the foot is held in fixed dorsiflexion with the patient walking on their heel alone.

Cavus: abnormally arched foot (the opposite of planus).

Coxa: referring to the hip.

Cubitus: referring to the elbow.

Diaphysis: the middle or shaft portion of a long bone.

Dorsal: when referring to the spine, dorsal means the same thing as thoracic.

Dorsiflexion: referring to extension at the wrist or ankle (see Extension).

Epiphyseal Growth Plate: the growth plate, or **physis**, separates the epiphysis from the metaphysis and represents the site of primary longitudinal growth.

Epiphysis: present at the ends of long bones (the phalanges have only proximal epiphyses), the epiphyses are sites of secondary ossification which participate in a joint and become apparent radiologically at different ages, depending on the epiphysis involved. The proximal epiphysis of the femur (really the cartilaginous femoral head) is not visible radiologically at birth, though the distal one is. The epiphysis of each long bone is eventually fused to the metaphysis at the time of skeletal maturity.

Equinus: referring to a plantarflexed position or deformity of the foot such that the individual in question walks on their toes.

Extension: in general, referring to the straightening of the two bones at a joint. However, sometimes used at the wrist and ankle to mean the opposite of palmar or

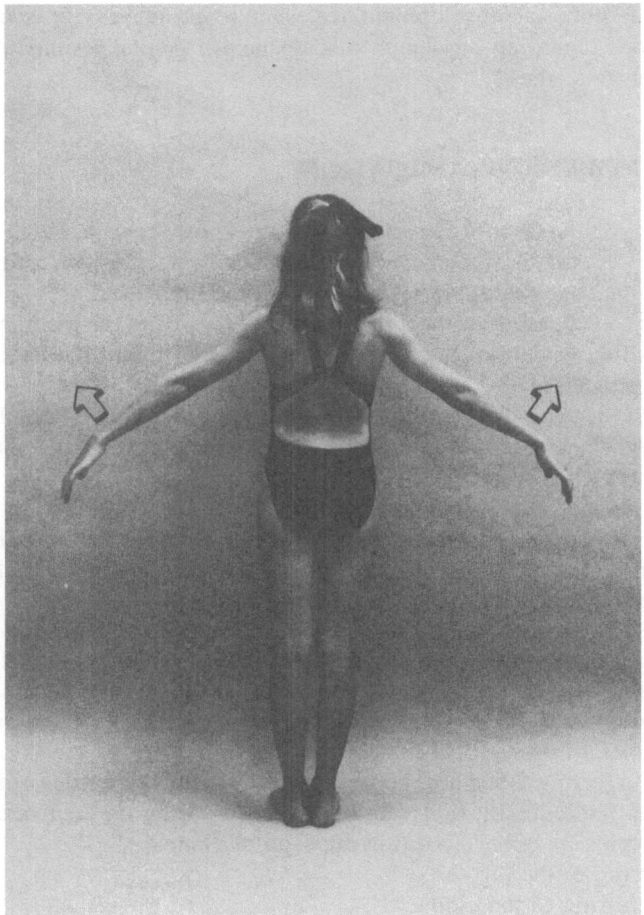

Figure 1.1. Abduction, in this case shoulder abduction, means movement away from the midline

plantar flexion (see Dorsiflexion). Extension of the spine is what you do when you bend backwards. Extension of the shoulder is movement of the arm posteriorly along a plane parallel to the sagittal plane.

   Flexion: bending at a joint or of the trunk. Implying palmarflexion or plantarflexion when referring to wrists or ankles, respectively. Flexion of the spine is what one does when bending forward. Flexion of the shoulders is movement of the arm anteriorly along a plane parallel to the sagittal plane.

   Genu: referring to the knee.

   Gibbus: a humpback deformity; an acute angular deformity of the spine.

   Hemimelia: a congenital longitudinal amputation of a limb, rather than a trans-

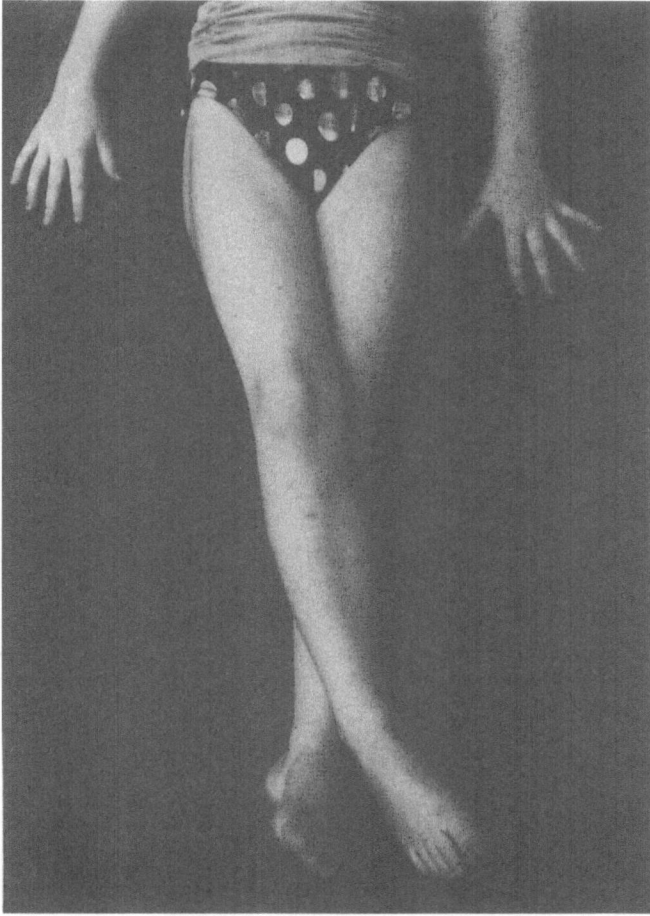

Figure 1.2. Adduction, here of the child's right lower extremity, means movement toward the midline

verse one. Fibular hemimelia is absence of the fibula, deformity of the tibia, and variable absence of the lateral rays of the foot.

Kyphosis: the posterior convex curvature of the thoracic (dorsal) spine. Everyone normally has some thoracic kyphosis. Kyphosis can be used to describe pathology if the curve is excessive or if it affects the cervical or lumbar spine, where posterior convex curves are abnormal.

Leg: that part of the lower limb from the foot to the knee.

Lordosis: the anterior convex curvature of the lumbar spine. Lordosis can be used to describe pathology if the curve is excessive or if it affects the thoracic spine (where there is normally a kyphosis).

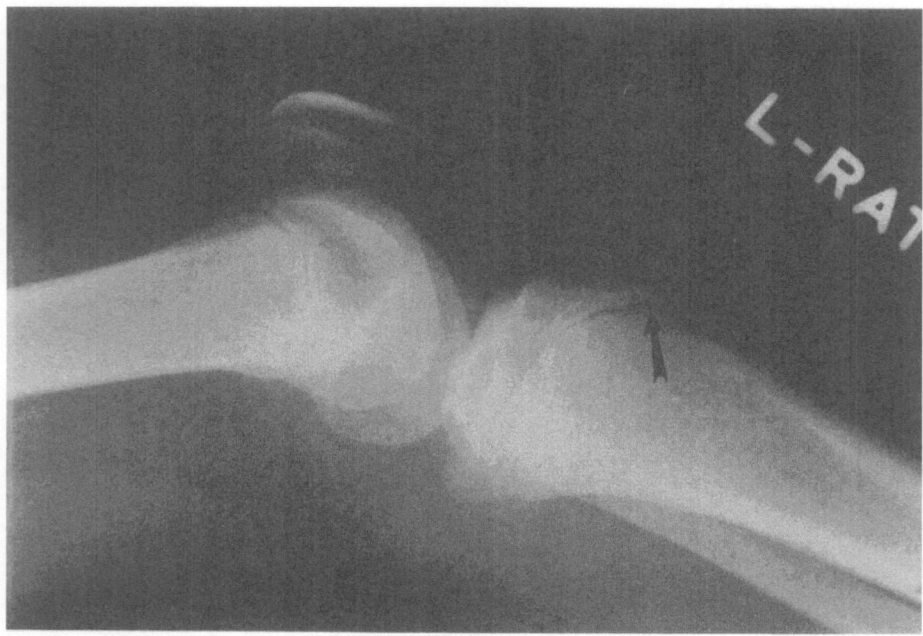

Figure 1.3. Tibial tubercle apophysis (arrowhead) here is more prominent than normal because this is a lateral radiograph of an adolescent with Osgood–Schlatter disease or traction apophysitis of the anterior tibial tubercle (see also Chapter 2)

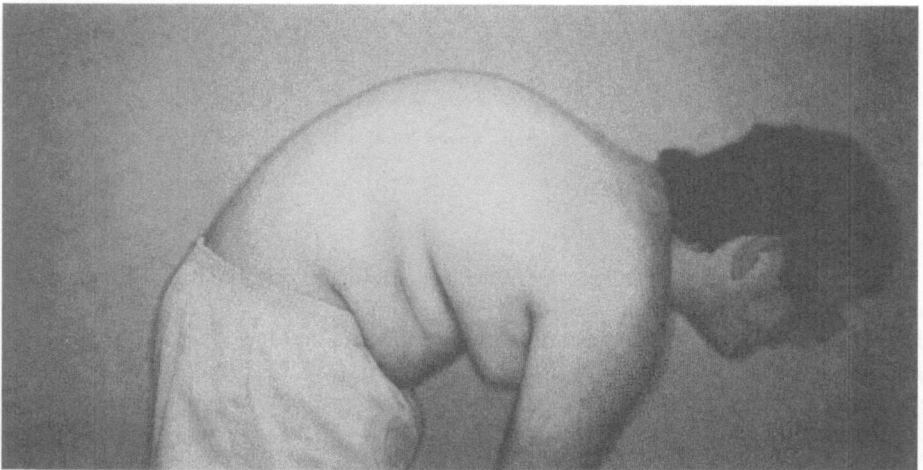

Figure 1.4. Thoracic kyphosis in an adolescent boy caused by Scheuermann disease Lots of adolescents have postural kyphosis or roundback If the kyphotic curve persists in forward bending, as pictured here, a true structural problem may be present (see also Chapter 9)

Mesomelia: one type of micromelia or short limb in which the deficiency is in the midsection of the limb; see also Rhizomelia and Acromelia.

Metaphysis: located between the physis (or epiphyseal growth plate) and the diaphysis, the metaphysis is the flared portion of the long bone in which the calcified cartilage from the physis is replaced by enchondral bone.

Pes: referring to the foot.

Phocomelia: a type of limb deficiency in which the proximal elements are missing and the distal elements arise directly from the trunk.

Physis: the preferred name for the epiphyseal growth plate. Located between the epiphysis and the metaphysis, the physis is the locus for longitudinal growth.

Planus: flat; as in pes planus.

Pronation: the act of becoming prone. When referring to the hand, pronation is turning the palm down; when referring to the forefoot, pronation basically means eversion.

Rhizomelia: one type of micromelia or short limb deformity characterized by maximum shortening of the proximal portion (or root) of the limb.

Supination: the act of becoming supine; when referring to the hand, the act of turning the palm up.

Talipes: the general term for foot deformities, the most prominent being talipes equinovarus (toe down, forefoot medially rotated, ankle in varus), the most well-known kind of clubfoot deformity.

Valgus: angulation of an extremity at a joint with the more distal part angled away from the midline.

Varus: angulation of an extremity at a joint with the more distal part angled toward the midline.

Volar: referring to palm or sole. Volar flexion is the same as palmar flexion or plantar flexion.

1.4.1. The Orthopedic Gestalt

Before we turn to the details of the local orthopedic exam, attention to some general aspects of the orthopedic exam is in order:

1. Is atrophy present? Is it longitudinal or circumferential? Sometimes it can't be seen by the naked eye and one needs a tape measure. Atrophy implies chronic disuse and should be looked for carefully in all children with extremity complaints.

2. Is asymmetry present? Remember that atrophy is not the only cause for unequal extremity sizes. Most times one leg is abnormally small but sometimes one leg is abnormally large. How to tell hemiatrophy from hemihypertrophy? This is difficult often (see below).

3. Are the extremities proportional to the child's size? Remember that the distance from the pubis to the floor (lower segment) should equal the distance from the pubis to the top of the head (upper segment) in all children age 11 years or older. The midpoint for younger children is more superior the younger the child. This upper segment/lower segment ratio changes from 1.7 at birth to 1.3 at 3 years to 1.0 at 11 years and beyond. In

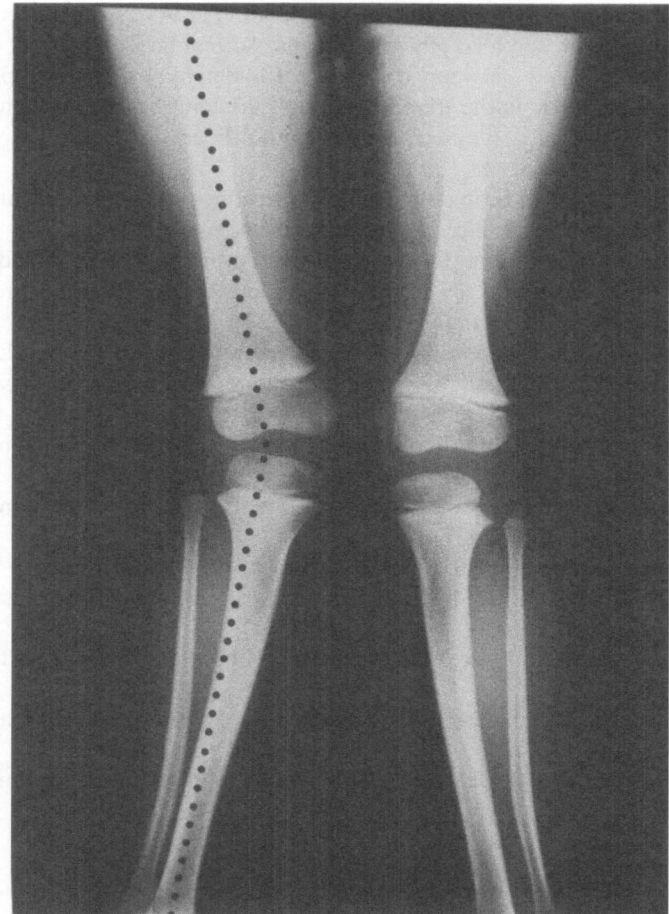

Figure 1.5. The genu valgum apparent on this radiograph measures 25° on the right, 15° on the left

school-aged children, therefore, pubis-to-floor distance should be roughly half of total height. If the asymmetrical lower extremity in question is compared with the expectable length (based on the above), it is possible sometimes to decide if the shorter extremity is atrophic or if the longer extremity is hypertrophic. Intervention in either case is different so the decision is not an academic one (see leg length discrepancy).

4. Also, remember that our arm span is roughly equal to our height (recall Leonarda da Vinci's drawing of the man in a circle?), though not quite. Our extremities are a little short early on (from birth to about 7 years) such that subtracting height from arm span equals about −3 cm. From 7 to 12 years, height and arm span are about equal. Thereafter, arm span is slightly greater than height, between 1 and 4 cm.

5. If the child is ambulatory, how does he walk? Ambulation can be somewhat simplistically divided into: **stance**, **push-off**, and **swing-through** phases. These are

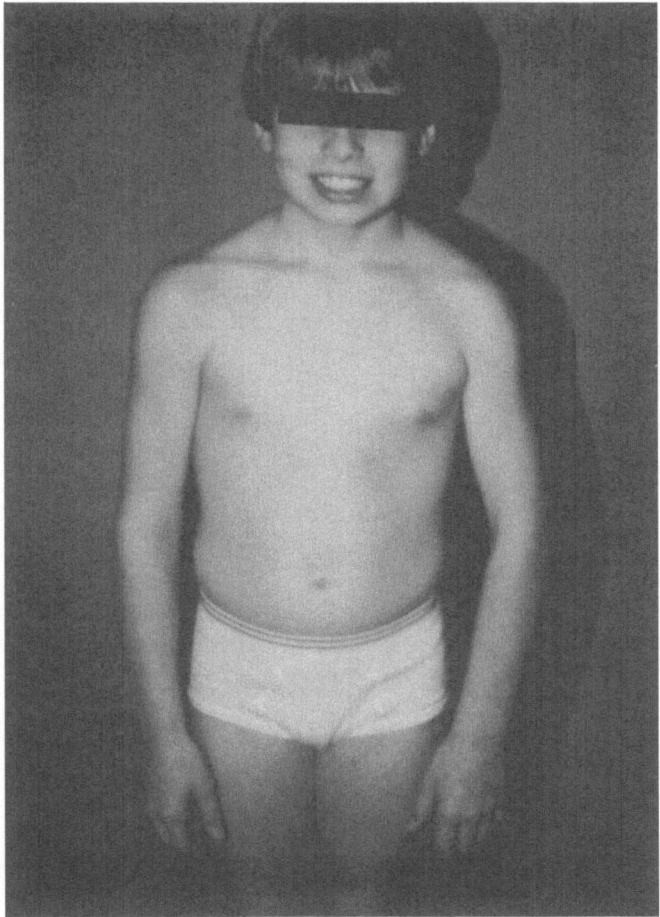

Figure 1.6. Atrophy is sometimes difficult to see unless you look for it This young man incurred a brachial plexus injury at birth, resulting in a flaccid weakness and both longitudinal and circumferential atrophy of the left upper extremity

obviously reciprocating motions such that when we are in the stance phase on one leg, we are swinging through on the contralateral leg

It's important to remember also that gait, like everything else in pediatrics, is a developmental process. The gait of a toddler is qualitatively different from that of an adult or even an older child. The toddler's gait is widely based, often with the feet placed lateral to the lateral margins of the pelvis. While the initiation of the stance phase in the gait of an adult begins with a heel strike, the toddler will instead have a midfoot or even a toe strike to begin the stance phase and may, in fact, remain on his toes throughout the stance phase.

Watch the child walk (a mandatory part of any pediatric exam). Is the gait smoothly

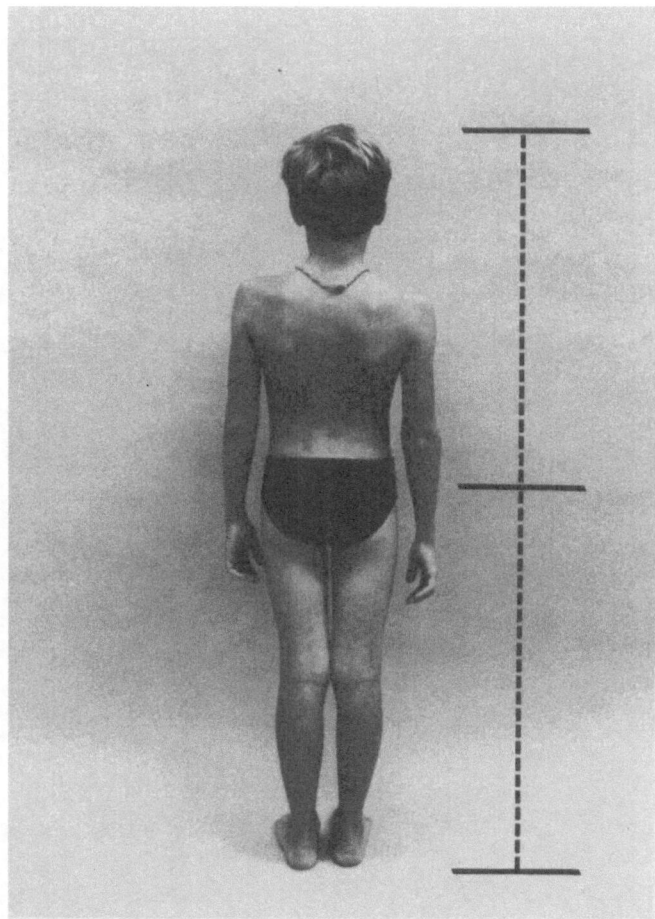

Figure 1.7. Note upper segment and lower segment symmetry. Note also that the shoulders, scapulae, and pelvis are horizontal and that the distances from the boy's sides to the inner aspects of his elbows are equal bilaterally

reciprocal? Is there any asymmetry? Having the child run may be useful since it will accentuate the gait abnormality. Abnormal gaits may be categorized as described below.

Abnormal Gait Patterns

Antalgic: to avoid pain during weight bearing the child may shorten the stance phase. This asymmetrical gait results from a large number of painful inflammatory, traumatic, or degenerative conditions and will result in an asymmetrical gait with a shorter stance phase on one side than the other.

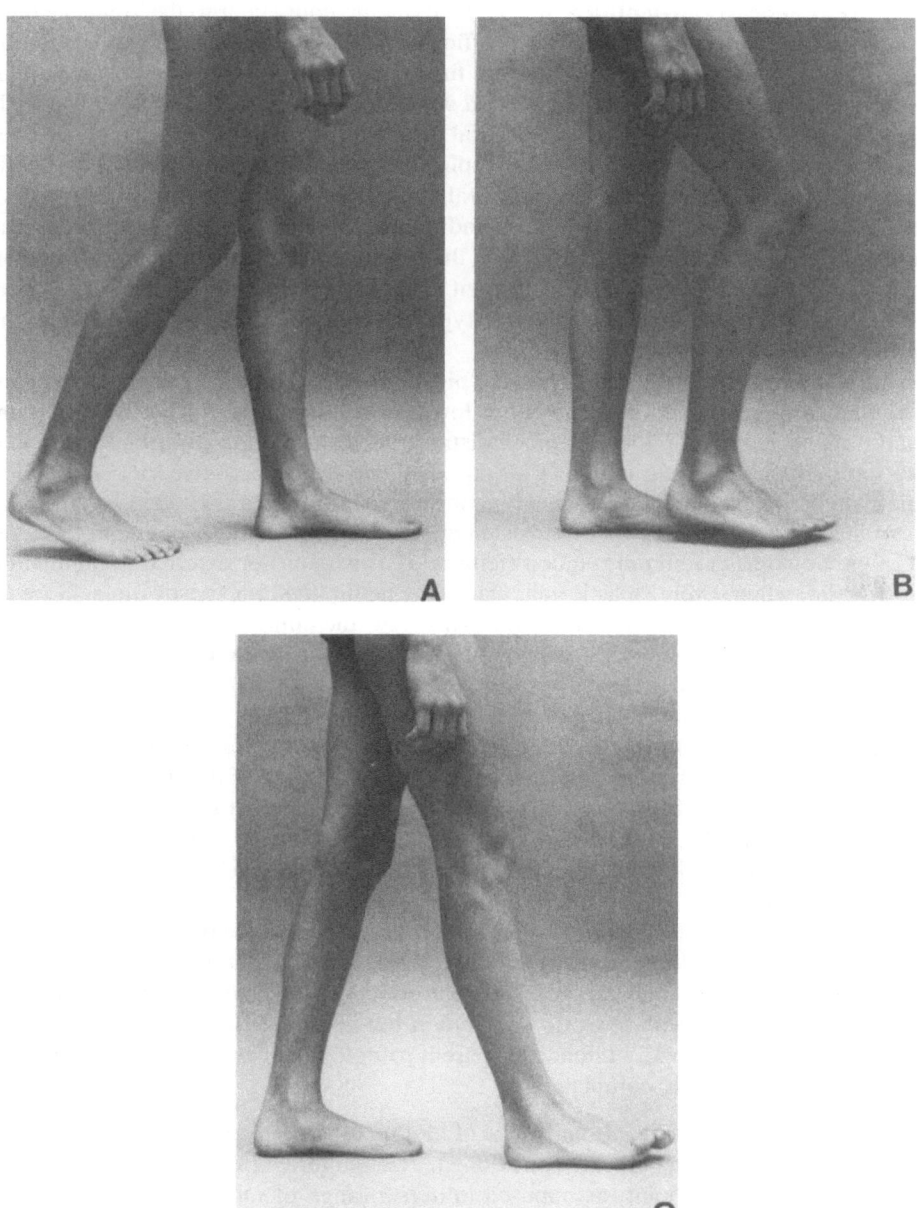

Figure 1.8. Normal gait exhibiting stance phase on the left and push-off on the right (A), leading to swing-through on the right (B) and heel strike on the right (C) Note active dorsiflexion of foot and ankle during heel strike (C) and reciprocal upper and lower extremity movements (A, B)

Lurching or Trendelenburg: this is the dynamic equivalent to the Trendelenburg test and reflects weakness or decreased efficiency of the hip abductors. When in the stance phase, the abductors on that side are firing maximally to keep the pelvis more or less horizontal and allow for unencumbered swing-through on the contralateral side. If the abductors for some reason (developmental dysplasia of the hip, Legg–Calve–Perthes disease, slipped capital femoral epiphysis, spina bifida) are less than effective, the pelvis will be inclined to droop and the contralateral leg will not be able to "pass underneath" without stubbing the toe. To avoid this, the individual will lean laterally during the stance phase *toward* the affected side to "hike up" the pelvis, allow the other limb to clear, and provide for a more favorable center of gravity over the affected hip. When this occurs bilaterally in such conditions as Duchenne-type muscular dystrophy or spina bifida, the child will exhibit a waddling gait.

Intoeing or outtoeing: if the child is "pigeon-toed," do the kneecaps point toward each other (implying rotation of the entire lower extremity at the hip) or do they point straight ahead (implying rotation more distally because of internal tibial torsion or metatarsus adductus)? If the child is walking, they will have a negative foot progression angle, which is the angle made by the line of direction the child is headed and the long axis of the foot. A positive foot progression angle means the child is outtoeing, as a result of either external femoral rotation (femoral retroversion) or external tibial torsion.

Spastic: when severe, spastic gaits caused by hemiparesis or spastic diplegia are no problem to identify. However, when mildly affected, the child may only demonstrate a stiff-legged or equinus gait. Upper extremity flexor posturing (wrist and elbow flexed) will only be apparent when they are stressed in some way, such as by running, walking rapidly, or walking on their heels or toes.

Steppage: under normal circumstances, active ankle dorsiflexion is required during swing-through, so that the toes will clear, and, at the beginning of the stance phase (heel strike), to keep the foot from flapping forcefully to the ground. If the ankle dorsiflexors are weak (Charcot–Marie–Tooth or other peripheral neuropathy, polio), the individual will need to lift his weak ankle high for clearance, resulting in a steppage gait or foot-drop type of gait.

Vaulting: when one extremity is considerably longer than the other, or functionally longer because of an abduction contracture of the hip, the patient will walk with this type of gait, hurdling or vaulting over the longer extremity during stance phase on that side.

Hysterical: hysterical gaits are uncommon but can be difficult to diagnose. The gait is bizarre, inconsistent, without an apparent pathological basis and often associated with other psychosomatic complaints.

6. When describing the normal range of motion of various joints, I will use passive range unless otherwise specifically mentioned. *Passive* range of motion is how far the examiner can move the joint, as opposed to *active* range of motion which is how far the patient can move their own joints. These two sets of measurements are usually, but not always, similar.

7. Remember that when assessing extremity or trunk problems, inflammation reveals itself in *five* ways. In addition to the usual tumor, rubor, dolor, and calor, reduced function or limitation of motion must be added to the list. For example, even in the

absence of redness, swelling, pain, or warmth, limitation of motion of a joint represents *objective* evidence for a pathological process.

1.4.2. Examination of the Spine

The spine has two major curves: a thoracic curve which is convex posteriorly and a lumbar one which is convex anteriorly. Abnormal accentuation of the thoracic curve is called *hyperkyphosis* and accentuation of the lower *hyperlordosis*. Either may be associated with pain and/or anatomical abnormalities of the vertebral bodies. Lateral curvature is called *scoliosis*. Structural, as opposed to postural scoliosis, is often

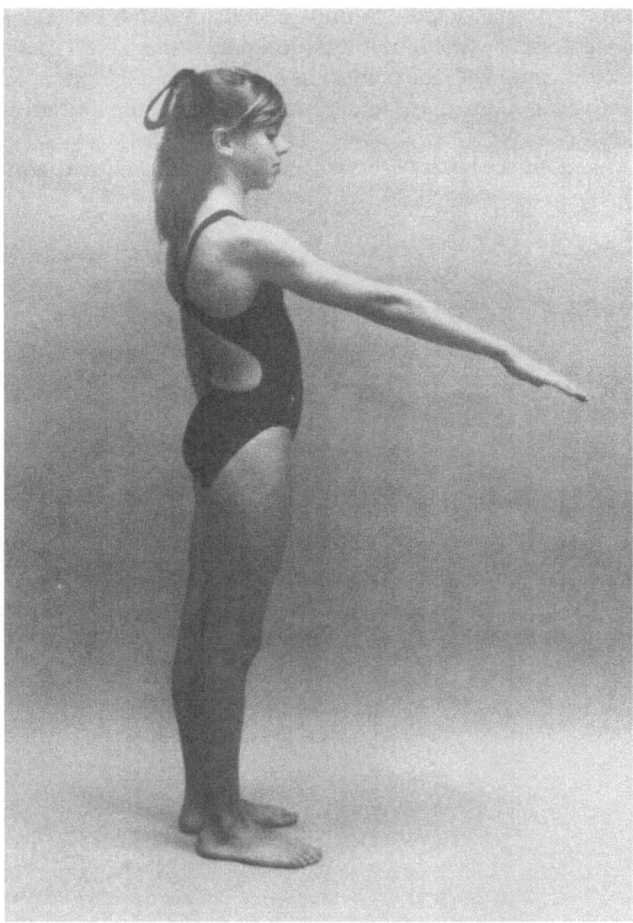

Figure 1.9. Normal lumbar lordosis and thoracic kyphosis. She is also exhibiting shoulder flexion

associated with a rib hump resulting from rotational as well as angular abnormalities of the vertebral bodies Rib humps can best be seen on forward bending

Lumbar scoliosis causes pelvic obliquity and thoracic scoliosis causes scapular obliquity when the patient is viewed from behind In addition, the distance from the patient's arms to the side of their thorax is asymmetrical

Although pelvic obliquity with the patient standing is most often a result of scoliosis, the combination of pelvic obliquity and an apparent scoliosis can also be caused by shortening of one of the lower extremities, resulting in a postural, but not a structural curve When this occurs, checking for scoliosis with the patient sitting will resolve the issue because the curve will then disappear An accurate measurement of the child's leg lengths from the anterior superior iliac spine to the ipsilateral medial malleolus will define the leg length inequity

If the curve is "decompensated" or unbalanced, a plumb bob dropped from the vertebral prominence of the neck will not fall along the gluteal cleft, documenting that the shoulders are not lined up with the pelvis but are displaced laterally Decompensated curves at any degree of curvature merit intervention earlier compared with compensated curves

Infants with idiopathic scoliosis deserve special mention and may present with their

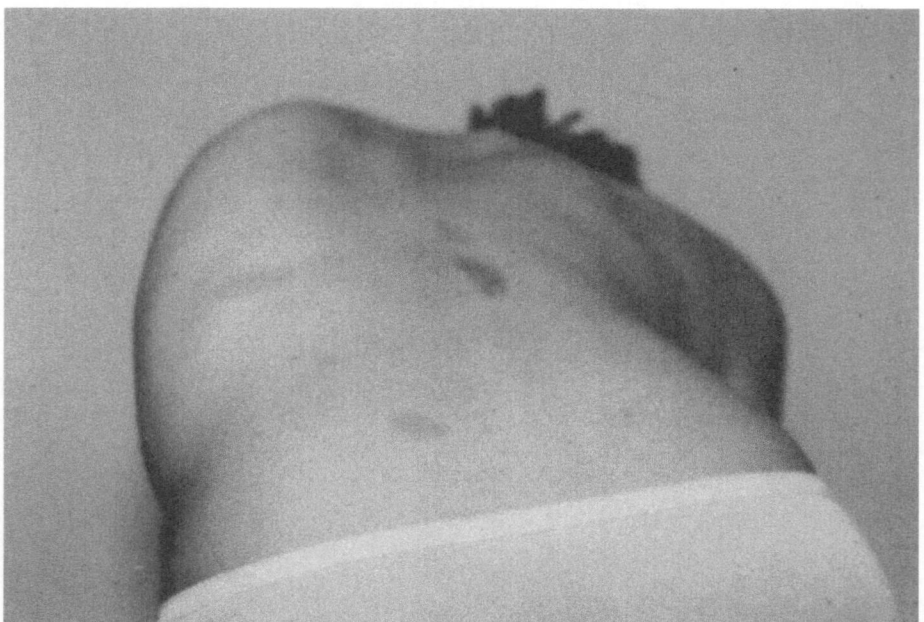

Figure 1 10   Thoracic prominence during forward bend in a young woman with scoliosis Note also the multiple cafe-au-lait spots Neurofibromatosis as seen in this patient often produces sharply angulated thoracic curves Rib humps in adolescents with typical idiopathic curves would likely be more subtle than those pictured here

curvature as part of a constellation of deformations, including metatarsus adductus (displacement of the forefoot medially) and developmental dysplasia of the hip. These curves are most often not rigid and will disappear if the infant is inspected when suspended by the armpits or when lying prone.

This is in contradistinction to congenital curves caused by anatomic abnormalities of the vertebral bodies themselves (like hemivertebrae) which are usually more rigid.

In either case, infantile curves frequently escape notice because we usually don't inspect the infant's back well and because babies are frequently so squiggly that it's difficult to know if their curve is a reality or not.

The spine should also be inspected for hairy tufts, hemangiomatosis, a mass, or sinus tracts over the midline, any of which might reflect an occult dysraphic process (spina bifida occulta).

Is the spinal segment overall short when compared with the height of the individual? Is the neck short or webbed as a result of fusion of cervical vertebral bodies (Klippel–Feil syndrome)?

The range of motion of the spine should be thoroughly tested. Rotational movement at the *cervical* spine should be close to 90° in either direction. That is, with the person facing due north, they should be able to turn and look almost due east and west. Lateral flexion occurs when the patient tries "to touch their ear to their shoulder" and should be about 75° from the vertical. Normal flexion at the cervical spine occurs when the

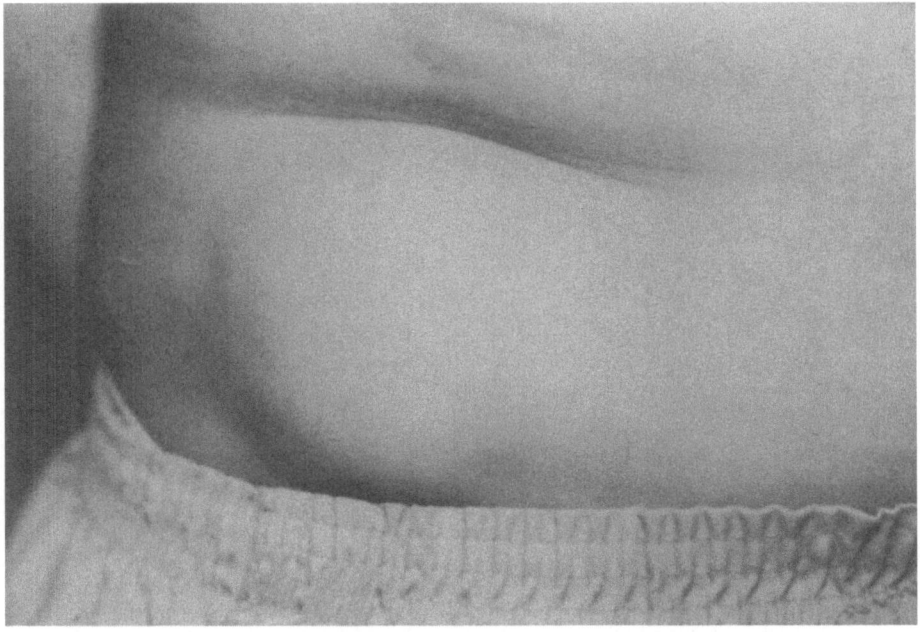

Figure 1.11. Lipomatous mass over the lumbar spine in this young man with spina bifida occulta.

patient is able to touch their chin to their chest Normal extension is almost 90°, such that with the patient looking "at the ceiling" the front of the face should be almost parallel to the ground **Torticollis** is present when the child holds their head in a tilted and rotated position and may be related to a variety of causes (see Chapter 9)

Check for normal flexion, extension, and rotation of the thoracolumbar spine remembering that good hip flexion can mask significant restriction of spinal flexion Children should pretty easily be able to touch the floor, most of that flexion coming from the lumbar, not the thoracic part of the spine Check for chest expansion From full

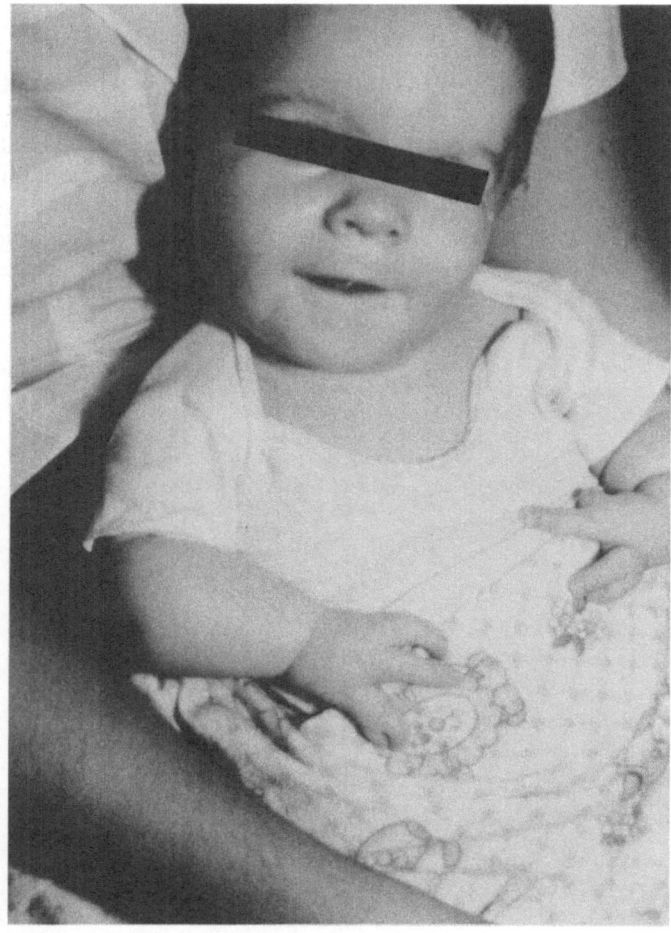

Figure 1.12. Congenital muscular torticollis on the left in this infant has been present long enough for there to be some hemifacial atrophy, including narrowing of the palpebral fissure on the left The head is held in left lateral flexion with rotation to the right Note also congenital digital abnormalities

exhalation to full inspiration, the chest circumference (in an adult) should increase by 5 cm when measured at the fourth intercostal space. Spinal rotation is mostly a function of the thoracic spine. Failure to elicit normal truncal rotation should prompt a search for thoracic spinal pathology.

Look for flattening of the lumbar spine (as a result of spondylitis, for example) with the patient in full forward bend. If apparent flattening is present, quantitate with the pediatric modification of the Schober test:

1. With the patient standing erect, locate a point on the midline of the back 10 cm superior to a horizontal line through the dimples of Venus (the surface markers for the sacroiliac joints).
2. Locate a second point 15 cm inferior to the first point in the midline (5 cm below the horizontal through the dimples of Venus).
3. Ask the patient to bend forward as much as they can. The distance between the superior and inferior points should increase from 15 to 21 cm approximately.

The adult variation on this theme is similar. Instead of measuring inferiorly 15 cm from the first point, measure down only 10. The second point will therefore be midway between the two dimples of Venus. With full forward flexion the increase normally will then be from 10 to 16 cm.

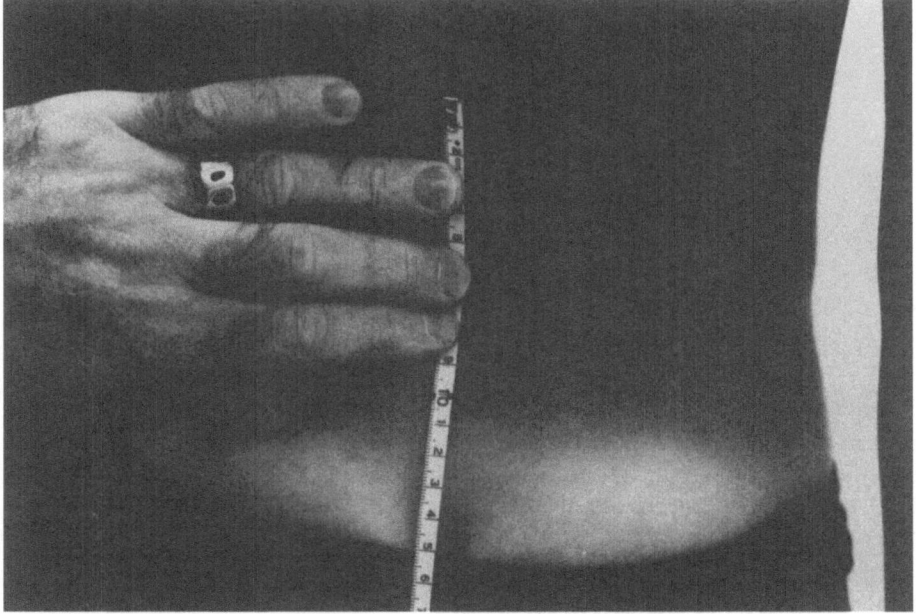

Figure 1.13. The pediatric Schober test is useful in the quantitation of restricted lumbosacral flexion, as might occur with ankylosing spondylitis. Point A is 10 cm superior to a horizontal line through the dimples of Venus (cutaneous markers for the sacroiliac joints).

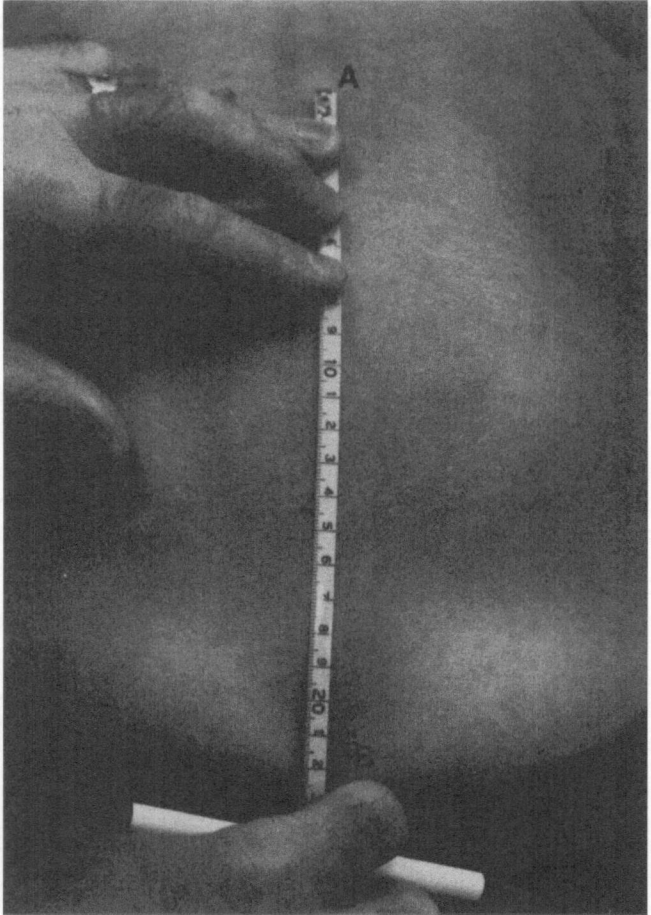

Figure 1.14. Point B is 5 cm below the same horizontal line. With maximal forward flexion, the 15 cm distance, from A to B, should increase to at least 21 cm, though normal is not well established.

Look for the opposite of lumbar flattening: lumbar hyperlordosis. A hip flexion contracture can cause this, which will then go away when you check the spine with the patient sitting. Don't forget to percuss for spinal tenderness (diskitis, spinal osteomyelitis) and for tenderness over the sacroiliac joints, lying immediately under the dimples of Venus on either side of the lumbar spine.

1.4.3. Examination of the Shoulder

The shoulder is a complex joint. Movement at the shoulder is affected not only by the adequacy of the glenohumeral joint but by the scapula and the clavicle as well.

Inspect the shoulder for proper positioning of the scapula (high in Sprengel's deformity) and clavicle (abnormally prominent in acromioclavicular or sternoclavicular dislocations) Is there webbing of the skin at the base of the neck as occurs with Klippel–Feil? Is there any atrophy of the deltoid which would occur with disuse caused by pain or as a result of axillary nerve palsy?

Intraarticular effusions are difficult to pick up when the shoulder is affected by arthritis because of the surrounding musculature. Determining range of motion is therefore important when evaluating the shoulder for inflammatory or degenerative

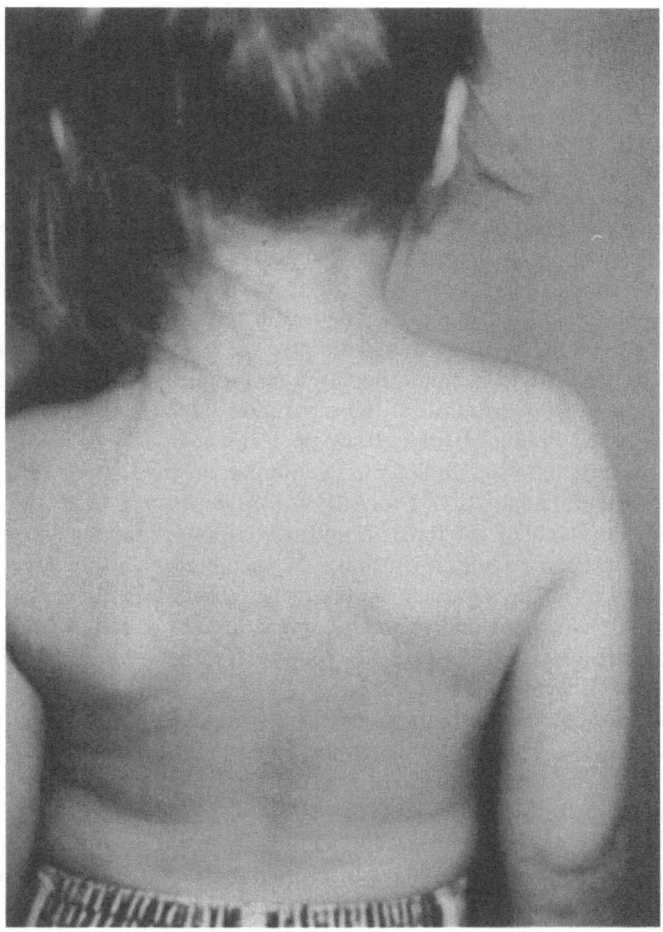

Figure 1.15. Sprengel deformity, as demonstrated in this young girl on the right, represents embryologic failure of the scapula to rotate and descend to its expectable position The child will also manifest decreased shoulder abduction on the affected side and may have other birth defects, including Klippel–Feil syndrome and renal anomalies

disease. First examine the active range of motion. Ask the patient to abduct the upper extremity with the elbow extended from the side to the overhead position. Should the patient elevate the shoulder on one side more than the other, it indicates that the patient is substituting scapulothoracic motion for glenohumeral motion. To check true gleno-humeral motion, examine the shoulder from the back. With one hand hold the inferior angle of the scapula and then passively abduct the arm with the other. Normally the arm can be abducted 90° before the scapular angle starts moving laterally. When the glenohumeral joint is affected, this motion is limited and the true range of motion is recorded as soon as the scapula begins to move.

The most important indication of shoulder pathology is the loss of external rotation. This is tested by having the patient hold both elbows close to the sides with elbows flexed 90° and the hands forward. Now ask the patient to actively move the hands away from the midline. This is external rotation of the glenohumeral joint. In males the normal range is 30 to 45°, females 60° or more.

1.4.4. Examination of the Elbow

The elbow is a well-machined joint with the proximal ulnar "jaws" (olecranon) fitting snugly over the distal humeral trochlea. This tight fit plus well-placed collateral ligaments provides for considerable stability but also makes for trouble if the tolerance of the close-fitting parts is exceeded by even a small derangement of the articular mechanism. Look for signs of intraarticular swelling by carefully inspecting the joint and by feeling for swelling or bogginess in the grooves formed by the olecranon and the medial and lateral epicondyles. Should this area feel doughy and/or tender, it indicates elbow joint irritation. Any irritation of the olecranon bursa should be obvious by the swelling evident at the "point" of the elbow posteriorly.

Often, significant elbow pathology is accompanied by loss of full extension or abnormal medial–lateral angulation. Normally the angle formed by the long axis of the humerus and the long axis of the forearm with the elbow in extension is about 15° of valgus. Excessive angular deviation is known as an increase in the carrying angle (or cubitus valgus) and occurs in a variety of syndromes (including Turner's). If unilateral, it may be the result of an old lateral condylar fracture. It is called "carrying angle" because it helps one to carry a bucket full of water without banging one's knee and getting one's clothing wet.

As a result of some fractures the normal carrying angle is lost and the elbow is straight in full extension. This is cubitus rectus. Supracondylar fractures of the humerus frequently result in the forearm angling toward the midline, referred to as cubitus varus, a "gunstock deformity."

The elbows flex from 0 (fully extended) to 140°, with enough flexion to easily touch the shoulder. The elbow also participates in pronation and supination. With the elbow flexed at 90°, ask your patient to assume the neutral position with the palm in a vertical (thumb up) position. Normal supination then involves 90° of rotation so that the palm is facing up (looking for a tip) and normal pronation involves rotation 90° in the opposite direction (palm facing down).

Palpate over the lateral epicondyle and proximal radial head for tenderness at the insertion of the wrist extensors or over the medial epicondyle at the insertion of the wrist flexors. Confirm by eliciting pain with resisted active wrist extension or flexion.

1.4.5. Examination of the Wrist

Distinguishing the wrist, another hinge joint, from the hand is, by necessity, somewhat an arbitrary exercise. Look for deviation of the wrist from the long axis of the forearm as occurs with juvenile rheumatoid arthritis. Inspect for localized swelling (as might occur with a ganglion cyst) or generalized swelling (as might occur with arthritis). Wrist extension (dorsiflexion) should be close to 90° such that with the hands together, as if in prayer, the forearms can pretty easily form a line parallel to the floor. Palmar flexion should be roughly of the same magnitude, about 80° in most children. The wrist in neutral can also be angled 40° in the ulnar and 5° in the radial direction.

Check for hypermobility. Can the wrist be passively flexed to place the radial side of the thumb on the forearm (suggestive of Ehler–Danlos or one of the other connective tissue or hyperlaxity disorders)?

1.4.6. Examination of the Hand

The hand is the most complex of all of our bony machines, difficult to do justice to in a few short paragraphs. Look at the fingers. Are they long and thin (arachnodactyly), short (brachydactyly), fused (syndactyly), crooked (clinodactyly), or fusiform (arthritis/tenosynitis)? Inspect for abnormalities of the palmar creases (simian or transverse palmar crease) and the flexion creases of the fingers. Absence of the latter would result from symphalangism or fusion of two phalanges on the same finger.

Is there clubbing, edema, cyanosis, or joint swelling? Is there a boutonniere deformity (hyperflexion at the proximal interphalangeal joint with extension at the distal interphalangeal joint), a swan-neck deformity (hyperextension of the proximal interphalangeal joint with flexion at the distal joint), or a mallet finger (fixed flexion of the distal interphalangeal joint)? Are there trophic ulcerations or other derangements of vascular supply, as would occur with Raynaud's; nail pitting or dystrophy as would occur with psoriasis?

Is there normal range of motion? The metacarpophalangeal joints can be flexed to 90° and extended (hyperextended) to about 45°. The interphalangeal joints can be flexed to at least 90°. Ask the patient to make a fist. It should be tight enough to prevent passage of light. Thumb opposition should be easily made and should be strong enough to keep you from pulling through, at least in the older child. Is the hand hypermobile with hyperextension at the interphalangeal joints?

1.4.7. Examination of the Hip

An accurate and thorough examination of the hip is an absolute necessity in the diagnosis of lower extremity problems in children. Diagnosing hip disease is difficult because the hip is a deep structure and is hard to evaluate for such usual signs of inflammation as redness or swelling. Frequently children with hip disease will present

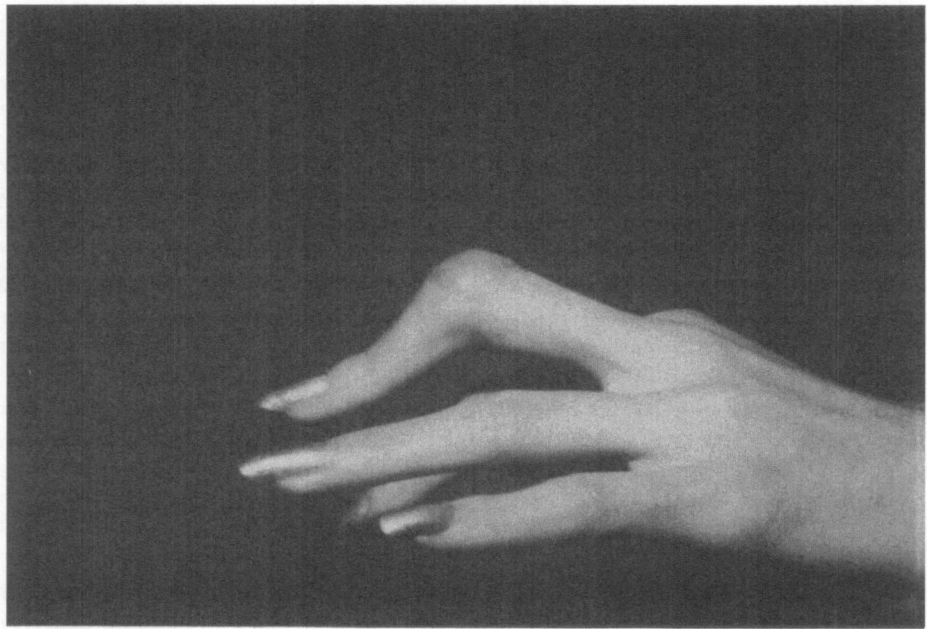

Figure 1.16. Typical boutonniere deformity in an adolescent with polyarticular form of juvenile rheumatoid arthritis. The extensor mechanism is affected by the JRA leading to fixed flexion at the proximal interphalangeal joint with hyperextension at the distal joint.

with referred pain to the knee or medial thigh, causing unnecessary and costly delays in the child's evaluation while exhaustive searches are made for knee pathology.

Assessing range of motion at the hip is also difficult because the patient will tend to compensate for any deficiencies in the mobility of the hip by moving the lumbar spine or the pelvis. Stabilizing the pelvis while checking for extremity movement is therefore very important. The patient is examined supine on the table with the buttocks and lower back flat on the table. The hips should range from at least full extension (0°) to about 140° of full flexion. Check range independently on each side. When a hip flexion contracture is present (patient lacks full extension), the tendency will be for the child to compensate for the lack of full extension with hyperlordosis of the lumbosacral spine. To keep from getting fooled, flex both extremities maximally (knee to chest), extend one with the other in full flexion to keep the back flat against the table (the Thomas test). Under normal circumstances, the extended extremity should lie comfortably on the table.

Abduction can be performed with the hip and knees flexed (frog-leg position) or with both in extension. Infants and small children can often attain 90° of hip abduction (knees to the table in the frog-leg position), older children at least 60°. With the knee and hip in extension, abduction may be somewhat less, perhaps 60° in the younger and 45° in the older child, because of the tightening of the soft tissues around the hip with

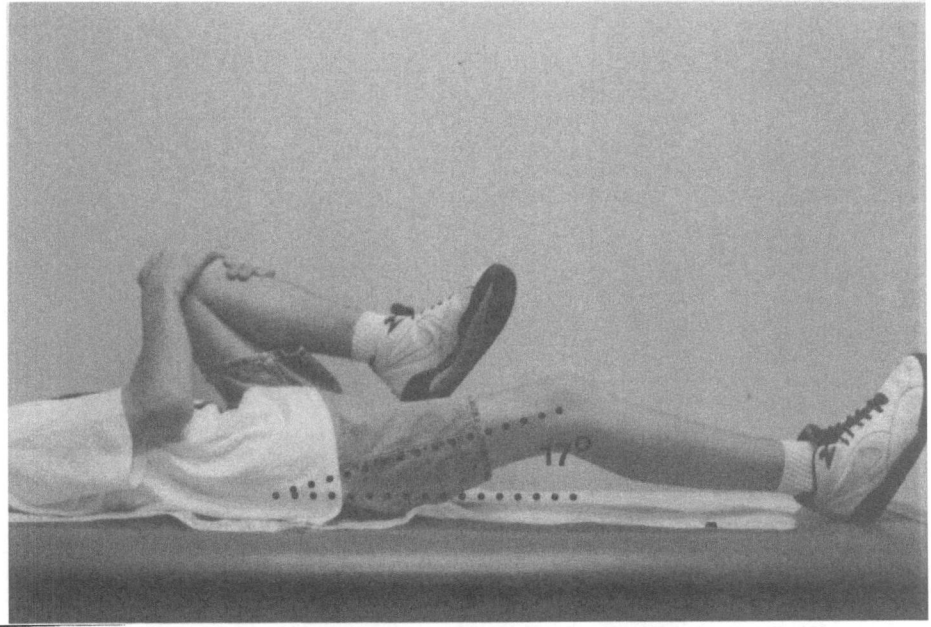

Figure 1.17. The Thomas test, with maximal hip flexion on the left and his back flattened against the table, this boy is unable to extend his right hip fully He has a 17° hip-flexion contracture

extension. Adduction is the opposite, bringing one extremity over the other, normally about 20°.

Internal rotation can be assessed with knees and hips flexed to 90° and the patient supine. With both knees together, the distal lower extremity is rotated cephalad and lateral, away from the sagittal plane of the body, normally to about 45°. Decreased internal rotation should be looked for carefully. **It is the most sensitive indicator of hip disease.** External rotation is performed similarly with each distal extremity rotated away from the sagittal plane but to the contralateral side, usually also about 45°. Internal and external rotation are usually equal to each other and, of course, should always be symmetrical as well, side to side. Rotation can also be evaluated with the hips in extension and the patient prone.

Check for weak hip abduction with the Trendelenburg test. With the patient standing, observe for a drop in the contralateral hemipelvis when the patient stands on one leg. Most children can hold their pelvis straight for 30 seconds. Any assistance to help the child balance must be given only on the side the child is standing on. Checking for a Trendelenburg is a problem for children under 5 or 6 years because of normal problems with balance in younger children but, when present, is a useful demonstration of weak hip abductors (see Trendelenburg gait, above).

Ortolani's test for hip dysplasia must be performed when the infant is happy, warm,

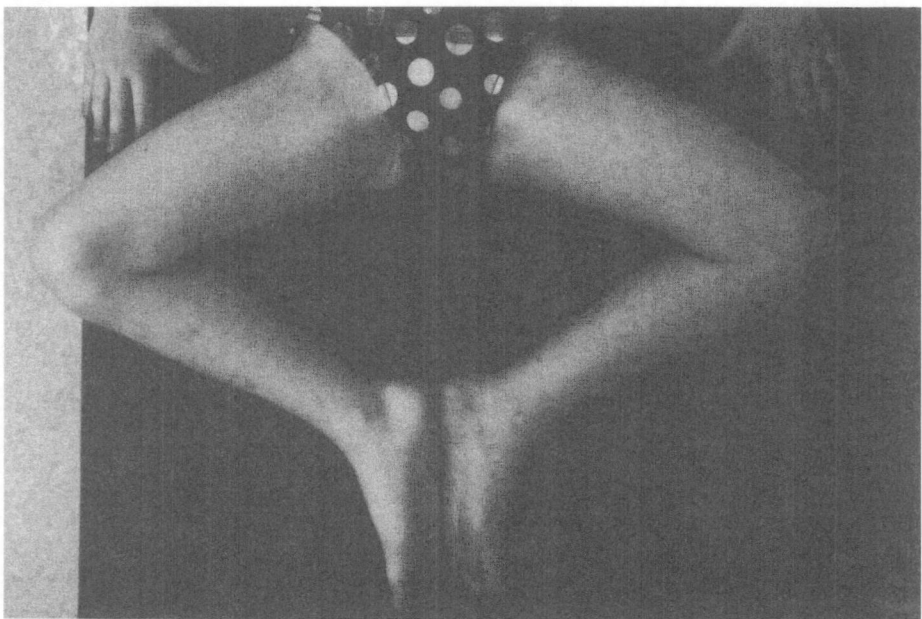

Figure 1.18. Most young children can abduct their hip to 90° with their knees and hips in flexion That is, in the frog-leg position, they can put each knee on the table

and well-fed, if possible. With both hips flexed to 90°, hold each knee in the palm of each hand, with the thumb along the medial aspect of each thigh, the fingers along the lateral aspect of each thigh, and the distal fingers over each greater trochanter. As one slowly and *gently* abducts and lifts, if a dislocation is present, the femoral head will be felt slipping over the posterior rim and into the acetabulum with a palpable clunk. Barlow's test uses the same principles but in reverse: as the hip is adducted, with slight thumb pressure from above, the femoral head can be felt slipping out posteriorly. Because the flexible soft tissues of the newborn and young infant tighten up in the months after birth, the Ortolani or Barlow may no longer be positive after 2 or 3 months in the child with a dislocation. It is also becoming clear that at least some of the infants who eventually are found to have hip dysplasia have normal hips at birth and, therefore, the term *congenital hip dysplasia* has been abandoned in favor of *developmental dysplasia of the hip*. Since not all dysplasia is present at birth, every child should have their hips examined and the results recorded at every well-child visit until the child is walking well.

To identify hip dysplasia in the older child, look for foreshortening of the femoral segment (since the dislocation is posterior and superior). The Galeazzi (or Allis) sign is positive when the heights of the knees, with knees and hips flexed and feet on the table, are unequal as a result of the shorter femoral segment on the affected side. Check the posterior flexion creases, particularly those of the knees and immediately below the buttocks, which will be asymmetrical for the same reason. Examine carefully for any

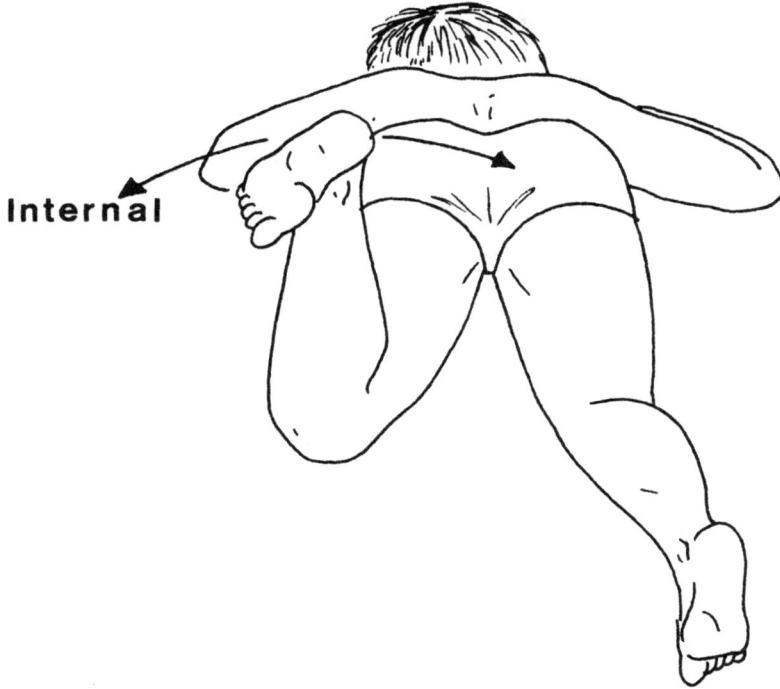

Internal

Figure 1.19. Internal rotation of the hip is one of the most sensitive indicators of hip pathology. It can be performed with the patient prone with the hips in extension or supine with the hips and knees in 90° of flexion.

diminution in range of motion, particularly in abduction, and look for abnormal telescoping in the anteroposterior dimension as one pushes and pulls the femoral head in and out of the acetabulum.

When bilateral disease (about 25% of the total) is present, all of the above may be less useful. Bilateral hip dysplasia produces a widening of the perineum as a result of lateral hip displacement as well as hyperlordosis of the lumbar spine. In toddlers look for a lurching Trendelenburg gait. Not surprisingly, many of these children are diagnosed late.

1.4.8. Examination of the Knee

The nice thing about the knee, unlike the hip, is that it's there for all the world to see. Look for swelling, redness, feel for warmth and tenderness. Small amounts of fluid in the joint will result in obliteration of the normal dimpling on either side of the patella. A larger effusion will result in expansion of the suprapatellar bursa with obvious swelling above the patella. If uncertain about intraarticular fluid, attempt to compress the suprapatellar area, forcing the fluid more inferiorly. The patella will then "float" on the

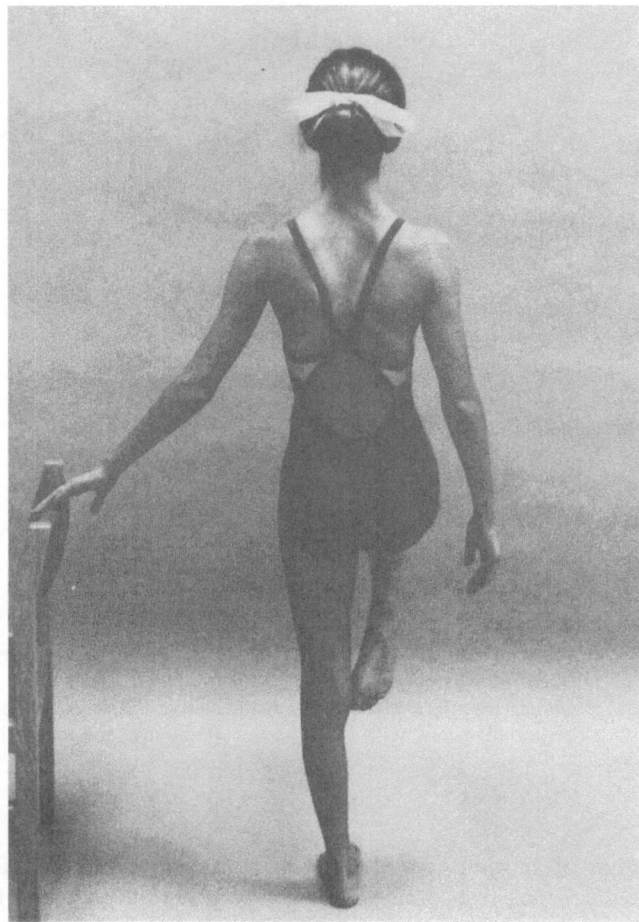

Figure 1.20. Professor Trendelenburg has a position, two different operations, two different physical examination tests, and a gait named after him The Trendelenburg test pictured here demonstrates adequacy of the abductor mechanism of the left hip in this case

increased joint fluid and will be ballotable by the examiner Excessive accumulation of fluid in the joint will sometimes result in the development of a synovial cyst posteriorly, in the popliteal fossa

Check for thigh and/or calf atrophy Specific painful pathology involving the knee will rapidly result in muscular atrophy as the affected extremity is favored Get in the habit of measuring with a tape

Most children have a few degrees of hyperextension (recurvatum) with full flexion of the knee to about 140° Most children can place, with a little help, the posterior aspect of their heel on the posterior aspect of their thigh To look for subtle knee flexion contractures or excessive recurvatum, have the child lie supine on the table and lift the leg by the foot while restraining the thigh against the table with the opposite hand. The heel can normally be lifted 1–2 inches from the table.

Find the joint line by looking for small indentations on either side of the patellar tendon when the knee is flexed. Joint line tenderness may result from meniscal or collateral ligament injuries. Tenderness over the tibial tubercle may be caused by Osgood–Schlatter's disease. Tenderness over the femoral condyles (on the proximal side of the joint line), particularly on the medial side, may result from osteochondritis dissecans. Check for pain with patellar compression with the knee extended and the quadriceps contracted, caused by chondromalacia patellae.

The angulation of the femur with the tibia changes over time. We are all normally born with a little genu varum (perhaps 10°) which straightens (by 18 months) and then transitions to valgus which is at its greatest between 3 and 4 years (about 15°). More straightening occurs with growth, leaving adults with a small valgus angulation of between 5 and 10°. Check for excessive angulation with the patient standing. Excessive valgus angulation at the knee is thought to contribute to abnormalities of patellar tracking, with resulting patellar subluxation or chondromalacia patellae.

Look for abnormalities in patellar tracking. The patella should track smoothly and without lateral or medial excursion in the intercondylar groove of the distal femur. Compare each side individually by observing patellar movement as the patient, in the sitting position, extends at the knee. Feel for crepitation. Is the patella riding high with the knee in extension (patella alta)? Is there excessive lateral/medial or superior/inferior mobility? The "apprehension test" attempts to measure patient anxiety over imminent patellar subluxation. With the knee in extension, try to displace the patella laterally while flexing the knee slightly. Patients who have experienced subluxation will become acutely apprehensive if they feel subluxation is about to occur again.

Check for excessive valgus or varus instability. With the knee in 20 or 30° of flexion and the examiner at the bedside, place the ankle under the examiner's arm and apply lateral and then medial stress to the knee. A small "jog" of motion is normal. Experience and side-to-side comparisons will help to define normality. Instability in slight flexion often is a result of collateral ligamentous injury. If lateral–medial instability also exists during full knee extension, cruciate ligamentous injury must be suspected.

With cruciate ligament injuries, excessive anteroposterior instability will result. With the patient supine and the knee in about 90° of flexion, stabilize the foot with one hand (or by sitting on it) and try to move the proximal tibia in an anterior direction (the anterior drawer test). Excessive displacement (again difficult to define but probably 1.5 cm or more in an adult) anteriorly is likely to be associated with an anterior cruciate tear. Similarly, a positive posterior drawer test is likely to be the result of a posterior cruciate ligamentous tear. Additionally, with posterior tears or injury, the tibia at rest will subluxate backwards, producing a deformity obvious by inspection with the knee in flexion.

The Lachman test is similar to the anterior drawer test but with the knee in about 10° of flexion.

Additionally, when confronted with perplexing knee discomfort, always examine the hips and think about the possibility of hip disease. Innervation to the hip joint is by the obturator nerve which sends a branch to the medial aspect of the distal thigh. Hip disease will often present as knee or thigh discomfort as a result of this referral pattern.

1.4.9. Examination of the Ankle and Foot

Check for signs of inflammation and range of motion. To check the ankle joint itself, grasp the foot proximal to the midtarsal joint and check for normal dorsiflexion (15–20°) and plantarflexion (50–55°). If restricted dorsiflexion is improved with knee flexion, look for tightening of the Achilles tendon; if not improved, look for intrinsic joint pathology.

Check for restricted subtalar motion by inverting and everting the heel underneath the talus. Arthritis of the talocalcaneal joint will result in decreased motion as will a coalition or fusion of any of the tarsal bones.

Remember that the foot is designed (wondrously) to work as a tripod. The tripod is comprised of the calcaneus posteriorly and the first and fifth metatarsal heads anteriorly. Limitation of subtalar motion or other rigid deformities of the foot or ankle may cause weight to be unevenly borne by two rather than the normal three points of the tripod with resulting pain and inappropriate wear and tear. Look for signs of skin callus buildup,

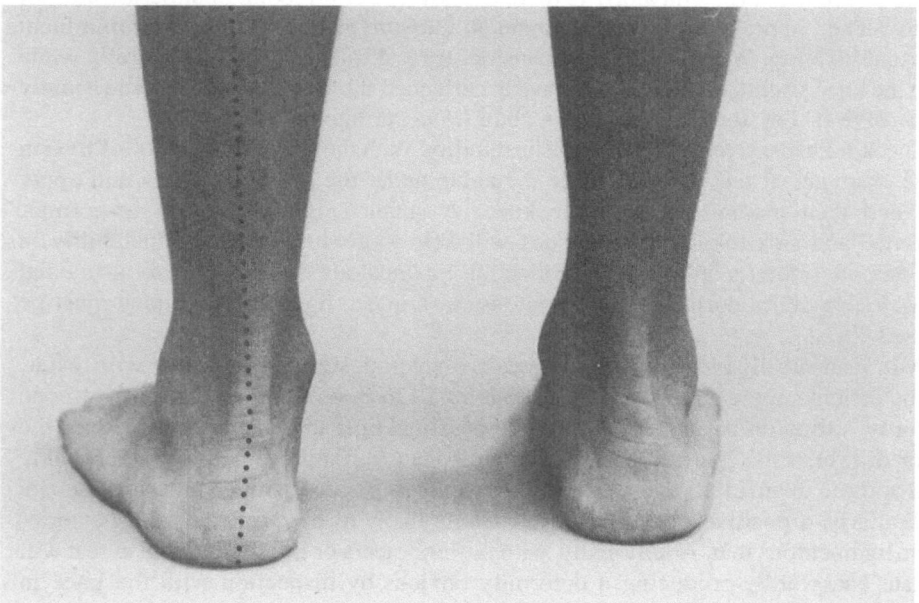

Figure 1.21. With the ankle in neutral (no dorsiflexion or plantarflexion), there is normally about 10° of ankle valgus, as demonstrated here. The heel normally goes into varus when the patient stands on their toes.

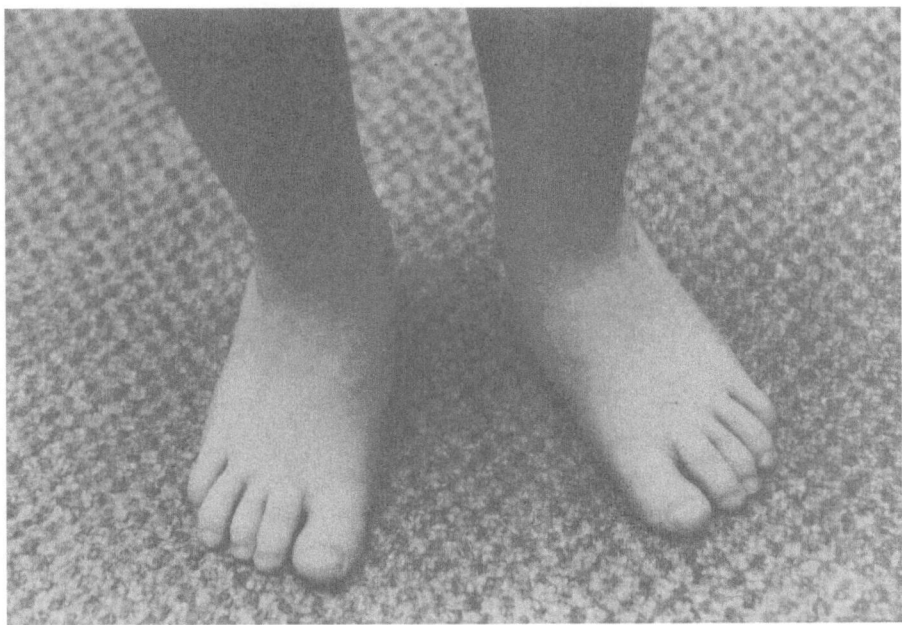

Figure 1 22   Typical pes planus also known somewhat less grandly as flat feet

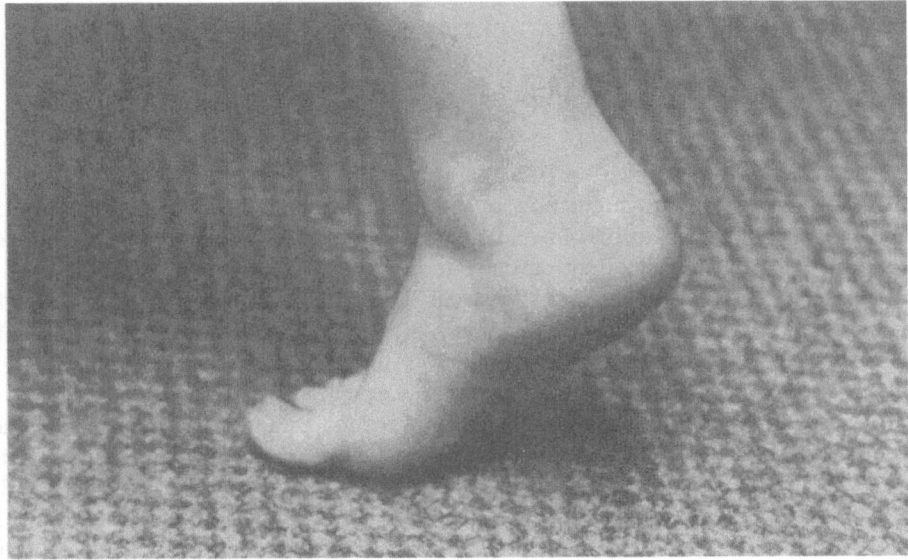

Figure 1.23. Most flat feet are flexible and do as well as feet which are not flat To prove it, have the child stand on their toes and the arch will appear If they're too young to stand on their toes, put them on their parent's lap

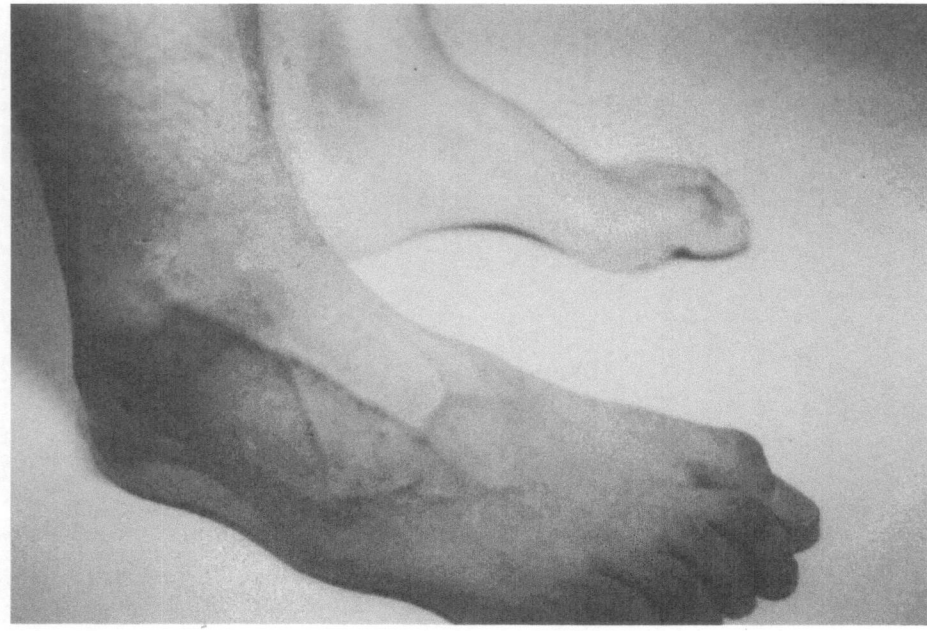

Figure 1.24. These feet belong to a patient who has Charcot–Marie–Tooth Note the typical claw foot deformity, the ankle varus, and the high arched (cavus) foot Charcot and Marie were French Charcot has a joint, a disease, a fever, a crystal, and an artery named after him Marie has two diseases, the one pictured above as well as Marie–Strumpell (ankylosing spondylitis) Tooth was English and has only one disease

tenderness or non-weight-bearing (silky) skin resulting from tripod failure. Check for abnormal varus or valgus angulation at the ankle, remembering that under normal circumstances there is about 10° of heel valgus at the ankle with the foot on the floor and about 10° of varus when standing on one's toes.

Similarly, check for abnormal shoe wear. Under normal circumstances we strike with our heel (slightly lateral aspect) and push off with the ball of our foot. This results in normal wear posterolaterally and anteriorly. Abnormal pronation or supination will result in excessive medial or lateral shoe wear, respectively.

Ligamentous laxity resulting in flattening of the longitudinal and transverse arches is frequent enough to be considered normal. Does the arch re-form when the child is not weight-bearing or when standing on tiptoe (implying flexible flat feet) or does the flat foot persist regardless of weight-bearing, because of an intrinsic bony abnormality?

Does the child have the opposite problem? Since the spectrum from planus to cavus feet is a continuum, moderate cavus positioning is no more abnormal than moderate planus. However, if acquired or progressive, particularly when associated with claw toes (metatarsal–phalangeal hyperextension with interphalangeal flexion), consideration

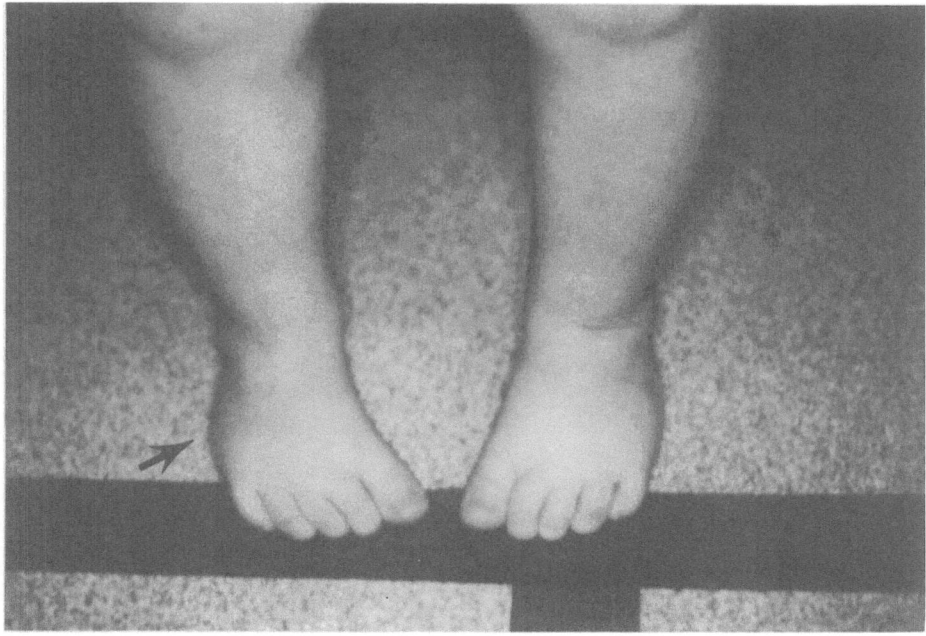

Figure 1.25. *Metatarsus adductus, worse on the right.* Also known as metatarsus varus, it is associated with convexity of the lateral border (arrow) of the foot (see also Chapter 4).

must be given to such neurological pathology as a peripheral neuropathy (as in Charcot–Marie–Tooth) or a spinal cord lesion (spina bifida occulta or tumor).

Is the foot normally oriented, one part with the other? Is the forefoot rotated medially (metatarsus adductus)? Is the first toe displaced laterally (hallux valgus)? Does the child walk on their toes (an equinus gait) or only on their heel (a calcaneal gait)?

2

Evaluation of the Child with Extremity Pain or Limp

2.1. INTRODUCTION

The child presenting to the physician with a limp or extremity pain is usually accompanied by anxious parents who are concerned not only about the cause but also about the permanency of the problem. Evaluation is often challenging since younger children cannot communicate verbally about their pain and may have trouble localizing it for the examiner. It is the physician's task to solve the mystery by accumulating as many clues as possible and analyzing them correctly.

This chapter will deal with this process in a general way, excluding children with arthritis. Disease descriptions below are included because they are relatively common causes of extremity pain. We are trying here to be practical rather than encyclopedic. Many other parts of this book also concern themselves specifically with problems that may cause pain in an extremity. For a discussion of the child with arthritis, see Chapter 11. For the child with a sports-related injury, see Chapter 8. For suspected child abuse, see Chapter 3. For other types of pediatric traumatic injuries, see Chapter 10.

Be prepared for diagnostic uncertainty in many cases. Physicians are usually pretty good at making sure that the symptoms of childhood extremity pain are not the result of anything serious. They are much less able to specify exactly what the pain is caused by.

2.2. PRESENTATION

In addition to limp and pain, children may present with a pseudoparalysis as a result of a painful extremity process. The infant, particularly, will manifest pathology by refusal to use the extremity in question.

An antalgic gait is a limp in which the patient reduces the time spent in stance phase on the affected limb. However, not all limps are **antalgic**. Some have nothing to do with a painful process. These include Trendelenburg, vaulting, spastic, steppage, and foot-drop gaits among others (see also Chapter 1).

2.3. THE HISTORY

As with many childhood medical problems, the most significant information is obtained by listening to the story. Sometimes complaints are intermittent and physical findings are absent at the time of the visit. Control the initial impulse to pass off the parents' concerns as nothing. This may be a particular temptation if a grandmother is present. Grandmothers may be overly concerned and protective, but somehow they are endowed with a sixth sense that must be respected. Their concerns should be weighed heavily in the physician's mind. Ask specifically why the parent or grandparent is worried (cancer?, crippling arthritis?, polio?). They may not tell you unless you ask and if you don't address their concern, you can't solve their problem.

In addition to the obvious issue of the child's age, the history should obtain information regarding the following:

- Fever, weight loss, rash, or other systemic symptoms.
- Focality. Does the child repeatedly touch, hold, or rub a particular part of the anatomy or does the pain seem to be multifocal or migratory?
- Are the symptoms chronic or acute?
- Trauma. This is not an accusatory question but is an attempt to get the parent to recall a specific incident.
- Are the symptoms worse in the morning or in the evening? Do they wake the child up?
- How much dysfunction do the symptoms cause? Does the child mention them in passing or do they prevent normal activity?
- Has there been any tenderness, redness, swelling, heat, or bruising?
- Has there been a recent viral infection?
- What makes the pain better? What makes the pain worse?
- Are there social or psychological stressors that may be contributing?

2.4. THE PHYSICAL EXAMINATION (see also Chapter 1)

Do the gestalt things first. Is this an ill-appearing child? Are they short? Are they thin? Are they obese? All physicians recognize that the examination is best done when the child is cooperative. Therefore, it is usually prudent, when examining a child for limp, to inspect the child's gait first before proceeding with the hands-on part of the examination. The child should be undressed down to diapers or undergarments. Having different sizes of inexpensive gym shorts for the children to put on helps to preserve modesty and assure a cooperative patient. The shoes and socks should be removed. Toddlers can be taken from the mother by the nurse and removed a short distance from the mother and, when released, will usually run back to the parent. Such brief glimpses

Table 2.1. Important History Features in Extremity Pain

Fever	What makes pain better
Rash	What makes pain worse
Weight loss	Dysfunction
Loss of energy	Missing school
Focal/multifocal/migratory	Missing play/sports
Acute/chronic	Social stressors
Morning/with activity/at night	Move
Swelling	Death
Warmth	Parental depression
Redness	Family history of chronic pain
Bruising	Other ill-defined somatic complaints
Recent infection	Symptoms of depression
Sore throat	Isolation
Skin infection	Sad
Viral infection	Poor school performance

are about all the physician gets to see with 12- to 18-month-olds. Older children can be encouraged to walk in the hallway. Having the child run a short distance is also helpful. The examiner is looking for asymmetry of gait. It is antalgic if the child does not spend as much time on one extremity during the stance phase as on the other.

In addition to a good general examination, look for focal signs of inflammation or bruising. Remember that intervertebral disc disease will cause referred pain to the lower extremities, that hip disease will cause pain over the medial thighs or knees, and that sacroiliac joint disease will cause buttock pain. Examine for decreased range of motion, particularly at the hips. Look for flexible or rigid flat feet deformities and check for generalized hyperlaxity. Examine the knees well. Is there patellar pain on compression, joint crepitus at the knee, apprehension with lateralization of the patella? Is there anteroposterior or lateral instability?

2.5. EXTREMITY PAIN WITHOUT SYSTEMIC SYMPTOMS

A good way to separate children with extremity pain is by the presence or absence of systemic symptoms like fever, weight loss, or malaise. This is a spectrum from traumatic injuries exhibiting little systemic symptomatology, to acute osteomyelitis with lots of systemic symptomatology. Included below is a list of relatively common causes of leg pain without such systemic symptoms.

2.5.1. Nighttime Thigh and Calf Pain ("Growing Pains")

This is one of the most frustrating complaints of all, for patient, parents, and physician. This is most commonly seen in 4- to 10-year-olds who may awaken in the night and demand massage or a warm bath to alleviate the problem. The distribution is symmetrical and is unaccompanied by such systemic symptoms as fever or weight loss. Examination is almost always unrevealing. Labeled "growing pains," it is hard to explain these symptoms on the basis of growth. Adolescents, growing faster than anyone, don't usually complain of these pains.

2.5.2. Painful Heels in 10-Year-Old Boys

A peculiar, unexplained complaint of pain in the plantar surface of the heel occurs in boys who are often overweight at about 10 years of age plus or minus a few months. It may be severe enough to cause an antalgic gait. There are no other complaints. Examination reveals the lad to be tender to deep palpation of the plantar surface of the heel. Stressing the foot into dorsiflexion does not cause pain along the plantar fascia as one would see in true plantar fasciitis.

X-ray examination of the foot is normal. It is important to recognize that sclerosis and irregularity of the calcaneal apophysis (see Fig. 2.1) is normal and is not a radiologic sign of calcaneal apophysitis (Sever disease).

The differential diagnosis of heel pain is extensive. It includes such inflammatory or overuse processes as Achilles tendinitis, retrocalcaneal bursitis, calcaneal apo-

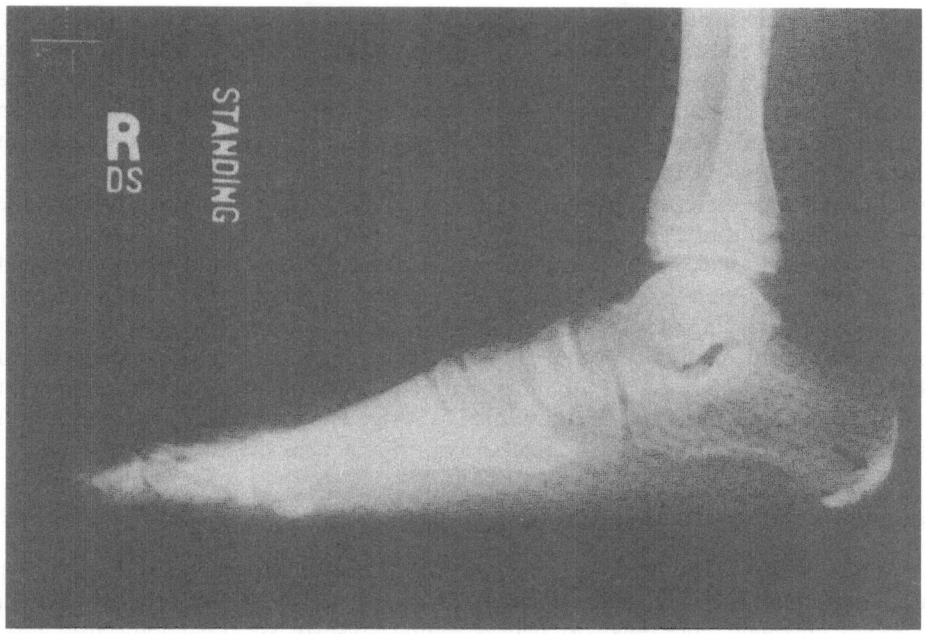

Figure 2.1. Plain lateral radiograph of the foot. Note the normal sclerosis and irregularity of the calcaneal apophysis (arrow) which is not a sign of calcaneal apophysitis (Sever disease).

physitis, and plantar fasciitis (see also Chapter 8). All generally respond to symptomatic treatment including activity modification and a heel cushion for the shoe.

Calcaneal apophysitis (Sever disease), in particular, is not uncommon in active children in late childhood or early adolescence. It is similar in etiology to apophysitis of the tibial tubercle (Osgood–Schlatter disease). Repeated stress of the Achilles tendon at its insertion onto the calcaneal apophysis results in microfracturation, inflammation, and pain. Pain is worse after exercise or with ankle dorsiflexion. Tenderness is present over the heel posteriorly and inferiorly. Plain films are normal and therapy is symptomatic, with emphasis placed on good heel cord stretching prior to any athletic activity.

Occasionally more significant pathology makes itself manifest, including calcaneal osteomyelitis, tarsal coalition, and osteoid osteoma. Usually, however, heel pain is an unexplained complaint and is happily self-limited, lasting for 6 to 12 months.

2.5.3. Snapping Hips in Adolescent Girls

As girls mature into teenagers they may present to the physician with the complaint that "my hip goes out of its socket." By this the young woman means that when she walks, and particularly when she walks in an exaggerated feminine style, a snapping can be felt lateral to the greater trochanter, considered by most people as the hip joint. This is rarely painful but sometimes the snapping is audible and the parents become concerned.

Physical examination reveals that the adolescent has a normal gait but when she stands on one foot and moves her pelvis anteriorly and posteriorly, a "clunk" can be felt over the trochanter. Even on inspection something is seen to suddenly move over the trochanter. Passive examination of the hip joint reveals the motion to be normal but, on occasion, the examination is very dramatic indeed and an initial impression of recurrent dislocation might be entertained. When one coolly considers such a possibility, however, it would have to be extremely painful except when it really does occur as a result of the tabes dorsalis of tertiary syphilis.

X-rays are always normal. What is occurring is the iliotibial band moving back and forth across the trochanter as the normal swaying motion of walking is accentuated by the young woman trying to appear more mature than she really is. This snapping motion can become a tic and, if repeated often enough, can cause a painful superficial trochanteric bursitis just deep to the iliotibial band. The treatment is simply to point out to the family and the adolescent that this is not significant pathology and that all that is required is to purposefully avoid the behavior that causes the snapping.

2.5.4. Reflex Sympathetic Dystrophy

Reflex sympathetic dystrophy (RSD), also known as reflex vasomotor dystrophy or Sudeck atrophy, is a chronic and potentially disabling pain syndrome of older children and adolescents which presents with pain, swelling, dysesthesia, vasomotor instability, or unusual posturing in an extremity. The extremity is also often either cold and mottled or warm and red. Dermatographism is often present, but only in the affected extremity. In adults, it often occurs as a consequence of an injury. In children, this is less often so and may occur bilaterally (Dietz *et al.*, 1990). Girls are more often affected than boys.

Though the etiology of RSD in children is unknown, psychosocial factors are thought to play a significant role in causation. Sherry and Weisman (1988) found an overly close, enmeshed relationship between affected children and their parents in the 21 families they studied. Overt or covert marital discord were also common as were school problems. They found the typical RSD patient to be a preadolescent girl, compliant and overachieving, trying her best to deal with excessive stress related to family dynamics or school problems or both.

Treatment is centered around sympathetic support and physical therapy, including mobilization, range of motion, and massage. Gentle but persistent urgings to use the affected extremity are necessary, often in an inpatient setting. Individual or family therapy is also often necessary. Severe muscle atrophy and osteopenia may occur if the above is not effective and more aggressive intervention must then be considered, including regional anesthesia and sympathetic blockade.

2.5.5. Fibromyalgia

This controversial syndrome of diffuse pain is characterized by discrete, predictable tender points ("trigger points") associated with anxiety, symptoms of depression, nonrestorative sleep, and other somatic complaints. School refusal may be a particular problem. Objective signs of systemic inflammatory disease are lacking. Its presence in children is just now beginning to be defined. Fibromyalgia may be primary or secondary to another musculoskeletal condition such as juvenile rheumatoid arthritis.

Tenderness must be present in three predictable "trigger point" locations and absent over other areas in order to make the diagnosis. Interestingly, the pain the children complain of is not localized to the tender points. The tender points are located at the midpoint of the superior border of the trapezius, at the second costochondral junction, over the upper medial border of the scapula, slightly distal to the lateral epicondyle of the elbow, at the upper outer buttock, at the medial knee, at the posterolateral neck, and over the lower lumbar region. More girls are affected than boys and treatment is centered around warm soaks, physical therapy, stretching exercises, massage, and, if necessary, antidepressants (Yunus and Masi, 1985).

2.5.6. Spiral Fracture of the Tibia (see also Chapters 3 and 10)

This injury, also called toddler's fracture, is seen in children 12 to 30 months of age. It is caused by a rotatory stress applied to the tibia occurring during a fall. The fall does not have to be impressive and may occur during play. The rotational stress causes a nondisplaced, long, spiral fracture of the tibia that does not cause deformity and the child is usually rather quickly pacified. They simply refuse to walk.

On examination, there is surprisingly little found. The child may or may not show discomfort with deep palpation of the tibia. There is no significant swelling. Sometimes a twist applied to the foot causes the child to wince but this does not localize the pain. The diagnosis is made after excluding other possibilities. A child who refuses to walk, is afebrile, and has normal range of motion must be considered to have a nondisplaced spiral fracture of the tibia until an X-ray proves otherwise.

X-ray examination is the definitive diagnostic procedure but the standard antero-posterior film of the tibia may not always demonstrate the fracture. A 45° oblique film usually will. If not, a technetium bone scan should be considered. External immobilization in a plaster cast for 3 or 4 weeks is all the treatment required.

Though not an injury specific for child abuse, other evidence for abuse should be sought in order to exclude this possibility (see Chapter 3).

2.5.7. Toes Hyperextended in the Shoe

Strange but true is the fact that occasionally a parent will bring you their child who cries and limps when they put their shoes on. The parent is usually pretty embarrassed when it's pointed out that the toe, usually the fifth, is inadvertently hyperextended as the shoe is slipped on. A variety of other "shoe" syndromes also occur. Beware.

2.5.8. Legg–Calve–Perthes Disease

This is a disease of the hip joint that occurs most commonly in boys aged 3 to 7 years. At the turn of the century the most common cause of hip disease in this age group was tuberculosis and the condition was called "coxitis." The disease led to permanent loss of hip function and significant disability. Three different observers (Legg of Boston,

Calve of France, and Perthes of Germany) more or less simultaneously recognized that some of these children were not systemically ill and after a period of time developed relatively normal hip function. It was learned that the nontubercular coxitis, now known as Legg–Calve–Perthes disease (LCP), is caused by spontaneous idiopathic ischemic necrosis of the capital femoral epiphysis. It occurs more often in boys with a M/F ratio of 5. Hips are bilaterally affected about 10% of the time. It is rare in African-Americans (Wenger and Rang, 1993) and uncommon in native Americans (Weinstein, 1990).

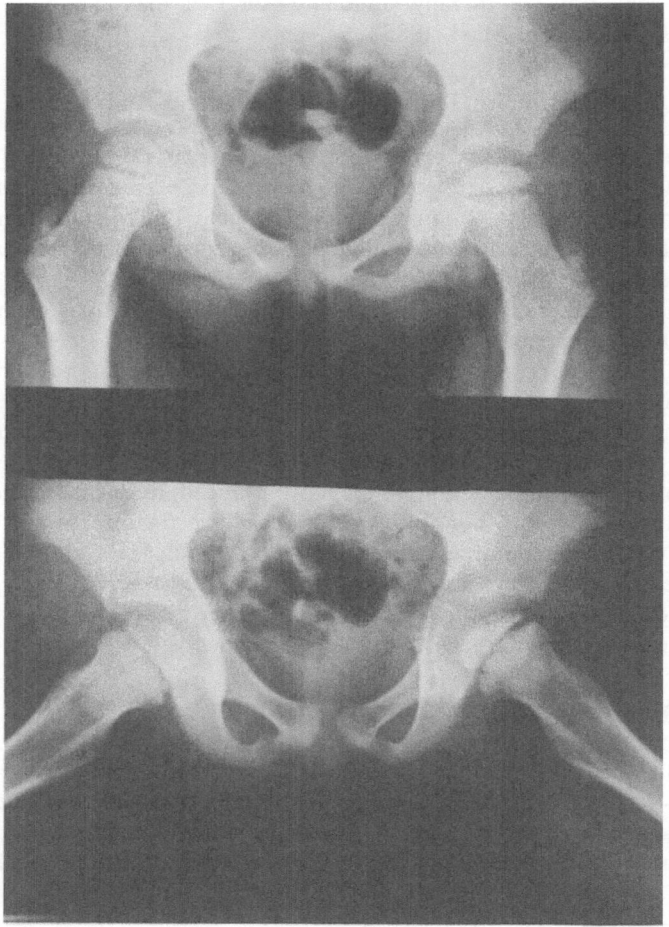

Figure 2.2. Early Legg–Perthes demonstrates itself in this left hip by a mild increase in radiodensity and loss of height of the proximal femoral epiphysis. Note also subchondral fracture and subtle ¹ ⁻ralization of femoral head, implying increased fluid in joint space (lower, frog-leg lateral film) ᴡn also as femoral head osteochondrosis or idiopathic osteonecrosis of the femoral head epiphysis, Legg–Perthes was originally described at about the same time by Calve (French), Legg (American), Perthes (German), and Waldenstrom (Swedish, but not of macroglobulinemia fame)

Children with sickle-cell disease and children on glucocorticosteroids are particularly predisposed to all types of aseptic necrosis, including LCP.

The usual presentation is that of an antalgic gait in which the involved hip is held flexed and externally rotated with the knee flexed. There may be a trunk lurch to the affected side when in stance phase. Medial thigh or knee pain may be prominent complaints and may erroneously take the physician's mind off the hip. Don't blame knee pain in a little boy on a sprain or strain. Check to make sure the hip examination is normal. If internal rotation or abduction is reduced or if a flexion contracture is present, anteroposterior and frog-leg lateral X-rays of the hip should be obtained. If initial films are negative but the diagnosis remains a possibility, repeat the X-rays in 1 month. Technetium bone scanning or MRI may be useful as well for early lesions. MRI is now considered by some to be the more sensitive imaging technique for these early lesions.

Differential diagnosis includes a variety of structural lesions which are usually apparent on X-ray, like residual from old hip dysplasia, idiopathic chondrolysis of the hip, slipped capital femoral epiphysis, spondyloepiphyseal dysplasia, or a variety of inflammatory processes which should be demonstrable with a CBC and sedimentation rate, like osteomyelitis or septic arthritis. JRA only rarely presents as monoarticular disease of the hip, though it can. Toxic synovitis should last only a few days. Persistent

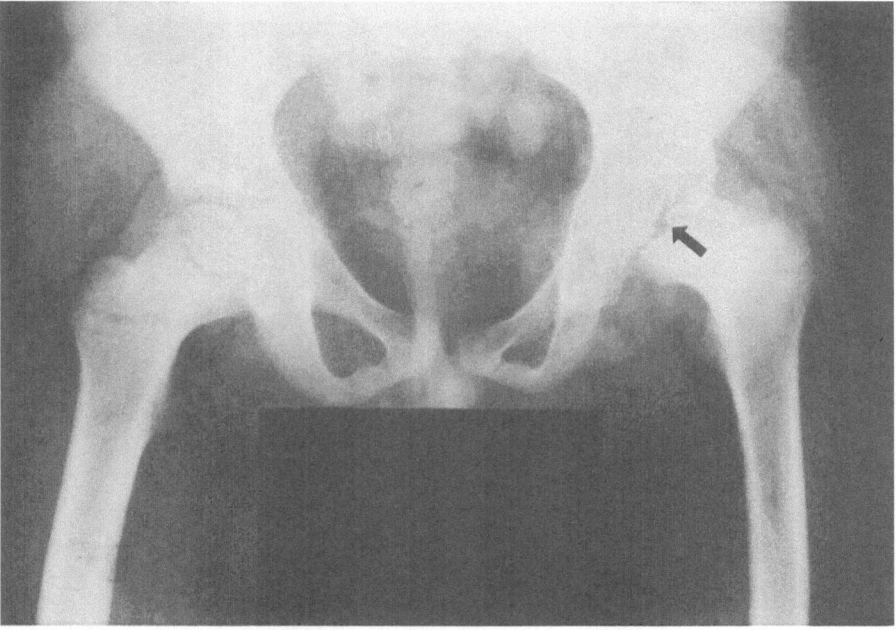

Figure 2.3. More advanced Legg–Perthes on the left with almost complete resorption of femoral head. Metaphyseal changes are also evident as well as irregularity of the acetabulum. Ossification lateral and superior to femoral neck implies extrusion of weakened cartilage likely to cause problems with fit as reossification occurs. Physeal line is marked with an arrow.

pain in the face of normal X-rays and blood work would lead to consideration of a neoplastic process and a technetium bone scan.

Healing occurs through replacement of the necrotic bone of the head of the femur and takes usually from 2 to 4 years. This new femoral head rarely appears the same as the original one but hopefully is concentric enough to result in normal function. Treatment must be individualized but always includes referral for orthopedic consultation, preferably with someone experienced in the care of childhood hips. In very young children with almost normal range of motion initially, the child can be treated by careful observation only. In older children, the treatment is aimed at containing the head of the femur within the acetabulum by various braces, casting, or surgery until the replacement process is completed. In general, boys younger than 8 years at presentation will ultimately have functional hips. For unknown reasons, girls with LCP have a worse prognosis, as do older boys.

2.5.9. Osgood–Schlatter Disease (OSD)

OSD is one of the two most common osteochondroses, the other being LCP. The term *osteochondrosis* refers to any of a large number of eponymously named diseases

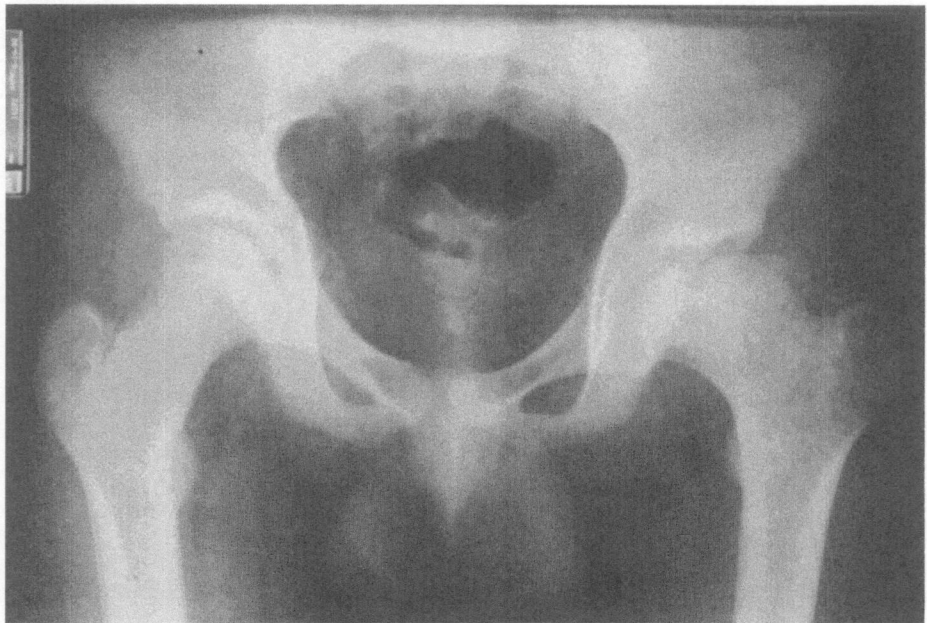

Figure 2.4. Well-healed Legg–Perthes on the left (not the same patient as in fig. 2 3) with shortening of the femoral neck, widening and flattening of what's left of the femoral head (coxa plana), and irregularity of acetabulum.

characterized by pathological changes in a secondary growth center (either epiphysis or apophysis) resulting from ischemic necrosis or traction.

OSD is a disease of the tibial tubercle that occurs most commonly in boys and quite predictably becomes symptomatic in early adolescence. The onset of symptoms is gradual and appears to be related to strenuous physical activity and rapid growth. The adolescent usually complains of knee pain to the parents after playing games like basketball or after prolonged running. During activity, the discomfort is not as severe as after resting for about an hour. The pain disappears completely after resting for a few days only to recur with renewed activity. By the time the patient is brought to the physician, the tibial tuberosity is more prominent than normal. Sometimes both tibiae will be involved. Pain is most severe if the tibial tuberosity is banged up against something or with kneeling. Girls may also develop OSD, though less frequently, and will present somewhat earlier, in keeping with their earlier age of puberty.

Physical examination reveals a normal range of motion of the knee joint without instability or swelling. There may be a prominent tibial tuberosity and, prominent or not, it is tender to palpation or percussion.

X-rays are not necessary for diagnosis. X-ray findings depend on the stage of the disease. Early, during the first few months, only soft tissue swelling is noted at the attachment of the patellar tendon to the tibial tuberosity apophysis. Later, after 6 to 12 months of symptoms, the tibial apophysis appears to fragment. Much later, after 2 to 4 years, small bony ossicles may appear within the distal portion of the patellar tendon.

The history of the treatment of OSD by physicians is one of overtreatment. The normal course is persistence of symptoms for about 2 years. Thereafter, the tibial tuberosity continues to have a beaked appearance but the symptoms diminish. Should the individual continue strenuous physical activity, the patellar tendonitis may persist until the mid-20s only to disappear when more normal activity is resumed. The primary care physician should restrict physical activity only if redness about the tuberosity or severe pain occurs. Cold compresses and 2 or 3 days of rest will allow the acute symptoms to subside so that the child can resume normal activities. Should the adolescent wish to participate in athletic activities enough to endure the discomfort, he or she should be allowed to do so. No permanent disability occurs from this condition. The parents should also be informed that if it does not hurt this 13-year-old boy too much to play basketball, it hurts no more to take out the garbage or mow the lawn!

On rare occasions, an adolescent can avulse the tibial tuberosity when jumping from a height, such as a wall. This causes acute pain and may require that the knee be immobilized in extension for a couple of weeks until the symptoms subside.

2.5.10. Slipped Capital Femoral Epiphysis (SCFE)

SCFE is also an adolescent disease and is an inferior and posterior slippage of the head of the femur off the neck. That is, the femoral neck goes north and the femoral head goes south. Slips can be either chronic or acute. SCFE occurs in young adolescents who complain of thigh, knee, or groin pain and who limp. SCFE most commonly presents in the summertime apparently as a result of increased physical activity with the warm weather months.

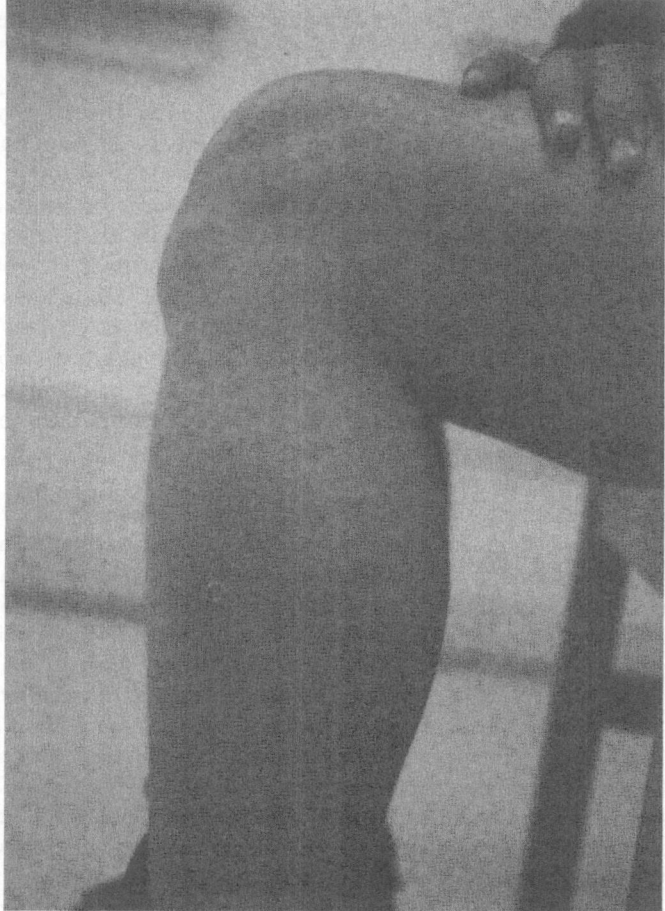

Figure 2 5 The bump over the tibial tuberosity caused by apophysitis of the tibial tubercle (Osgood–Schlatter disease) is tender There should be no intraarticular joint swelling, however, or any internal derangement of the knee Osgood (American) and Schlatter (Swiss) both more or less simultaneously described this problem in 1903

Acute slips present like any other fracture of the femur, with severe pain The blood supply to the proximal femoral epiphysis runs along the femoral neck and is particularly likely to be compromised with an acute slip, with resulting avascular necrosis superimposed SCFE occurs more often than expectable in African-American children and in obese children, though half of the children affected are of normal weight The disease usually presents unilaterally, though 30 to 40% of children with one slip will develop bilateral disease eventually and therefore must be seen at regular intervals to follow the

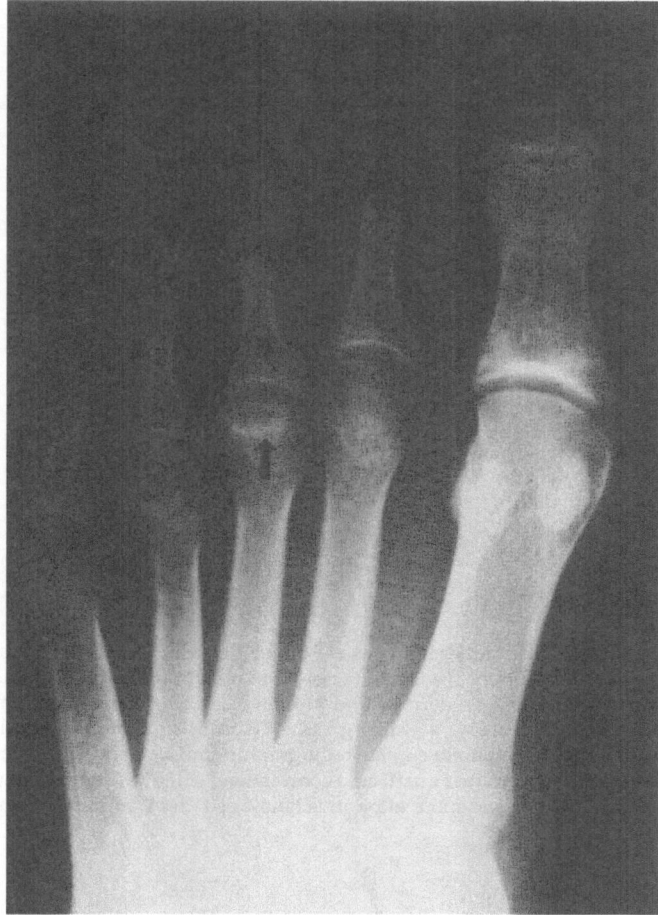

Figure 2 6 There are a large number of eponymously named osteochondroses mostly of obscure etiology including such clinically important ones as Legg–Perthes disease Freiberg infraction or disease is pictured here (arrow) and represents sclerosis, partial collapse, and eventual flattening of the head of the second or, less commonly, third metatarsal head in young adolescent girls It causes local pain and tenderness may be a stress fracture, is less common than Legg–Perthes or Osgood–Schlatter disease and is treated by putting a cushioned metatarsal bar inside the shoe to take the weight off the sensitive metatarsal head

"normal" hip Delays in bony maturation, sometimes associated with frank endocrine abnormalities, have been described (Morrissy, 1990) Early recognition and prompt treatment result in an excellent prognosis

Physical examination shows a typical hip limp (antalgic, flexed and externally rotated), with a lateral lurch (Trendelenburg) gait When the child lies supine on the examining table, it will be noted that the involved lower extremity is externally rotated

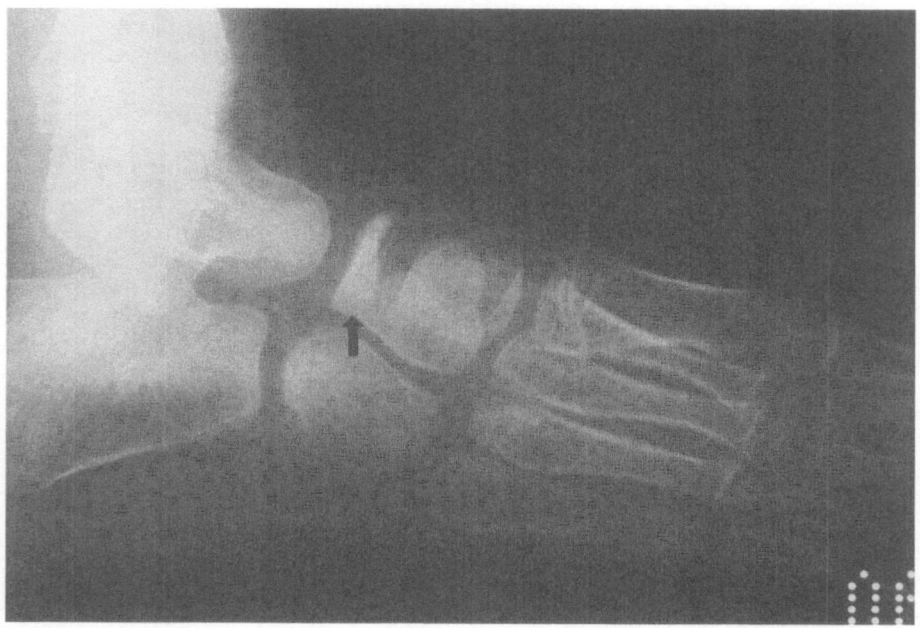

Figure 2.7. Still another of the osteochondroses is Kohler disease, which is represented by the sclerosis and collapse of the tarsal navicular (arrow) demonstrated on this radiograph. It is associated with pain with activity, tenderness and swelling and is treated symptomatically with activity modification or, if necessary, a walking cast. Diagnosis is problematical since many asymptomatic children will demonstrate similar radiographic findings and symptomatic children may have abnormal radiographs on their unaffected contralateral side. It is somewhat unique among the osteochondroses in that it occurs more often in school-aged children rather than adolescents.

and cannot be internally rotated, an external rotation contracture. When the hip is passively flexed, the thigh externally rotates more, in some cases to 45°. There may also be a flexion contracture at the hip early on in the disease as well as loss of abduction.

An X-ray examination of the hip is required with emphasis on the lateral projection (frog-leg lateral). Since the slip is often in the anteroposterior dimension, slips often don't project well on standard AP films of the pelvis.

SCFE is one of only a few pediatric orthopedic emergencies. Weight-bearing must cease completely at diagnosis because partial slips sometimes become complete slips if the patient is allowed to continue to ambulate. Complete slips carry an increased risk of vascular compromise, aseptic necrosis, and persistent and potentially debilitating hip disease. Some children get to definitive therapy too late because they have been treated for a "groin pull," imagined knee problems or arthritis for many months. Remember that monoarticular arthritis of the hip is an uncommon way for JRA to present.

Therapy is surgical pinning to prevent further slippage, usually without reduction.

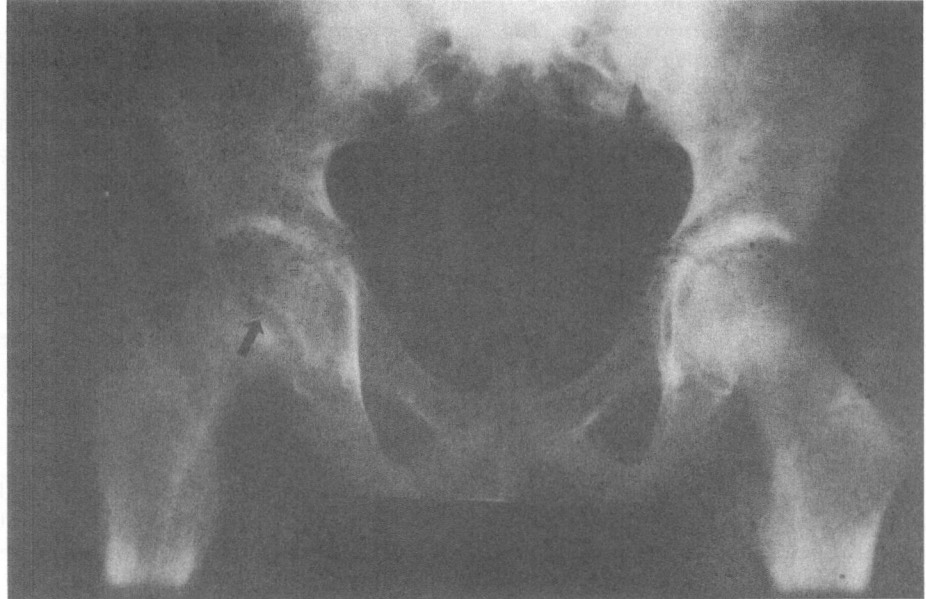

Figure 2.8. Anteroposterior hip film of an adolescent boy with right-sided slipped capital femoral epiphysis (SCFE). To rule out a slip, a frog-leg lateral film (abducted, externally rotated) is essential since most slips are in an anteroposterior direction and may therefore be missed on an AP film. In this case, however, a line along the superior aspect of the femoral neck on the right doesn't pass through any of the femoral head; compare with normal left hip. Additionally the physis is clearly widened on the right (arrow) compared with the left, both of which are abnormalities suggestive of SCFE

2.5.11. Overuse Injuries, Shin Splints, Stress Fractures

These and other causes for extremity pain associated with athletic endeavors are discussed in Chapter 8, Sports Injuries in Children.

2.5.12. Flat Feet

Flat feet, both the everyday flexible variety and the rigid variety, may cause foot and extremity pain. They are discussed in Chapter 4, Developmental Orthopedics.

2.5.13. Hypermobility

A variety of well-defined genetic syndromes are associated with joint hypermobility. They include Marfan syndrome, Down syndrome, Ehlers–Danlos syndrome, and osteogenesis imperfecta, among others. Many more children, however, are at risk for joint injury and extremity pain as a result of a general predisposition to hyperlaxity.

This may present as pain and limp or even joint effusion after vigorous physical activity. They may be able to perform entertaining "double-jointed" tricks for their friends with their fingers. Family history is often positive for similar problems. On physical examination such children may demonstrate recurvatum, the ability to hyperextend the elbows or knees more than 10° beyond straight, neutral extension. They usually can put the radial border of their thumb on the flexor surface of their forearm. Hypermobility may also predispose to the development of other deformities which independently may cause limp or painful extremities, including developmental dysplasia of the hip and recurrent patellar dislocation.

Treatment is directed toward protecting chronically injured joints. This may be accomplished by exercises to improve the strength of opposing muscles to the joint in question. Joints may have to be rested if symptoms persist. We become less flexible as we age, luckily, and problems associated with hypermobility improve with age as well.

2.5.14. The Patellofemoral Syndrome

The patellofemoral syndrome represents a spectrum of dysfunction from mild problems of patellar tracking between the condyles of the distal femur to recurrent episodes of patellar dislocation. Chondromalacia patellae is the term used to describe anterior knee pain in adolescents presumably resulting from malalignment, overuse, direct trauma, recurrent dislocation, or some combination of more than one of the above. It is one of the most common causes of adolescent knee pain. Despite its name, the articular surface of the patella is normal and any degenerative changes present are found deeper within the patella. Typically, patellofemoral pain occurs with stair walking, sitting for long periods, or any other activity which increases compressive forces on the patella. Stiffness or even locking are also sometimes described. Bilateral pain is frequent. Effusions are uncommon.

On physical examination, pain or crepitus is found on patellar compression with the knee in extension. Patient apprehension as the patella is moved laterally or medially should raise the question of recurrent subluxation in addition to any tracking problem. X-rays (AP and lateral) should be obtained to eliminate other pathological processes involving the knee. "Sunrise" or patellar views may demonstrate patellar lateralization or irregularities.

Treatment consists of exercises to increase overall quadriceps strength, hopefully improving tracking through the intercondylar groove. This should be done isometrically or by knee extension against mild resistance but only through the last few degrees before full extension is reached. To extend through the entire movement arc of the knee puts excessive compression on the patella and may exacerbate the problem. Limitation of pain-producing activities is warranted during periods of increased discomfort. Mild analgesics, like acetaminophen, used judiciously or ice packs may also be helpful.

2.5.15. Other Mechanical Knee Problems

Other painful intraarticular problems involving the knee are handled in other parts of this book. See Chapter 6 for a discussion of such birth defects involving the

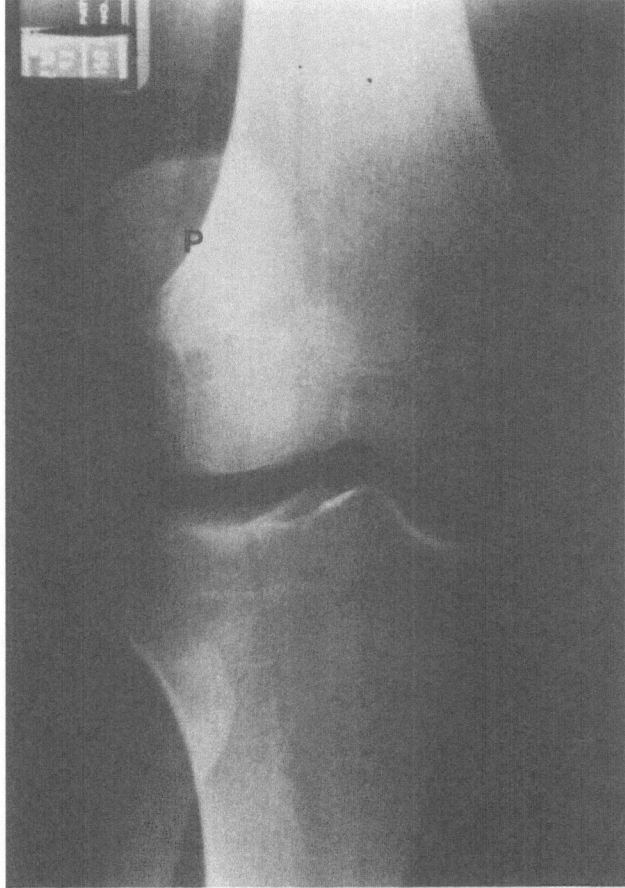

Figure 2.9. Patella alta is demonstrated in this AP knee film, with the patella (P) high-riding and laterally deviated

knee as discoid meniscus. See Chapter 8 for overuse or ligamentous injuries affecting the knees of young athletes.

2.5.16. Osteochondritis Dissecans (OD)

OD is a local degenerative lesion of articular cartilage and bone which generally affects adolescents and older children. It may occur in any joint but is most common in the knee, affecting usually the lateral side of the medial condyle of the femur. Other areas such as the lateral femoral condyle and the patella are also affected and have, in general, a less favorable prognosis. Boys are three times more likely to be affected than girls.

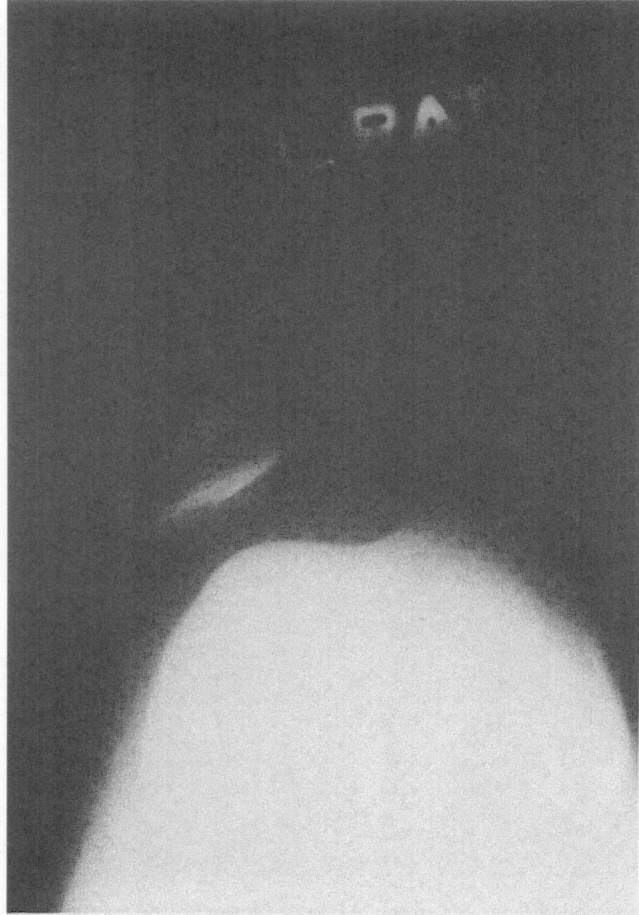

Figure 2.10. Axial or "sunrise" view of same patient as in Fig. 2.9 demonstrating shallow femoral sulcus and lateral subluxation.

Bilateral disease is not uncommon (Ozonoff, 1992). Prognosis is generally good with most healing without difficulty after minimal intervention.

OD causes pain and swelling and can cause locking of the knee as well if the injured fragment of articular cartilage separates from the underlying bone to form a loose body within the joint. The etiology of OD is unknown though trauma or inadequate blood supply are often mentioned as possibilities.

Radiologically, OD is associated with a lucent semicircular lesion of the medial femoral condyle. It often involves the intercondylar notch and is bordered with a sclerotic edge. A small bony fragment may be situated within the fossa of the lesion. Beware of a similarly appearing normal variant evident posteriorly in the condyles of younger children. Lateral views should help differentiate anteriorly located OD from these posterior normal condylar irregularities. "Notch" views may be necessary if standard AP films of the knee are negative and OD is suspected.

Patients with open growth plates seem to do well with only a decrease in activities. Immobilization for a short period of time may be beneficial and crutch walking may be useful if symptoms persist.

In adolescents or in children who have failed a conservative approach for 6 months, surgical evaluation, either arthroscopically or open, is appropriate. Drilling of the intact

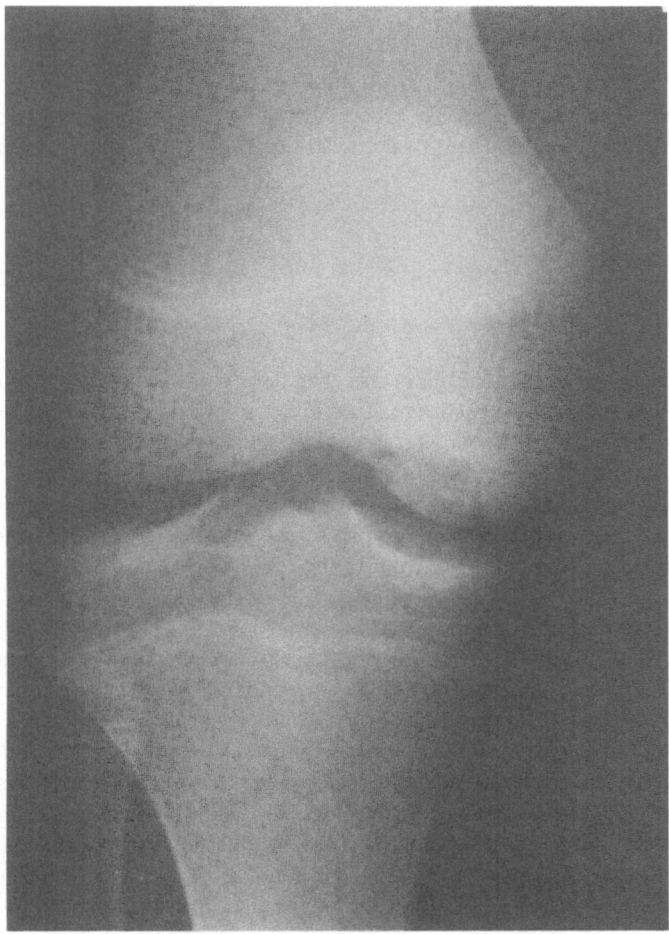

Figure 2.11. Osteochondritis dissecans is clearly seen in this 15-year-old male. It is present in the typical location, the lateral aspect of the medial femoral condyle. When not seen on AP projection, a notched or tunnel view is sometimes useful to detect lesions located more posteriorly. However, normal ossification variations occur posteriorly as well, sometimes leading to confusion

Table 2.2. Common Causes of Extremity Pain without Systemic Symptoms

Nighttime calf and thigh pains ("growing pains")	Osgood–Schlatter disease
Painful heels	Slipped capital femoral epiphysis
Snapping hips	Overuse, shin splints, stress fractures
Reflex sympathetic dystrophy	
Fibromyalgia	Hypermobility
Spiral fractures of the tibia	Patellofemoral syndrome
Poorly fitting shoes	Osteochondritis dissecans
Legg–Calve–Perthes disease	

injured area may be useful to increase blood supply. Partially separated fragments may be drilled and fixed with either pins or screws. Completely detached fragments should be excised.

2.6. EXTREMITY PAIN WITH MODEST SYSTEMIC SYMPTOMS

2.6.1. Transient (Toxic) Synovitis of the Hip

The time from 3 to 7 years of life is one of the more rowdy ages of childhood and is associated with two causes of limp, more often in boys. The first is Legg–Calve–Perthes and is described above. The second is transient or toxic synovitis of the hip (TSH). It is associated with sudden hip, knee, or medial thigh pain and occurs most often in the spring of the year. Although a low-grade temperature may be present, the child really is not systemically ill and is brought to the physician with decided antalgic hip limp with hip and knee flexed and the child walking on the toes of the affected extremity, if walking at all.

Physical examination will generally show a well-looking child with, at the most, a low-grade fever. The child will prefer to hold the hip in flexion, abduction, and external rotation, presumably in an attempt to reduce intracapsular pressure and thereby reduce discomfort. Careful examination of the hip will demonstrate a hip flexion contracture (see Thomas test, Chapter 1), diminished internal rotation, and limited abduction. The CBC and erythrocyte sedimentation rate are generally normal and X-rays of the hip prove unrevealing. The author has aspirated the hip joint of such children on several occasions and has obtained only a few cubic centimeters of clear sterile synovial fluid.

The cause of this malady is not known. It occurs most often in the same sex (boys) and age group (3 to 7 years) as LCP but there is no apparent relation between the two diseases. Large series of patients with transient synovitis have been followed and only 1% have developed LCP. Even this modest, apparently increased, predisposition to aseptic necrosis with TSH may be phony since distinguishing early LCP from TSH may be difficult.

The child with TSH is easily treated by bed rest at home for 3 to 5 days. One follow-up visit should be made in about 2 weeks. At that time, no limp and a normal range of motion are expectable outcomes. If the child does in fact have early LCP, symptoms of hip irritation and signs of reduced hip motion will persist.

The diagnosis of transient synovitis of the hip is a diagnosis of exclusion. Humility, circumspection, and insecurity are important emotions to harbor when making the diagnosis of TSH. Significant fever, persistent or worsening signs of symptoms, leukocytosis, or increased acute phase reactants should make one consider strongly a true septic arthritis and a hip aspiration.

2.6.2. Tumors and Other Neoplastic Processes

Tumors of the skeleton may be primary or secondary, benign or malignant. They present as pain or as a mass or they may be picked up incidentally on an X-ray done for some other purpose. Pain may result from osseous invasion, and is often worse at night, or may be a result of a "pathologic" fracture through weakened bone.

2.6.2.1. Primary Malignant Tumors

Fortunately, primary malignant tumors of bone are rare in children. They include osteosarcoma, Ewing sarcoma, and a variety of other, even less common neoplasms. They most often occur in the metaphyses or diaphyses of long bones during adolescence, more often in males than females. The femur, pelvis, and humerus are common sites. Half of all osteogenic sarcomas occur around the knee.

The presenting complaint is constant, dull, well-localized pain of several weeks' duration. The pain is unrelated to activity and the hallmark is nocturnal pain. The complaints are usually well-localized to the affected area. If the tumor is in the metaphysis of bone, the adjacent joint motion is usually decreased.

A deep, firm, rather painful mass may also be noted by the patient and parents. All too often these complaints are brushed off as a muscle pull though the latter should not cause pain for long, does not hurt at night and, is usually related to activity.

Weight loss may also be present. Ewing sarcoma in particular is associated with systemic symptoms of fever with leukocytosis and elevated ESR. Metastases are often to the lungs.

Radiographically, osteosarcoma produces an ill-defined lesion most often at the metaphysis of a long bone, combining elements of bony destruction and formation. Soft tissue swelling may be present as well as soft tissue calcification in a diffuse, scattered "sunburst" pattern. Periosteal elevation caused by tumor expansion may result in Codman's triangle.

Ewing's sarcoma is more likely to be diaphyseal, ill-defined, and with lots of periosteal elevation and reaction, sometimes resulting in a layered, onion-skin appearance (Springfield, 1990).

2.6.2.2. Primary Benign Lesions

A variety of benign, often cystic bony lesions have been described. They often are discovered incidentally or as a result of a pathological fracture. Nonossifying fibromas

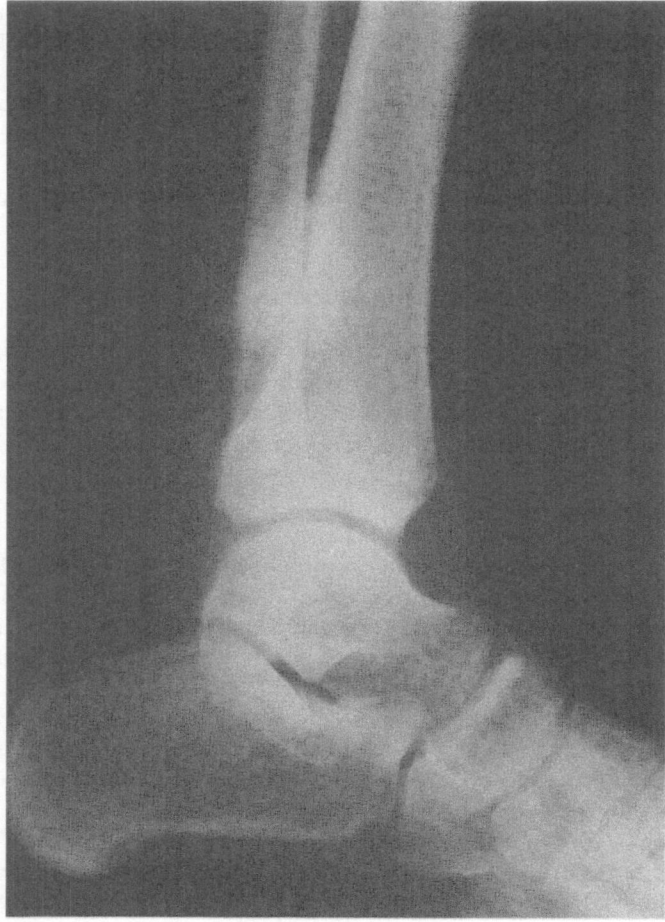

Figure 2.12. Osteogenic sarcoma of distal tibia in a teenager. X-ray courtesy of the Department of Diagnostic Radiology, University of Kentucky.

and fibrous cortical defects are well-defined islands of uncalcified fibrous tissue within the bone often seen incidentally around the knee.

Exostoses are bony outgrowths which may occur singly or, when inherited as a dominant trait, in multiple locations. The latter is associated with generalized short stature as well as localized growth abnormalities. Simple bone cysts, also known as unicameral bone cysts, are well-defined metaphyseal lesions filled with clear liquid. Pathological fractures are common. If at risk, the cyst can be treated with surgical curettage with grafting or steroid injection into the cyst.

Aneurysmal bone cysts are full of blood and may cause aching pain because of their tendency to expand, even if they don't fracture.

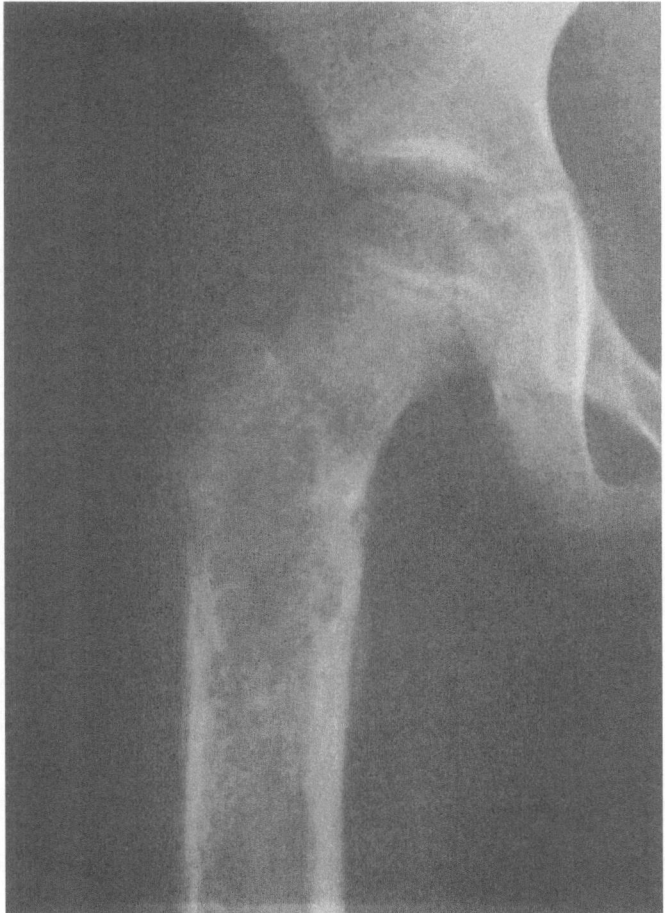

Figure 2.13. This is an X-ray of far-advanced Ewing sarcoma in an 8-year-old girl from Guatemala Note medullary infiltration, cortical destruction, and periostitis Ewing sarcoma occurs most frequently in the femur, pelvis, and humerus, but can involve any part of the skeleton

Osteoid osteomas cause nighttime bone pain which is very focal and is classically described as relieved with aspirin. When present in the spine it is an important consideration because it causes painful scoliosis. Radiologically there is a small, 5- to 10-mm nidus surrounded by densely sclerotic bone. The nidus is usually radiolucent on plain radiographs but may be calcified on CT. On technetium bone scan it produces intense local uptake at the lesion layered on top of diffusely increased uptake in the region (Ozonoff, 1992). A similar, but larger lesion (greater than 20 mm) is called an osteoblastoma.

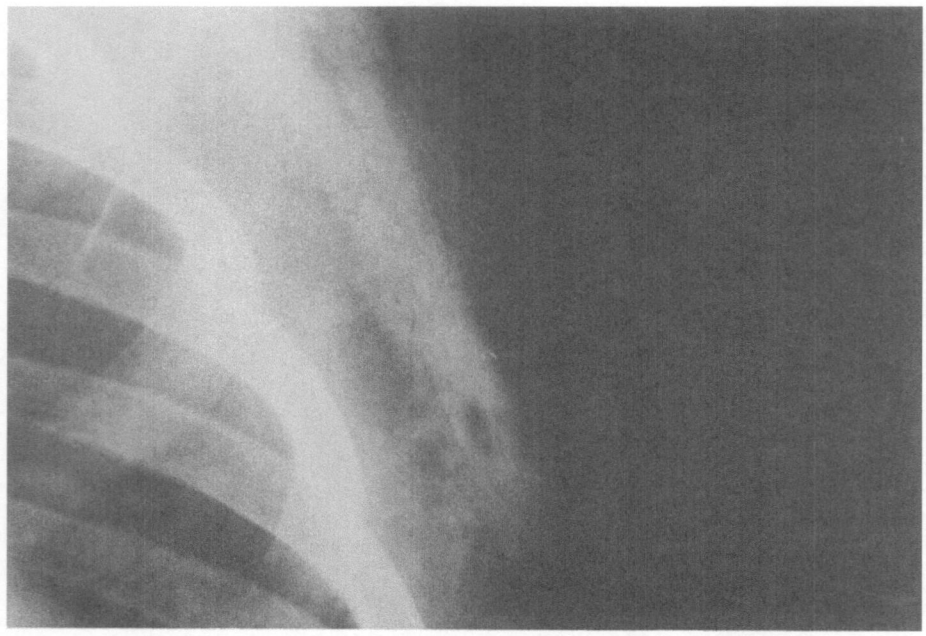

Figure 2.14. Ewing sarcoma of the scapula Note periosteal "onion skin" appearance which is typical X-ray courtesy of the Department of Diagnostic Radiology, University of Kentucky

2.6.2.3. Secondary Neoplasia

Two secondary neoplastic processes are worth mentioning, namely acute leukemia and neuroblastoma. Both cause infiltrative disease of the skeleton, usually with diffuse pain, sometimes with joint effusions. Dramatic systemic symptoms are most often absent though low-grade fever, malaise, and anorexia are common.

Up to 50% of children with leukemia will have musculoskeletal symptoms at the time of presentation. Often they are thought to have some form of JRA. Hematology evaluation may show elevated ESR and may be indistinguishable from JRA. Ostrov *et al.* (1993) found that only children with leukemia, as opposed to JRA, had nighttime pain and nonarticular bone pain. Plain radiographs in children with JRA generally showed only joint effusions, while children with leukemia had periosteal elevation, metaphyseal rarefaction on X-ray, and more abnormalities on technetium bone scanning (Ostrov *et al.*, 1993). Serum lactic dehydrogenase (LDH) levels may be useful distinguishing between inflammatory and neoplastic causes of limb pain with neoplastic causes manifesting significant elevations in serum LDH levels (Wallendal *et al.*, 1992).

With neuroblastoma, X-rays will often demonstrate lytic lesions of the spine, skull, femur, ribs, or pelvis (Cassidy and Petty, 1990).

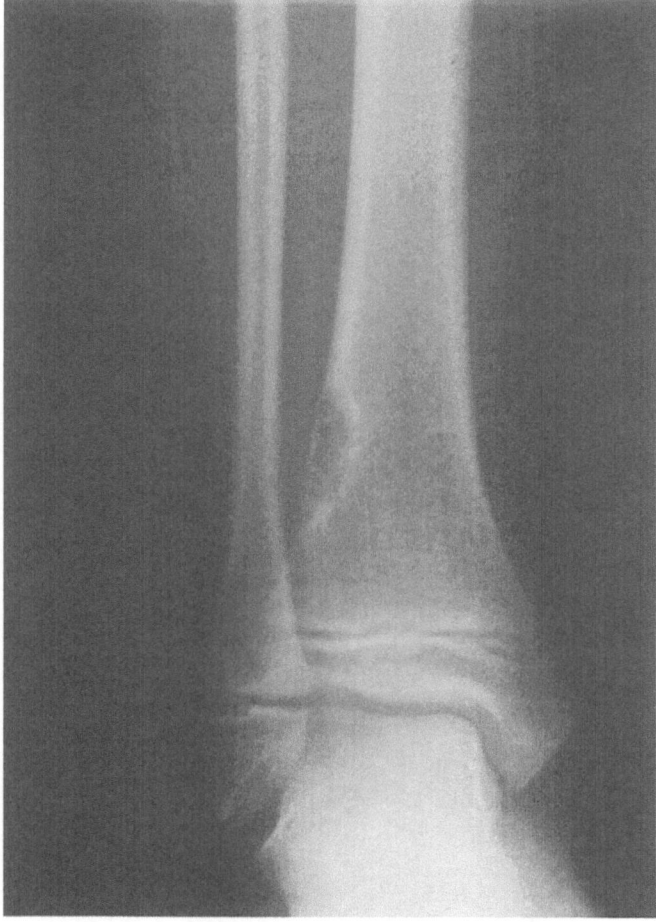

Figure 2.15. This is a benign cortical defect of the distal tibia They are common and benign except if very large and predispose to pathological fracture They start at the metaphysis and move toward the center of the bone shaft as growth occurs

2.6.2.4 Diagnosis

An X-ray examination (anteroposterior and lateral films at a minimum) should be performed on any child with persistent local complaints. The radiologist should be able to inform the primary physician if there are any osseous changes suggesting a malignancy. If the initial films are negative, obtaining films of the more proximate parts of the extremity should be considered since painful lesions sometimes produce symptoms referred distally.

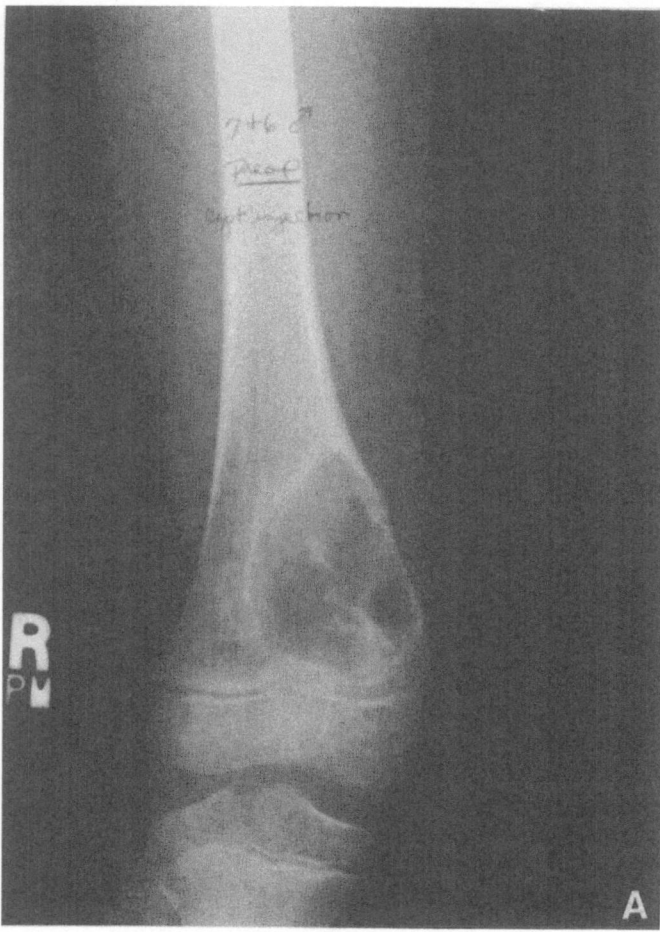

Figure 2.16. (A) Simple bone cyst of the distal femur, a somewhat unusual location since most are in either the femoral neck or proximal humerus These are also known as unicameral bone cysts though irregular septumlike structures are frequently visible (B) After successful steroid instillation, the cyst has healed in and the child has grown, with what remains of the cyst's walls moving centrally (arrow)

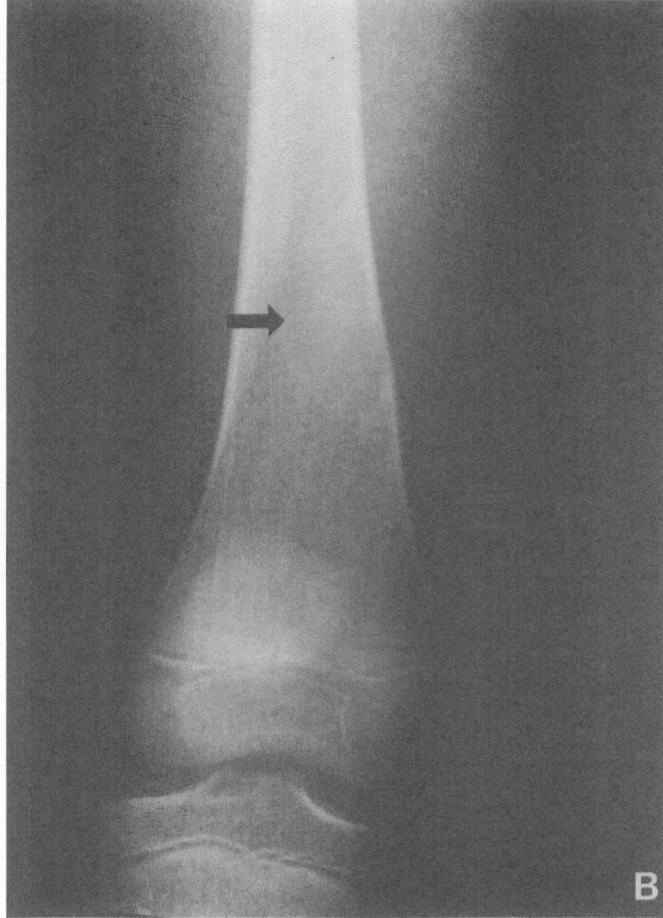

Figure 2.16. (*Continued*)

Radioisotope bone scanning or a repeat of the plain films after 2 weeks may prove useful in a child with persistent discomfort, systemic symptoms, or an abnormal CBC, platelet count, ESR, or elevated serum LDH level. A positive X-ray examination should result in an immediate referral to an orthopedist or oncologist expert at dealing with this type of pathology and other consultants as appropriate.

2.6.3. Discitis

Discitis is a low-grade and chronic inflammatory process involving an intervertebral disc occurring in infants and young children. Etiologically, its cause is obscure,

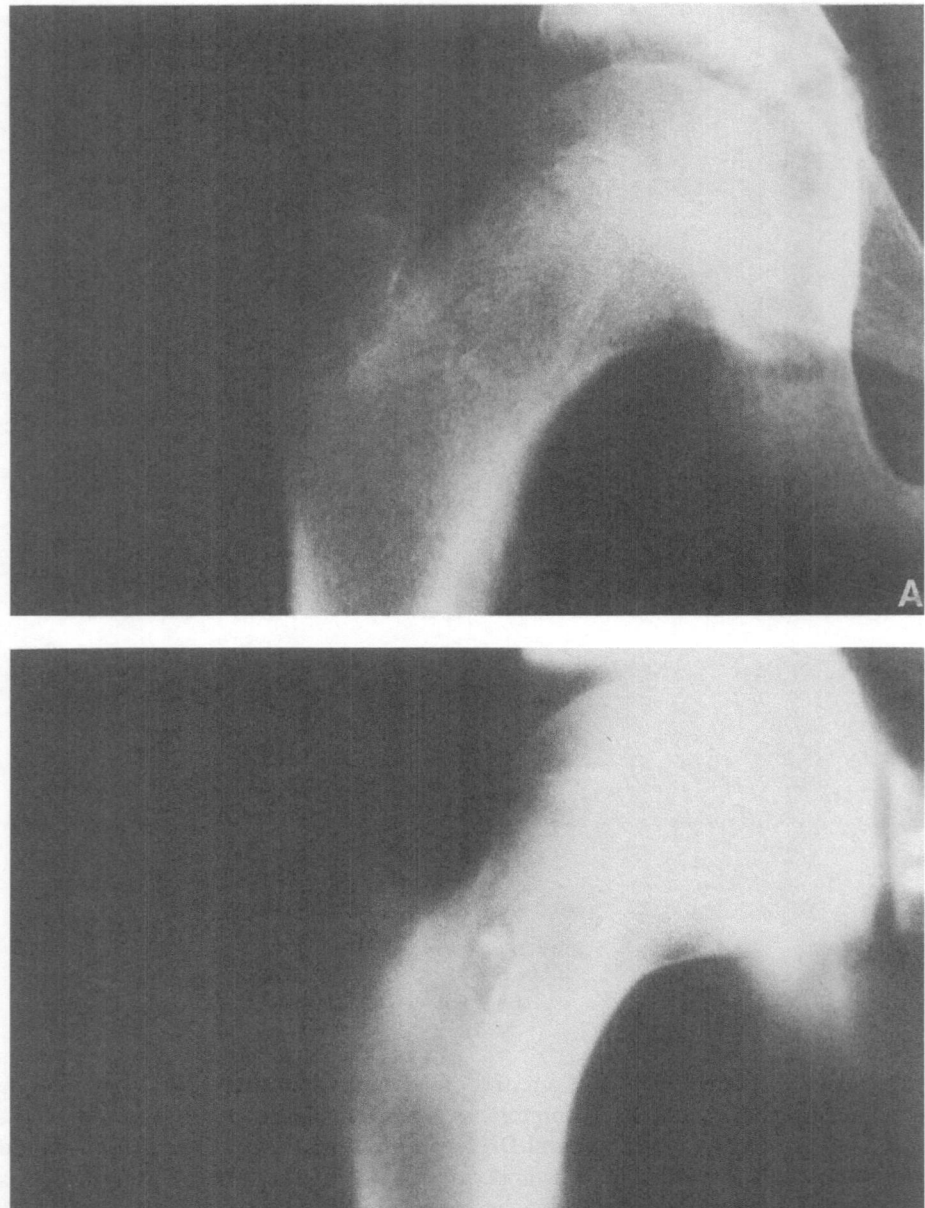

Figure 2.17. (A) Osteoid osteoma in a 14-year-old boy The plain radiograph shows only an ill-defined lucency with slight surrounding sclerosis (B) Tomogram shows central calcification of nidus and surrounding sclerosis Lesions, like this one, in cancellous bone excite less surrounding reactive sclerosis than lesions in cortical bone

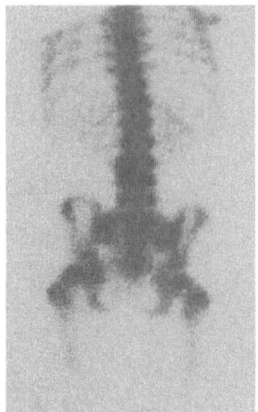

Figure 2.18. Osteoid osteoma in the neural arch of one of the midlumbar vertebrae. Such a lesion would be expected to cause painful scoliosis with the concavity of the curve on the same side as the lesion. Note corresponding "hot" spot on technetium bone scan as well as apparent mild scoliosis.

though sometimes *Staphylococcus aureus* can be cultured if the disc is aspirated. The lumbar spine is most frequently involved.

It remains unresolved whether this condition is a true infection or not. Discitis is quite different and much more benign than true vertebral osteomyelitis which presents with more dramatic systemic signs, symptoms, and loss of volume of the affected vertebral body radiographically.

Children with discitis will present with lower extremity pain, abdominal pain, or refusal to walk more often than back pain, which makes their diagnosis difficult. Stiffness of the back and localized tenderness, however, is typical if searched for. Either hyperlordosis or a loss of the normal curvature may occur. Low-grade fever is common.

The WBC count is most often normal though the ESR is usually moderately elevated. A radioisotope bone scan will often show increased uptake by the two vertebral bodies adjoining the inflamed disc. Eventually, after 3 or 4 weeks, radiographs will show intervertebral narrowing with sclerosis and erosions affecting the contiguous vertebral margins.

Tuberculin skin testing should be performed to exclude tuberculous disease as the spine. Aspiration or biopsy of the affected interspace is not often rewarding enough to balance the risks of the procedure unless complications or recurrent disease are manifest (Crawford *et al.*, 1991).

Treatment is supportive with activity limited as necessary. Anti-inflammatory analgesics may prove useful. Antibiotics are not often needed unless more conservative measures fail (Crawford *et al.*, 1991).

2.6.4. Viral Myositis

A variety of infectious agents can cause muscle aches or even myositis with elevation of muscle enzymes and ESR. Perhaps most common are the muscle aches which often occur during the recovery phase of influenza. These most often affect the

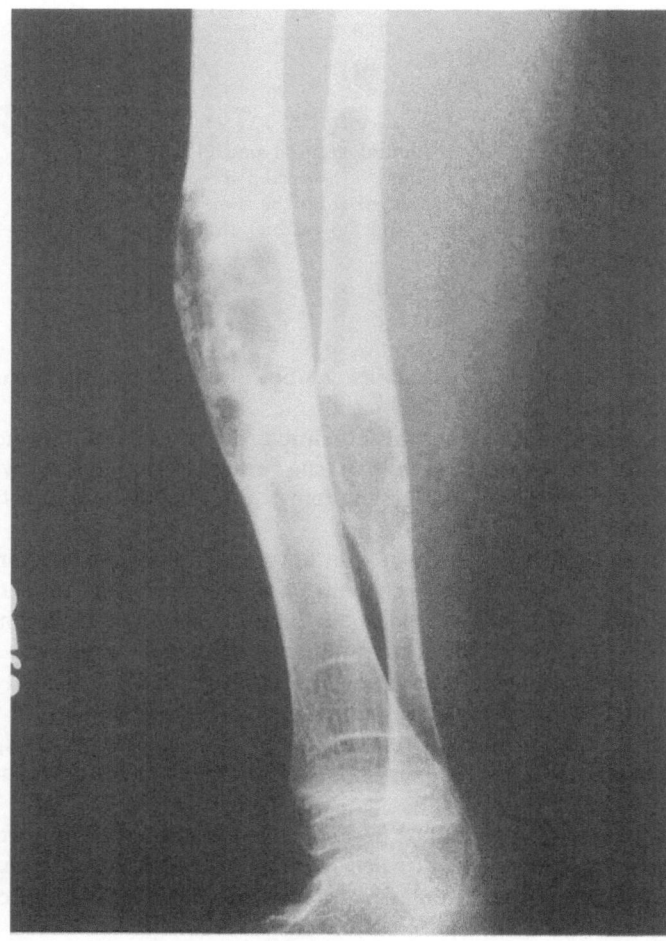

Figure 2.19. Campanacci disease, also known as ossifying fibroma or osteofibrous dysplasia. Typical location for this luckily uncommon lesion of unknown cause; likely to result in bowing and pathological fracture.

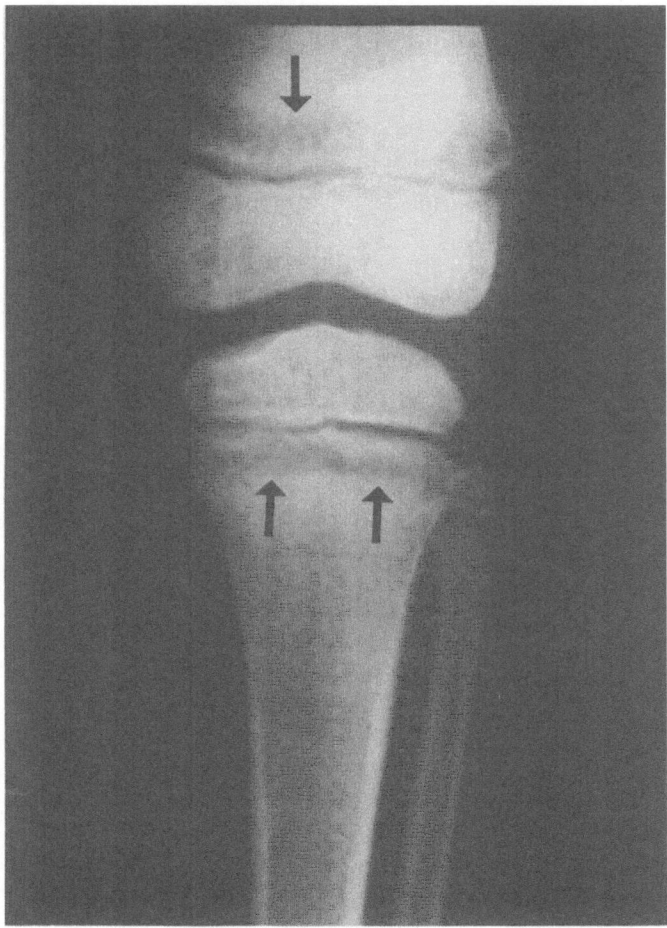

Figure 2.20. Typical metaphyseal rarefaction in child with acute leukemia (arrows). Generalized osteoporosis and periosteal elevation may also occur, causing radiologic changes, with any type of acute leukemia. X-ray courtesy of Dr. Vesna Criss, Department of Radiology, University of Kentucky.

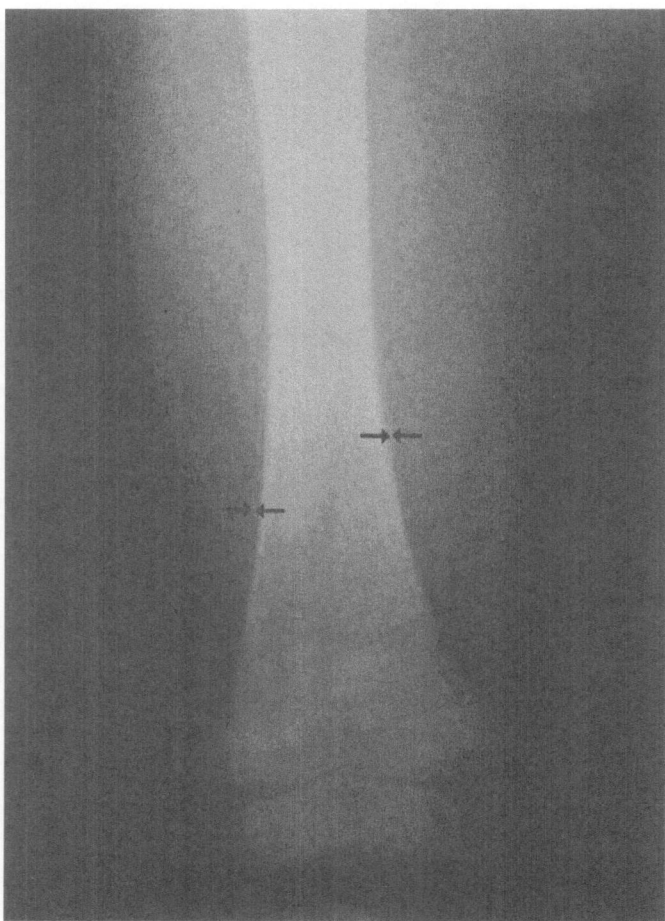

Figure 2.21. Periosteal elevation with new bone formation due to neuroblastoma (arrows). The same picture might also occur as a result of leukemic infiltration, sickle-cell disease, osteomyelitis, or trauma. X-ray courtesy of Dr. Vesna Criss, Department of Radiology, University of Kentucky.

calf muscles and can be severe. Many other viruses are implicated, as well as toxo-plasmosis and trichinosis. Bacterial infection of the muscle itself, often staphylococcal, has also been described, usually subsequent to muscle injury.

2.7. EXTREMITY PAIN WITH SIGNIFICANT SYSTEMIC SYMPTOMS

2.7.1. Acute Osteomyelitis

Hematogenous osteomyelitis is a metaphyseal disease. It seems to start as a result of bacteria taking up residence in one of the myriad of sinusoids that are present in the primary spongiosa of the metaphysis. These bacteria grow to form an abscess which subsequently decompresses by forcing the pus down the intramedullary canal, out through the surrounding periosteum, up through the epiphyseal plate (in infants) or into the adjacent joint. The child will therefore present with fever and pain in an extremity near a joint. This pain may cause the child to refuse to walk or move the extremity, termed *pseudoparalysis*. When the involved portion of the bone is palpated, exquisite tenderness will usually be apparent.

Staphylococcus aureus and group A streptococci are the most commonly found pathogens throughout childhood with *Haemophilus influenzae* making a contribution among patients 1 month through 5 years (Jackson and Nelson, 1982). Other organisms are occasionally implicated. *Pseudomonas aeruginosa*, for example, is frequently found causing infection resulting from puncture wounds incurred through the sole of a sneaker or tennis shoe.

Laboratory studies will generally show a leukocytosis with a shift to the left and an elevated ESR. On X-ray examination, soft tissue swelling will be the only finding for the first 10 days. Radioisotope bone scan will usually demonstrate increased uptake in the involved metaphysis. Blood cultures may be positive occasionally though the quickest way to obtain a specific diagnosis is to pass a needle down to the bone at the point of maximum tenderness. This will likely be the location where the perforating abscess has lifted the periosteum off the cortex and under which there will be pus to be aspirated, Gram-stained, and cultured.

Treatment consists of bed rest, specific antibiotic therapy given intravenously, and close monitoring. Pain and fever will decrease in the first 24 hours. Indeed, under optimal circumstances, within 3 or 4 days, the child may become so asymptomatic that it becomes difficult to obtain compliance for the recommended 6 weeks of antibiotic treatment.

Some children do not follow such a happy therapeutic course. Should the child's fever, pain, or tenderness persist or worsen despite antibiotics, the treatment physician should consider more active intervention. Sometimes the abscess ruptures into the adjacent joint which then demands treatment for a septic arthritis as described below. Surgical drainage of the metaphysis may also be indicated if the child does not improve after 3 or 4 days of antibiotics.

The physician should be a little cautious when indicating to the parents whether the child has been "cured" of the osteomyelitis or not. An old axiom, when chronic

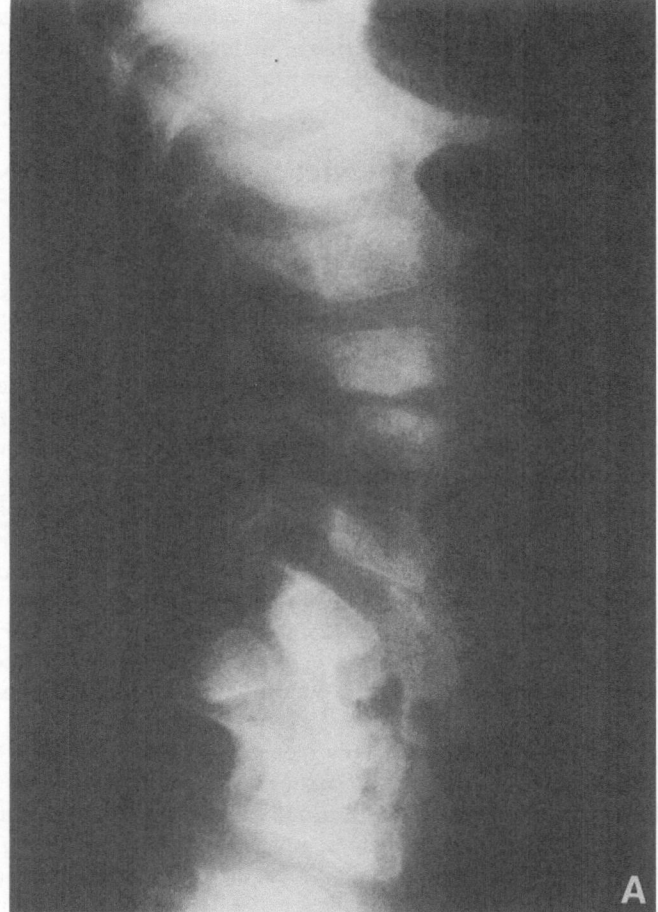

Figure 2.22. (A) Narrowing of L-3–L-4 disc space with vertebral end plate sclerosis was the result of discitis in this 33-month-old child. (B) A little less than a year later, the disc space has reconstituted itself to a considerable degree.

osteomyelitis was more common, goes "once osteomyelitis, always osteomyelitis." Under modern treatment we may be able to be more optimistic. Should the child be followed for a year or so and should X-ray examination reveal normal bone, then one may state that the osteomyelitis is gone forever (see also Chapter 11).

2.7.2. Septic Arthritis (see also Chapter 11)

Septic arthritis or pyarthrosis can occur in children of any age though after the age of 1 year or so it becomes increasingly uncommon. The child with a pyarthrosis will

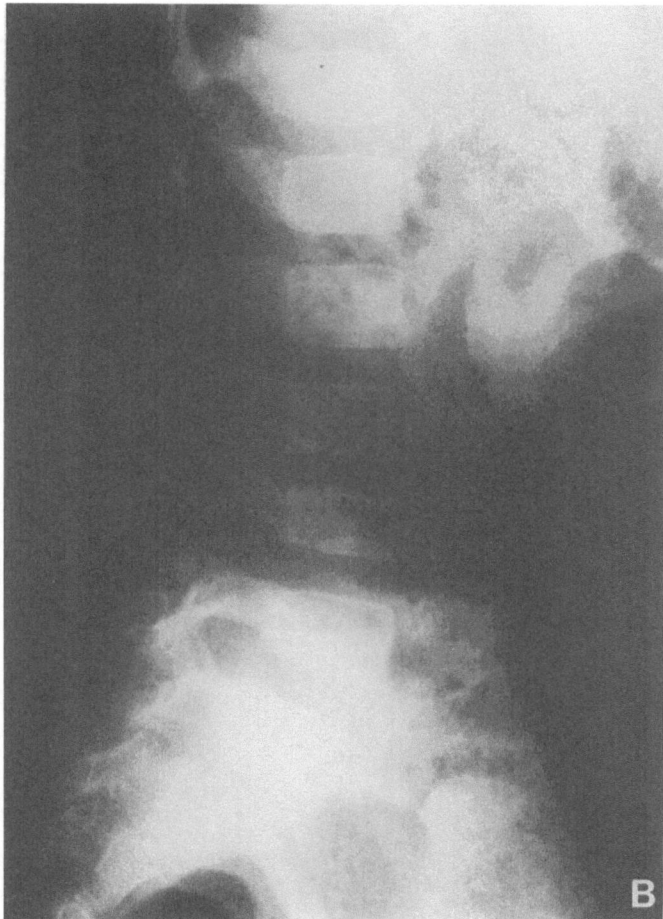

Figure 2.22. (*Continued*)

**Table 2.3. Extremity
Pain with Modest
Systemic Symptoms**[a]

Transient synovitis of the hip
Bone tumors, other neoplasia
Leukemia, neuroblastoma
Discitis
Viral myositis

[a]Arthritis excluded, see Chapter 11

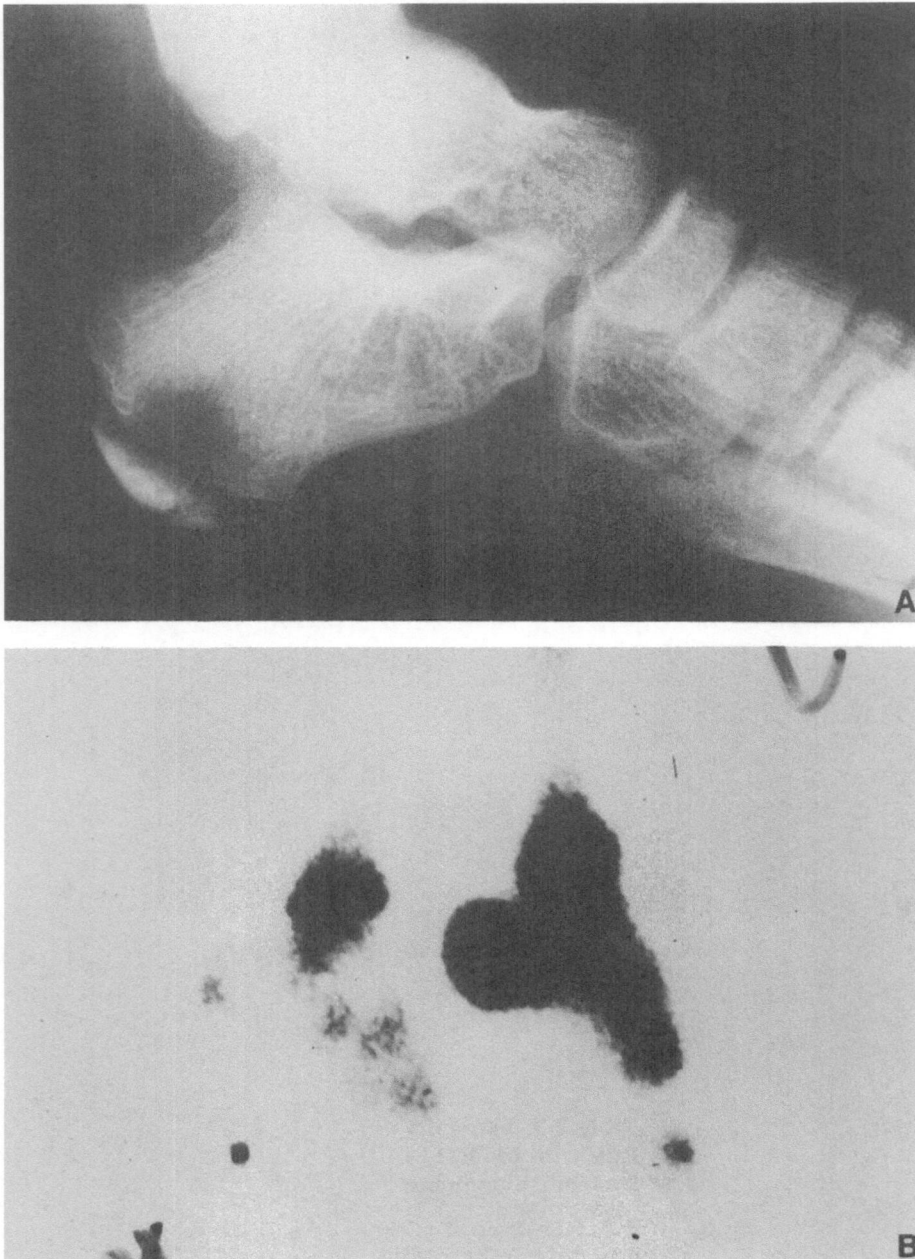

Figure 2.23. (A) Lytic lesion of heel in this 6-year-old boy with osteomyelitis of the calcaneus. (B) Technetium bone scan showing increased uptake; lateral of normal foot and ankle is to the left.

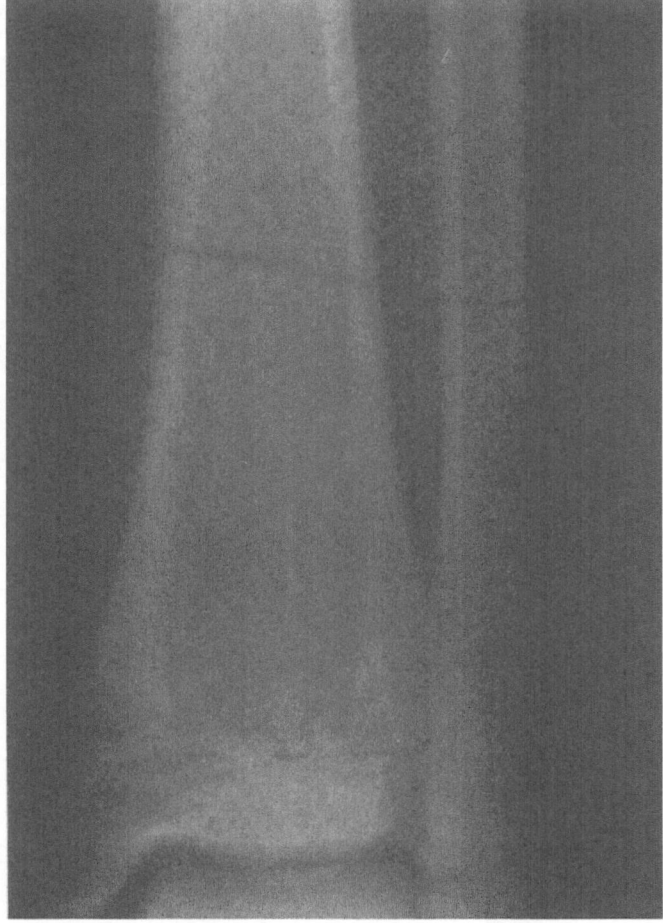

Figure 2.24. Osteomyelitis of the distal tibia in this 14-year-old boy demonstrating typical medullary damage and periosteal new bone formation. X-ray courtesy of the Department of Radiology, University of Kentucky.

present with fever and significant pain on motion of the joint. Joints most often affected include knee, hip, ankle, and elbow (Shaw and Kasser, 1990). The joint itself will usually be red, swollen, tender, and warm. *Staphylococcus aureus* and group A streptococcus are common throughout childhood. During the period between 2 months and 5 years, *Haemophilus influenzae* is found. Group B streptococcus and enterics (in newborns), pneumococcus, gonococcus, *Pseudomonas aeruginosa*, and meningococcus also occur, though more rarely (Jackson and Nelson, 1982).

Do not hesitate to aspirate a joint if the general signs of an acute infection with painful limitation of motion, swelling, or redness of a joint should suggest the diagnosis.

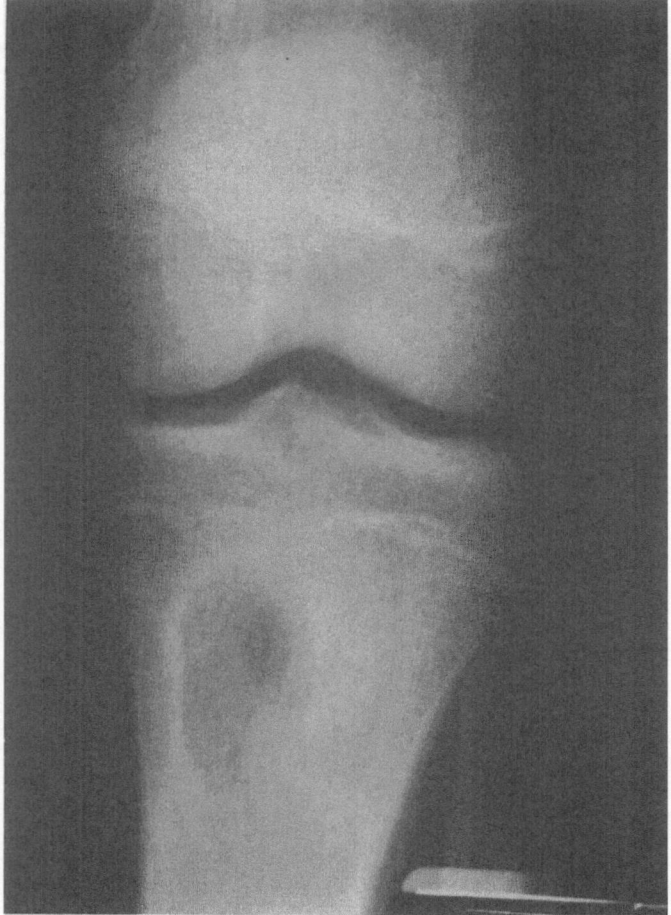

Figure 2.25. A Brodie abscess, of which this is an example, results from subacute or chronic osteomyelitis, often initially unrecognized. Bony metaphyseal destruction as a result of infection leads to a pus-filled, but often sterile, cavity; they are usually treated with surgical drainage and intravenous antibiotics. X-ray courtesy of the Department of Radiology, University of Kentucky.

Assuming that a sterile needle is used after proper skin preparation, there is very little risk of infecting the joint and the knowledge gained makes the effort well worthwhile (see also Chapter 11).

Early and energetic treatment with antibiotics is essential, usually for between 3 and 6 weeks. Surgical arthrotomy and drainage must be done for all septic hips because of the danger of septic necrosis of the femoral head with resulting permanent deformity. Optimum drainage of other septic joints remains somewhat controversial. Repetitive aspirations can be considered effective as long as clinical and synovial fluid improvement is apparent. However, repeated aspiration of a joint may be technically a problem as well as psychologically traumatizing for a child (Shaw and Kasser, 1990).

Neonatal Pyarthrosis

Septic arthritis or pyarthrosis of the hip in the neonate, in particular, is a potentially crippling and life-threatening disease. The time of onset is usually between day 7 and 14 of life and the most common source of the infection is hematogenous spread though direct inoculation does occur as a complication of femoral puncture.

The basic pathology is most commonly a hematogenous osteomyelitis on the medial side of the proximal metaphysis of the femur. An osseous abscess forms in this portion of the ossifying femur which is within the hip joint since the reflection of the joint capsule on the femur is distal to the proximal metaphysis. Within hours the abscess ruptures into the hip joint which causes the most dramatic signs and symptoms. The child may present systemically unwell, with lethargy, fever or hypothermia, and poor feeding though these symptoms may sometimes be absent. Almost always the mother notes that the child seems to be in pain when the diaper is changed. Should presentation be delayed a day or two after the onset of symptoms, swelling of the groin and buttock may be evident.

Inspection reveals that the child prefers to hold the extremity in external rotation, abduction, and flexion to reduce as much as possible the intraarticular pressure, thereby minimizing the discomfort. Examination of the child will reveal that passive motion of the hip, particularly internal rotation, results in pain. Palpation of the groin causes a painful response.

Should the physician suspect neonatal pyarthrosis of the hip, he should appreciate that this is an urgent problem. The infection increases the pressure within the hip and the inflammatory response soon results in thrombosis of the blood supply to the head of the femur. Untreated pyarthrosis of the hip joint results in dissolution of the head and a portion of the neck of the femur. The child will have a short lower extremity and an unstable hip with limp and disability all his life.

Aspiration of the hip joint should be done with some haste under fluoroscopic control. **This is true even if an orthopedic surgeon is not immediately available. Do not wait for the blood culture to come back. Do not order a radioisotope bone scan.** If a child presented with a stiff neck the physician would immediately stick a needle in the lumbar subarachnoid space. Pyarthrosis of the hip is a similarly urgent event and the diagnosis should be sought urgently. **Stick a needle in the hip joint.** Hip aspiration is done by inserting the needle in the groin starting a finger breadth lateral to the femoral pulse and directing it toward the neck of the femur. The needle can be felt to pierce the capsule of the hip joint and, once the bone or cartilage of the neck of the femur is felt, aspiration should reveal pus. If no pus is found, it is wise to inject 1 or 2 cc's of radiopaque dye to be sure the needle is in the hip joint.

If aspiration confirms the hip joint to be infected, immediate open drainage is indicated with supplemental antibiotic treatment. Even with early diagnosis and quick drainage of the hip, many infants will have permanent loss of function of the hip joint. The only way to give the child any chance for a normal hip is quick and effective action.

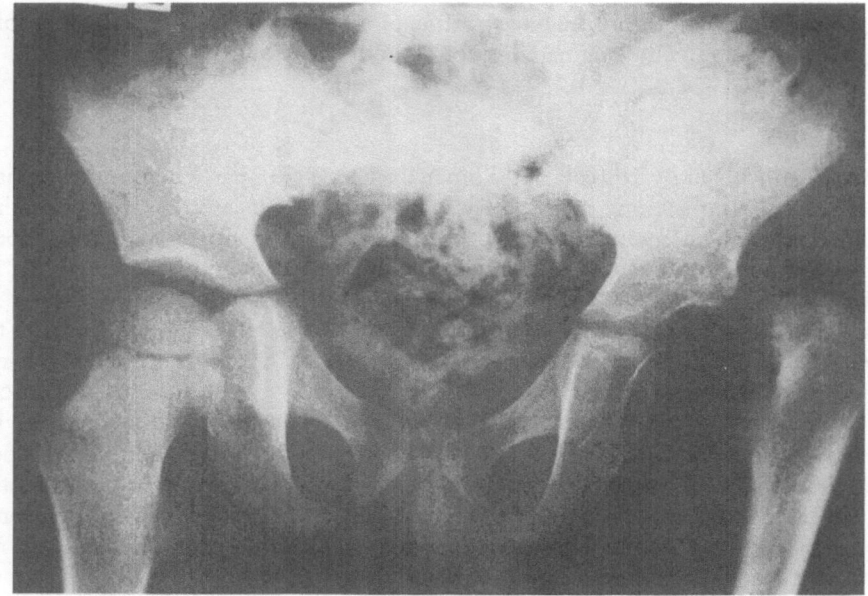

Figure 2.26. What we're trying to prevent, this young man from Poland was left this way after a septic hip in infancy destroyed his femoral head

Table 2.4. Extremity Pain with Significant Systemic Symptoms[a]

Septic arthritis
Acute osteomyelitis
Appendicitis/psoas abscess

[a]Arthritis excluded, see Chapter 11

2.7.3. Appendicitis/Psoas Abscess

Occasionally, an intraabdominal or pelvic process will mimic hip disease with hip flexion deformity and pain on ambulation. Abdominal examination may demonstrate signs of localized peritonitis or a mass. Abdominal ultrasound is also useful.

Case 1

J L is a 51-month-old male brought to your office by his mother for evaluation of leg pain of 2 weeks duration

His pain is mostly at night and usually affects the left calf, though he occasionally complains of pain in the right calf and in both thighs He most often begins to complain within 30 minutes of retiring and responds well to a dose of Tylenol and some massage He complains of pain not at all during the daytime He is active, eats well, has lost no weight, and does not have fevers or a rash

His initial physical examination is unrevealing His height and weight are appropriate for his age He is not ill-appearing His general examination is normal Specifically, there is no pathological lymphadenopathy or organomegaly On extremity examination there is no swelling, warmth, redness, or tenderness All joints demonstrate full range of motion His gait is normal There is no hyperlaxity His spine is normal with a normal range of motion and no focal tenderness

Comment: A child with a typical history of nighttime calf pain and a normal physical examination needs nothing further at the time of the first visit Reassuring the parent and child sometimes helps If the parents seem a little too attentive to the complaints, they might be counseled to be a little less so Follow-up should be arranged If symptoms worsen in general or localize, if the parent is particularly anxious, or if the child demonstrates anything on physical examination, workup with a CBC, ESR, platelet count, and X-rays should be initiated

Case 2

J J is a 7-year-old boy with persistent right knee pain

Previously well, J J was first noticed to be limping 2 months ago by his grandmother At about the same time he developed pain and some stiffness of the right knee, usually after he had been particularly active He was seen by another physician who diagnosed "growing pains" after anteroposterior and lateral knee films were unrevealing There is no fever, weight loss, rash, trauma, or other symptoms of a systemic illness There is no family history of significant rheumatologic or orthopedic difficulties He is described by his parents as healthy and well-adjusted

Physical examination reveals a healthy-appearing male who plots at the 25th percentile for both height and weight His general examination is completely normal Musculoskeletal examination reveals an antalgic gait with decreased stance phase on the right side Additionally, when in stance phase on the right he leans slightly to the right, a Trendelenburg gait He has decreased abduction and internal rotation at the right hip compared with the left

CBC, ESR, and platelet count are considered but are held pending X-rays Anteroposterior and frog-leg lateral films of the pelvis are obtained Both reveal concentric widening of the joint space on the right, presumably caused by an effusion, with mild, diffusely increased density in the femoral head and a linear subchondral lucency thought to represent a fracture line The diagnosis of LCP disease is made and the child is referred to a consulting orthopedic surgeon

Comment: Prognosis depends on the extent of bony necrosis, age (the younger the better), sex (boys do better), and how well the femoral head is "covered" by the acetabulum Treatment is oriented toward containing the femoral head within the mold of the acetabulum, leading to concentric and congruent reformation of the femoral head Don't forget that hip disease frequently causes pain referred to knees or medial thighs

Case 3

"Quentin" is an 18-month-old white male who refuses to walk

The patient was in his usually state of good health until about 1 week prior to presentation when he developed a low-grade fever (100 5°F, taken rectally) and increased irritability He was clingy, refused to eat, and insisted on being held On the day of presentation he refused to walk at all or even stand There was no history of rash, trauma, weight loss, or gastrointestinal symptoms His past medical history was otherwise unrevealing He has had all of his immunizations and his development was quite normal with walking beginning at about 10 months His parents had been bringing him to the practice ever since birth and seemed attentive and concerned There were no apparent social stressors

Physical examination revealed a healthy-appearing male toddler who is happy in his mother's arms When he is moved, however, or when his mother tries to put him down, he protests vigorously His temperature was 99 8°F rectally His general examination was normal

His extremity examination revealed only unhappiness when he was touched It was difficult, however, to localize this unhappiness to any particular part of the anatomy There was no swelling, warmth, redness, or severe limitation of motion

A CBC, ESR, and platelet count were obtained and revealed a WBC of 18,500 with a shift to the left, a normal hemoglobin and platelet count, and an elevated ESR of 45 mm/hr Lower extremity radiographs were obtained and were normal A radioisotope (technetium) revealed localized uptake in the vertebral bodies adjacent to the L_3–L_4 interspace Subsequent evaluation of the lumbar spine demonstrated localized tenderness over the area in question

Comment: The CBC, ESR, and platelet count were logical as a first step considering the history of fever

If they had been completely normal, an occult fracture (spiral fracture of the tibia) or some other form of traumatic injury might have been considered Other causes for leg pain unassociated with signs or symptoms of systemic inflammation (LCP, SCFE) would be unlikely considering his young age A bone scan might have been appropriate as a next step even if the CBC and ESR were normal since some occult skeletal trauma may not demonstrate itself on radiographs within the first 10 days after the injury but is apparent on technetium bone scan (periosteal strip injuries or a torus fracture, for example, see Chapter 3)

The elevated WBC and ESR open up a larger number of possibilities including osteomyelitis, discitis, juvenile rheumatoid arthritis, juvenile dermatomyositis, malignancy, viral arthritis, septic arthritis, and Kawasaki disease, among others Most can be excluded on the basis of the child's clinical presentation Certainly a septic arthritis would not be one to miss Septic arthritis of the hip is usually localizable to the hip on physical examination even in a child who is generally unhappy and who doesn't like any part of his body being moved

2.8. DIAGNOSIS

Diagnosis begins with a careful history and physical examination. In children with systemic symptoms, focal signs or symptoms, or persistent symptoms, a CBC, including a platelet count, ESR, LDH, and X-rays (AP and lateral) are indicated. An elevated serum LDH may be a result of a neoplastic process, including leukemia, neuroblastoma, or primary bony malignancies (Wallendal *et al.*, 1992) though a normal LDH does not rule them out. Technetium bone scanning may be useful if an inflammatory, neoplastic, or occult traumatic lesion is suspected. Other diagnostic tests may be indicated based on the child's clinical picture such as blood cultures or aspiration of the periosteum for suspected osteomyelitis or joint aspiration for suspected septic arthritis.

2.9. THERAPY

Specific therapy will spring from the diagnosis at hand. Describing the details of therapy for all of the conditions outlined above is beyond our scope here. Several general principles are, however, worth listing:

- Regardless of diagnosis, follow-up is essential. Many of the conditions responsible for extremity pain may manifest themselves subtly at onset Many others are diagnoses by exclusion. Patients should return in order to learn whether you were right when you told them not to worry.
- Oral or intraarticular steroids should be used only if the diagnosis is known and

only if the physician has had experience with their use in children with chronic rheumatologic diseases.

- Nonsteroidal anti-inflammatory drugs like aspirin, ibuprofen, naproxen, or tolmetin may have their place in the temporary treatment of acute extremity discomfort. They should not be used indefinitely without a diagnosis for which they are indicated.
- Normalizing a child's life is an important goal regardless of the child's problem. In general, "home-bound" educational programs should be avoided. This is, of course, true for children whose symptoms are really manifestations of school phobia but is also true for other children whose symptoms allow them to unreasonably duck their responsibilities if their parents or teachers permit it.

3

Musculoskeletal Manifestations of Child Abuse

3.1. INTRODUCTION

The notion that some children are injured by their caretakers and that intervention is therefore warranted is a relatively new one in this country It was not until 1946 that Caffey described the now well-known association between fractures of long bones and subdural hematomas and not until 1962 that Kempe and colleagues galvanized the medical world with their description of the battered child syndrome. Since then, a rapidly burgeoning literature has addressed an increasingly complicated field, with newly described manifestations of abuse, including sexual abuse, being brought to the attention of the medical profession and the public.

This chapter addresses the musculoskeletal manifestations of abuse. The reader is referred to other recent sources for excellent reviews of the general topic of child abuse (Kempe and Helfer, 1987).

3.2. EPIDEMIOLOGY

Epidemiological data vary from author to author though there is general agreement that child abuse is not uncommon. New cases of substantiated physical abuse occur in the United States at a rate of about 1200 cases per million population per year. Three percent of these children die, amounting to about 4000 childhood deaths per year in the United States (Schmitt and Krugman, 1992). Males are more frequently physically abused than females with a ratio of about 2 to 1 (Dalton *et al.*, 1990; Worlock *et al.*, 1986).

Younger children are more likely to be abused than older ones. Overall, about 10% of all injuries affecting children under the age of 5 years seen in hospital emergency rooms are the result of abuse. Two-thirds of abused children are under the age of 6 years and one-third are under 1 year (Schmitt and Krugman, 1992). Of all children who die as a result of abuse or neglect, 90% are younger than 5 years and 41% are younger than 1 year (McClain *et al.*, 1993).

Extremity or orthopedic injury as a result of abuse is common, with between 11 and 55% of physically abused children found to have fractures (Merten *et al.*, 1983; Chapman, 1990). As with abuse in general, skeletal injuries occur more frequently the younger the child (Chapman, 1990; Skinner and Castle, 1969).

3.3. RISK FACTORS

Risk factors include those social factors that increase isolation and reduce family support. Children are frequently abused as a result of adult caretakers being staggered by some new crisis such as loss of employment. A history of neonatal separation from the parents as occurs with prematurity is obtained more frequently than expectable.

Although most abused children don't grow up to abuse their children, there is an increased likelihood of this cycle of violence perpetuating itself if the caretakers themselves were abused, with one-fifth to one-third of abused children growing up to abuse their own children. Recently these data have been called into question (Widom, 1989). If the child is perceived as being demanding or hyperactive (perhaps related to previous central nervous system injury) or is unwanted, they may be at risk when the family is stressed or unbalanced by other factors (Kempe and Helfer, 1987).

3.4. THE PHYSICIAN'S ROLE

Like any other clinical problem, the physician's role in cases of possible physical abuse includes identification, immediate medical care, and appropriate follow-up. Unlike many other medical problems, child abuse is also likely to involve the physician in a forensic process in which he must collect evidence and think about the possibility that the injured child (or another child in the household) may be at risk of life-threatening injury if returned to the household.

Identification and Protection

When confronted with the complexity of a child who may have been the victim of nonaccidental trauma, it is important to remember that the responsibility of the physician does not include being a prosecutor or judge. It is not necessary to positively identify the child as abused. It is necessary only to raise the question. In fact, physicians are required by law in most states not just to report child abuse but also to report **suspected** child abuse.

Identification under these circumstances is essentially a two-phase process. Is this child injured? If so, is the injury the result of abuse? The initial phase is, of course, made easier for the physician if the child's injuries are apparent. However, this is not always the case. Instead, the child may exhibit only generalized irritability, decreased sensorium, poor feeding, dehydration, or reluctance to move the injured extremity (pseudoparalysis). The child may be growth retarded (failure to thrive) or dirty. Chronic subdurals will not likely be accompanied by overt signs of cranial trauma but instead may result in a large cranium with a tense fontanel and a shrill cry. The caretakers may be inebriated, combative, or not related to the child. The child may present dead on arrival apparently as a "sudden infant death syndrome" victim, without obvious traumatic injury. Kleinman *et al.* (1989) found 8 cases of abuse in their series of 12 cases of unexplained infant death.

Even apparent injury may be subtly manifested. Age is important here as usual. Bruising that would be insignificant in a 3-year-old may be a sign of abuse in a 6-week-old. Robertson *et al.* (1982) examined 400 normal nonabused children and recorded the extent and location of bruising of children of different ages. Only 4 of 60 (6.7%) children 2 weeks to 2 months of age had any type of bruising at all. Lumbar bruising, relatively more common in school-aged children (14%), was rare in normal children under the age of 3 years (0.8%). The opposite pattern existed for facial and head bruising which was considerably more common in normal children 18 months to 3 years than in children of school age. As might be expected, 34% of children between 18 months and 3 years had bruises over the anterior tibiae.

On the other hand, regardless of age, children diagnosed with suspected or definite physical abuse had a strikingly different pattern of bruising compared with the normal population of 400. Of the abused population, 59.8% exhibited head or facial bruising versus 6.5% of the normal population; regarding thigh and buttock bruising, arm bruises, and burns, the respective totals were 41.7 versus 9.25%, 38.1 versus 8.5%, and

11.3 versus 0.75% (Robertson *et al.*, 1982). Look for cord loop marks, bruises widely dispersed over the surface of the body, bruises over the posterior surface of the body rather than the anterior (little children fall forward usually). Look for bruises in the shape of a human hand.

Trying to decide if child abuse is a possibility requires not only physical examination skills and radiological expertise but interviewing acumen as well. There may be some injuries that are pathognomonic (see below), but many injuries require putting together the caretakers' stories (interviewed separately, if possible) with the child's injury, looking for an appropriate fit. Knowing "normal" childhood responses to accidental trauma is important. For example, Helfer and co-workers found that of 246 children younger than 5 years who fell out of bed at home or in the hospital, only 3 had skull fractures on X-ray and none had serious intracranial injury. Altogether, 4 more incurred other fractures, though none was femoral (Helfer *et al.*, 1977). This doesn't mean that an isolated skull fracture or even a femoral fracture allegedly resulting from a fall out of bed actually is a result of child abuse, but it does mean that care should be exercised in assigning accidental trauma as an explanation too readily. The child needs to be evaluated thoroughly.

A formal skeletal survey should be undertaken when nonaccidental injury has been demonstrated or is suspected, including cases of unexplained death. In general, it should be done with a "lower threshold" in children who are younger than 18 months because osseous injury is more common in younger abused children and because younger children are much less likely to provide information during the interview. "Babygrams" or "bodygrams" should not be done because the technical deficiencies which result often preclude diagnosis of the often subtle radiological manifestation of abuse. The survey should include: AP of the chest, lateral chest (with a good look at the thoracic spine), AP humeri, AP forearms, PA hands, AP pelvis, lateral lumbar spine, AP femora, AP tibiae, AP feet, AP skull, lateral skull including lateral cervical spine (Kleinman, 1990). All suspected neurologic injury merits appropriate imaging (CAT scanning in most hospitals).

Radioisotope bone scanning is an appropriate supplement to X-rays but should not be considered a primary screening tool. Radioisotope is normally taken up by tissues around the growth plate, making metaphyseal and epiphyseal fractures difficult to pick up. Bone scanning is less sensitive than X-rays for vertebra and skull fractures and it is difficult to estimate the age of the fracture from a bone scan. Bone scanning may be

Table 3.1. What a Skeletal Survey Should Include

AP chest	AP femora
Lateral chest	AP tibiae
AP humeri	AP feet
AP forearms	AP skull
PA hands	Lateral skull
AP pelvis	Lateral cervical spine
Lateral lumbar spine	

useful, however, in demonstrating early osseous injury in symptomatic patients with negative X-rays.

The responsibilities of the physician also require compulsive documentation of the child's injuries on the chart and reporting to the appropriate child protection agency. Coagulation studies should also be considered in a child with bleeding or bruising to document normal clotting since this may become an issue in court.

3.5. PATTERNS OF INJURY

The bony manifestations of child abuse result from the actual mechanism of injury, how it is done, together with the biological characteristics of the developing skeleton at the time the abuse occurs. Both vary with age.

3.5.1. Shaken Baby Syndrome

Preschool children are particularly vulnerable because they are small and because they are more likely to be inarticulate than older children. The extremities of young children make attractive handles to abusing caretakers and therefore lesions that are a result of torsional, tractional, or shearing forces are more common the younger the child. The shaken baby syndrome, a constellation of rib fractures, retinal hemorrhage, and subdural hematoma, results from the child being grasped about the thorax and shaken to and fro in an anteroposterior plane. Young infants are particularly vulnerable because of their small size and this pattern of injury is thus **not** often seen in children over 1 year (Kleinman, 1990). Infants often present with obvious CNS damage, including coma, seizures, and a tense fontanel.

3.5.2. Multiple Fractures

Because child abuse tends to be recurrent, multiple serious injuries occur to the same child over time, leading to one of the most specific radiologic manifestations of child abuse: multiple fractures in varying stages of healing. Similarly, the original pattern of lesions described by Caffey, long bone fractures associated with subdural hematoma, also is a very specific lesion. Finally, though not common, the presence of bilateral, symmetrical forearm fractures implies an attempt on the part of the victim to protect themselves against assault with a heavy, hard object and is occasionally seen in children old enough to try to defend themselves.

Table 3.2. The Shaken Baby Syndrome

Retinal hemorrhage
Subdural hematoma
Rib fractures

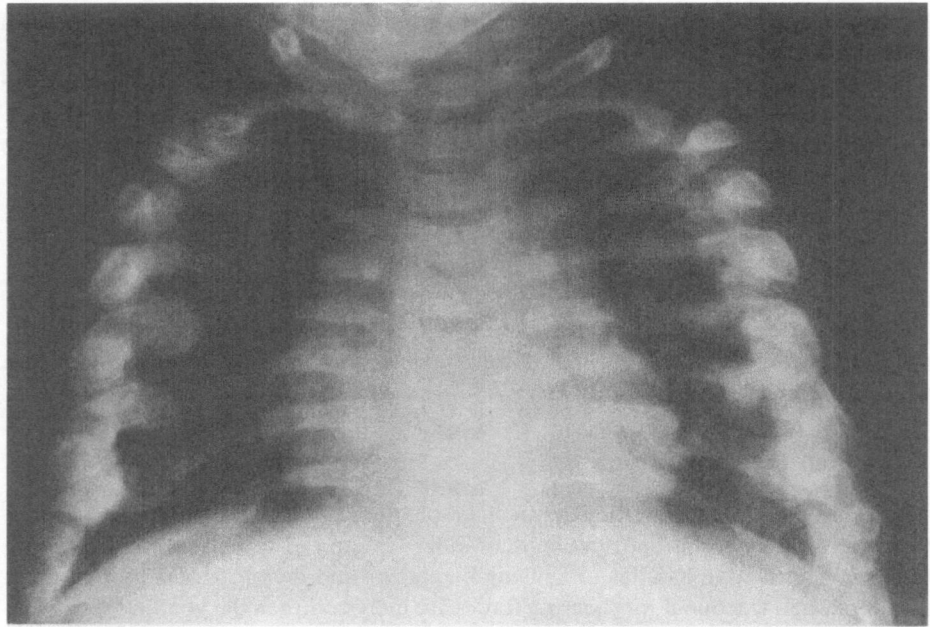

Figure 3.1. Multiple rib fractures in an abused 6-month-old female Same patient as in Fig. 3.2 X-ray courtesy of Dr Vesna Criss, Department of Radiology, University of Kentucky

3.5.3. Injuries Associated with Periosteal New Bone Formation

The developing skeleton itself will define the nature of injury. The periosteum in young children is much more loosely attached to the cortex than in older children or adults. Torsional or wringing injuries of long bones will result in detachment of the periosteum, subperiosteal bleeding, subperiosteal new bone formation and a typical, though nonspecific, "bone within a bone" appearance (Silverman, 1980). Unlike metaphyseal fractures (see below), periosteal new bone cannot be seen with X-rays until at least 5 days and frequently not until 10 days after injury (Merten and Carpenter, 1990). Radioisotope bone scanning, though not specific, may be useful in the detection of these early lesions.

Periosteal new bone formation may also be seen in many infiltrating, hemorrhagic, or infectious conditions, including osteomyelitis, acute leukemia, sickle-cell disease, congenital syphilis, pulmonary osteoarthropathy, scurvy, and hemophilia. The widespread, florid, and frequently symmetrical nature of the periosteal new bone formation in child abuse as well as the clinical presentation usually make the differential diagnosis relatively easy. When in doubt, laboratory evaluation, including complete blood count, sickle-cell test, and coagulation studies, may be needed.

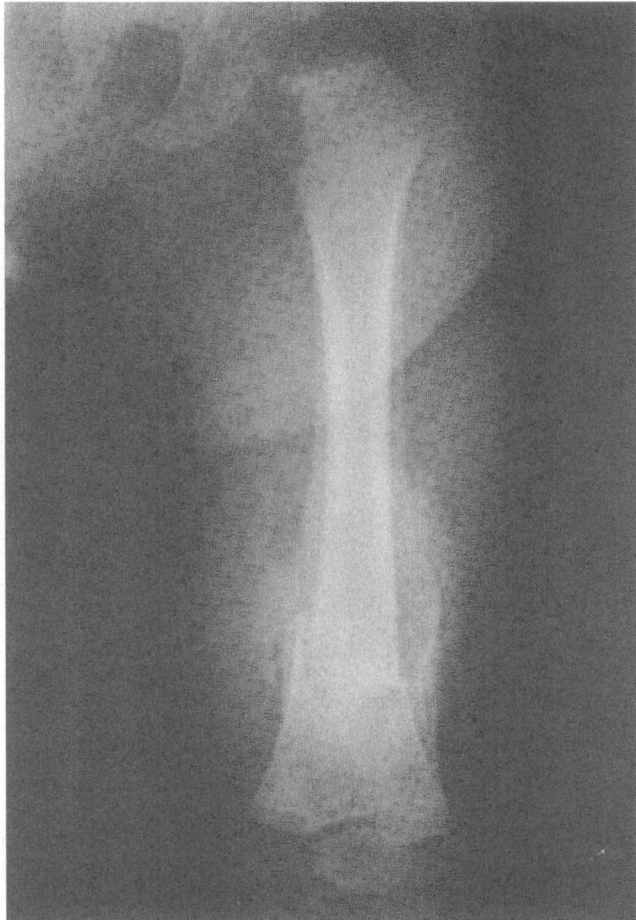

Figure 3.2. Fractured femur; same patient as in Fig. 3.1. Note periosteal elevation and healing callus. X-ray courtesy of Dr. Vesna Criss, Department of Radiology, University of Kentucky.

3.5.4. Metaphyseal Fractures

Twisting or pulling on the extremity of the young child will result in fracture through the primary spongiosa (the most immature layer) of the metaphysis, immediately central to the physis of the long bones. The fracture line will proceed transversely across the metaphysis except at the circumferential periphery of the metaphysis where the fracture line will turn centrally toward the diaphysis, leaving a small rim of metaphysis attached to the physis. These metaphyseal fragments don't require callus or bone repair to make themselves visible and therefore can be radiologically seen immediately after the traumatic episode (Caffey and Silverman, 1967). The adjacent

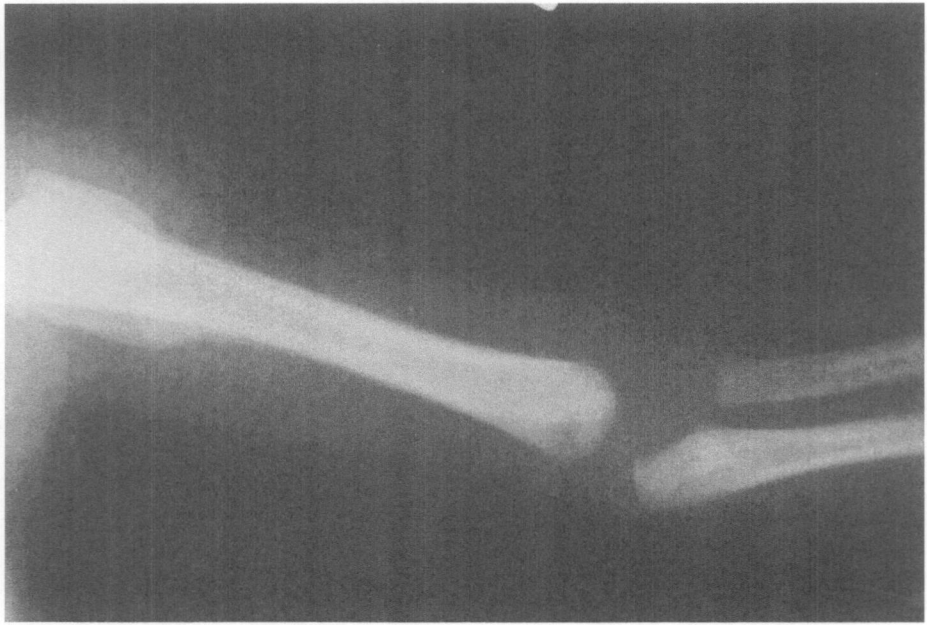

Figure 3.3. Healing avulsion fracture of proximal humerus in 3-month-old resulting from child abuse. Note periosteal elevation with "bone within bone" appearance. X-ray courtesy of the Department of Radiology, University of Kentucky.

physis is cartilaginous, and if the fracture is visualized by a true anteroposterior X-ray beam, only the silhouetted, most peripheral part of the rim of metaphyseal bone will be seen as a metaphyseal "corner" fracture. If the X-ray beam catches the fracture line obliquely, the fractured metaphyseal rim will appear as a curved semicircle of bone, a "bucket-handle" fracture. Like periosteal injury, metaphyseal fractures tend to be multiple and are frequently symmetrically present in the long bones of the extremities. Specific therapy is not normally necessary and the prognosis for normal growth with metaphyseal fractures is good since the physis is not involved. Important because of their specificity, metaphyseal fractures represent a minority of total long bone fractures in most abused children (Kogutt *et al.*, 1974; Worlock *et al.*, 1986) though they become more predominant in studies of abused infants (Kleinman *et al.*, 1989).

3.5.5. Growth Plate Injuries

The physis, or growth plate, is vulnerable to injury throughout childhood, particularly so across the middle zone of hypertrophic chondrocytes. Growth problems from growth plate fractures are the result of damage to the physis itself and, perhaps more importantly, to the local blood supply (Tachdjian, 1972). Such fractures are common in children with accidental injury. Their presence must be explained by an appropriate history of significant trauma.

3.6. BONY LESIONS SPECIFIC TO CHILD ABUSE

Specificity here of course is a spectrum with posterior rib fractures, acromio-clavicular fractures, metaphyseal fractures, multiple fractures of different ages, and the shaken baby syndrome all being the most specific. The latter three were discussed above and the other two will be discussed below.

3.6.1. Posterior Rib Fractures

Posterior rib fractures, most commonly seen near the costovertebral junction posteriorly, result from thoracic compression and are virtually pathognomonic of abuse. Fractures occur along the ventral aspect apparently as a result of levering the rib against the transverse process. They are usually multiple and bilateral and are often associated with CNS damage, subdural hematomas, and retinal hemorrhages (the shaken baby syndrome).

Because the fracture is of the ventral surface of the rib only, it is difficult to see by means of X-rays until callus formation begins. Bone scanning may be useful in the detection of early lesions (Kleinman, 1990). They have been variably reported in between 5 and 27% of abused children, almost always in infants and young children (Merten and Carpenter, 1990) and were the most commonly found fracture in one series of eight fatally abused infants (Kleinman *et al.*, 1989). Posterior rib fractures have not been described as a result of cardiopulmonary resuscitation (Merten and Carpenter, 1990).

Rib fractures other than those that occur posteriorly are also frequently associated with abuse although they are certainly known to occur as well with serious, well-documented accidental trauma. Sixty-three percent of such fractures in children under the age of 3 years were the result of abuse in one series. The authors found a high mortality rate overall (43%) with mortality increasing with the number of fractured ribs (Garcia *et al.*, 1990).

3.6.2. Acromioclavicular Fractures

Though uncommon, avulsion fractures of the acromion and/or lateral clavicle are thought to reflect abuse. The pathogenesis of these lesions is similar to that of metaphyseal fractures: violent traction or twisting of the upper extremity.

3.7. INJURIES SUGGESTIVE OF CHILD ABUSE

Slightly less pathognomonic of abuse than the above are the following lesions: periosteal separation injuries, fractures through the physis (growth plate), and spinal,

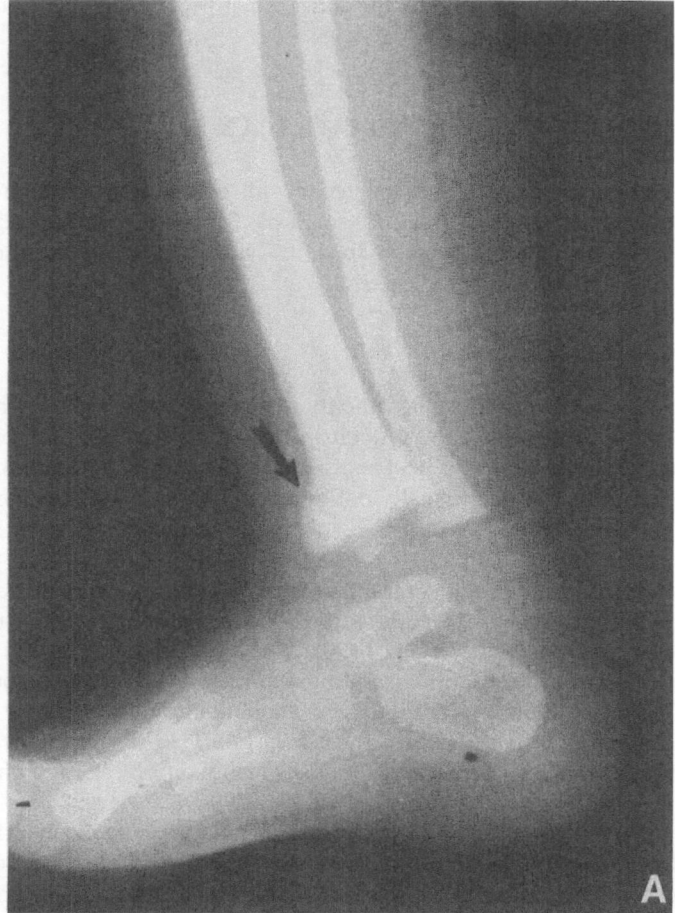

Figure 3.4. (A) Metaphyseal "corner" fracture, note fracture line (arrow) angling proximally as fracture line extends to the surface of bone, producing distinctive radiologic appearance (B) When X-ray beam is not perpendicular to long axis of bone, the circumferential nature of a metaphyseal fracture becomes apparent, producing "bucket-handle" appearance X-ray courtesy of Dr Al Selke, Department of Radiology, University of Kentucky

skull, scapular, sternal, and digital injuries The first two were discussed above, the remainder will be discussed below

3.7.1. Vertebral Fractures

In the absence of an appropriate explanation, vertebral fractures may represent abuse Violent hyperflexion as would occur with the shaken baby syndrome may lead to

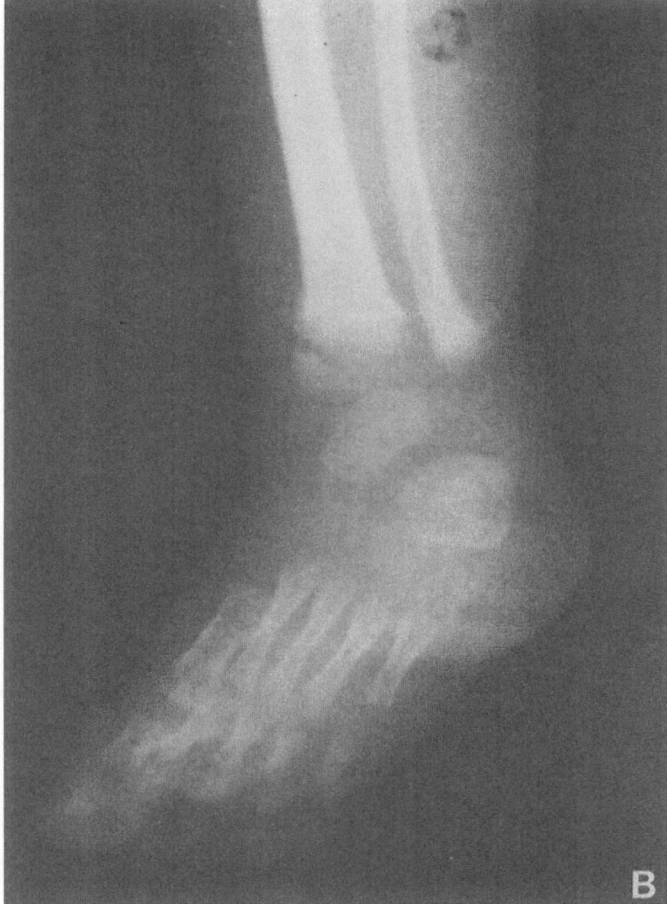

Figure 3.4. (*Continued*)

anterior notching or even to frank compression of the vertebral bodies, most often seen in the lower thoracic or upper lumbar spine (Kleinman, 1990). A similar pathogenetic process may be operational in the development of avulsion injury to the spinous processes, described by Kleinman in 16% of one series of abused children. Areas of irregular calcification seen on X-rays adjacent to spinous processes do not represent the spinous processes themselves but rather ossification secondary to myositis ossificans or cartilaginous calcification resulting from disruption of the interspinous ligamentous attachments (Kleinman and Zita, 1984). They may coexist with compression fractures. Radiologic evidence for any of the injuries discussed above can frequently be seen at several consecutive vertebral levels.

Fracture dislocation injuries occur as well, often with spinal cord trauma, and

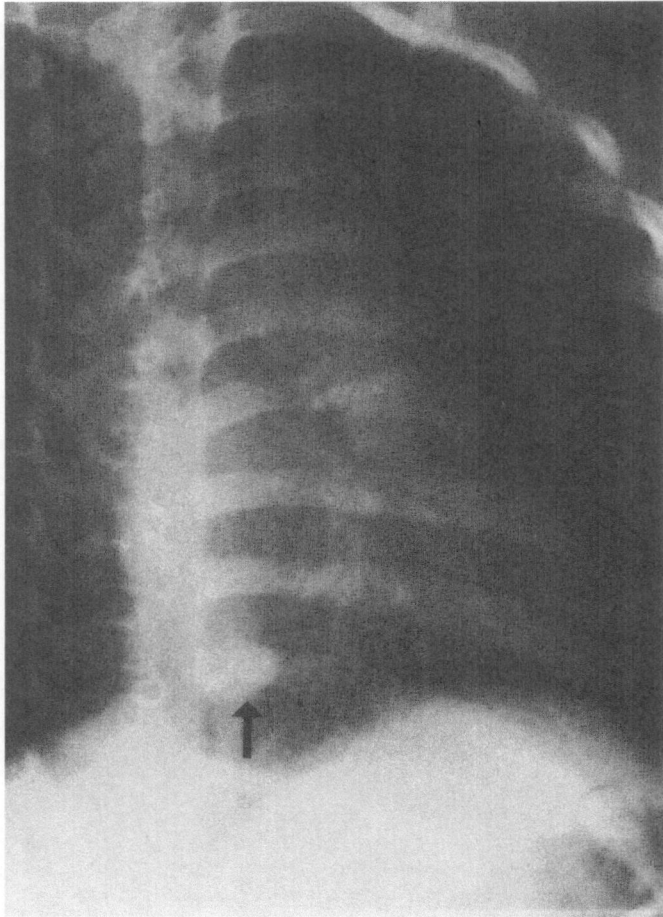

Figure 3.5. Typical posterior rib fracture (arrow) in 1-year-old abused male. X-ray courtesy of Dr Vesna Criss, Department of Radiology, University of Kentucky

Table 3.3. Traumatic Bony Lesions *Specific* for Child Abuse

Metaphyseal fractures
Posterior rib fractures
Acromioclavicular fractures
Multiple fractures of different ages
Shaken baby syndrome

represent the result of violent injury as might occur if the child was thrown against a hard, immobile object.

3.7.2. Skull Fractures

Skull fractures are common in child abuse, occurring in 22% of physically abused children in one series and representing one-third of all radiologically proven fractures. Most were linear, mostly in the parietal or posterior parietal areas, and most (82%) had spread sutures (Kogutt *et al.*, 1974).

Under ordinary circumstances, skull fractures would not be expected as a result of falls of less than about 3 feet (Helfer *et al.*, 1977). Accidental skull fractures are most often linear, narrow, and uncomplicated by intracranial bleeding or other CNS complications such as seizures, apnea, or extreme lethargy. Strongly consider abuse if any of the following are present: multiple fractures, diastatic or growing fractures, complex or branched fractures, nonparietal fractures, or depressed fractures. Some authors consider a depressed occipital fracture virtually pathognomonic of abuse (Chapman, 1990).

3.7.3. Other Suggestive Injuries

In addition to acromial avulsions, transverse fractures of the scapula have been described in abused children and are usually secondary to direct trauma. Sternal

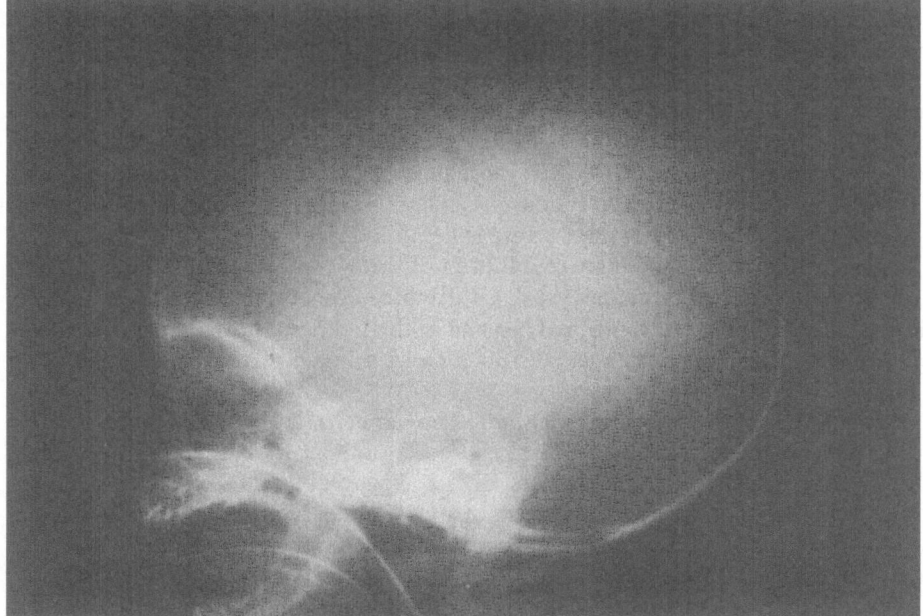

Figure 3.6. Complex skull fracture, with significant diastasis of fracture lines, in male infant who was abused. X-ray courtesy of Dr Vesna Criss, Department of Radiology, University of Kentucky

Table 3.4. Traumatic Bony Lesions
Suggestive **of Abuse**

Periosteal separation	Complex skull fractures
Spinal fractures	Scapular fractures
Digital fractures	Sternal fractures

fractures and mandibular fractures should be considered to be abuse unless an appropriate explanation of serious, forceful accidental trauma is forthcoming, such as an automobile accident.

Hands, because they are so accessible to potentially abusing caretakers, are frequently the site of nonaccidental injury, 10% in one series.

3.8. NONSPECIFIC INJURIES

Relating relatively nonspecific fractures to abuse is important and challenging. Many abused children are likely to have been seen by physicians before for "accidental" injury (Skinner and Castle, 1969) and, like so many other difficult problems, the earlier the diagnosis, the more likely the child and their siblings are to survive without sequelae.

Diagnosis here is challenging because the majority of injuries suffered by physically abused children are no different from injuries suffered by children involved in serious, accidental trauma. Seventy-seven percent of fractures incurred by abused children in one series were of long bones, with nonspecific diaphyseal fractures the most common (Merten and Carpenter, 1990).

When present, a spiral fracture may provide some indication that abuse has occurred because of its association with torsional forces (Worlock *et al.*, 1986; Chapman, 1990). This is particularly so in children under 15 months of age (Dalton *et al.*, 1990) who are nonambulatory. However, most abusive fractures are not spiral and many spiral fractures are not the result of abuse (Dalton *et al.*, 1990; Worlock *et al.*, 1986).

Sometimes the location of the fracture is helpful. Thomas *et al.* (1991) reported 14 children with fractures of the humerus. Eleven of these were thought to be caused by abuse. All were midshaft or metaphyseal. Of the three humeral fractures resulting from accidental trauma, all were supracondylar and all had occurred after traumatic events consistent with the injuries such as falls off a rocking horse, off a tricycle, and down the stairs.

Age is also important. In the same study, Thomas *et al.* (1991) found that 36% of 25 children with fractured femora had been abused. However, looking at the 10 children below 1 year of age with fractured femurs, 60% had been abused. Worlock *et al.* (1986) compared children with fractures as a result of abuse versus accidental trauma and found that all of the abused children were younger than 5 years compared with only 15% of the group with accidental fractures.

The presence of more than one fracture was found by Worlock *et al.* (1986) to also be important. Of the 35 abused children, 7 (20%) had two fractures and 19 (54%) had three at the time of presentation compared with only 19 (16%) with two fractures of 116 in the group with accidental fractures. There were, additionally, no children with more than two fractures in the accidental group. Bruises about the head or face in association with any fracture or over widely disparate body parts may be important, particularly so as they are uncommon in normal preambulatory infants and in children with accidental fractures (Worlock *et al.*, 1986; Robertson *et al.*, 1982).

3.9. ASKING QUESTIONS

Other questions must be asked when confronted with the potentially abused child manifesting nonspecific injury:

1. Is the injury consistent with the caretaker's story and with the child's developmental age? Are there inconsistencies over time or differing stories from different family members? Who was caring for the child when the injury occurred?
2. Is there a history of previous serious traumatic injury affecting this child?
3. Are there any social risk factors evident such as recent family discord, homelessness, alcoholism, or other abused persons in the family?
4. Is there something about this child which makes them "at risk," such as a handicapping condition, hyperactivity, or other behavioral problem?

When dealing with nonspecific injuries, whether associated with fractures or not, the physician must rely on these historical features. As mentioned above, the legal responsibility of the physician is to report all cases of **suspected** abuse. By nature of the complexity of this problem the physician will often not be certain that abuse has in fact occurred. However, because of the significant possibility that the abused child will return at some subsequent point with an even more significant injury, even a suspicious trivial injury must be evaluated thoroughly at the time of presentation.

The social service evaluation is not the responsibility of the examining physician. However, child protection workers must be acquainted with your concerns. Physicians, and others, are specifically protected from liability in the courts even if the social service evaluation or further forensics prove that abuse has not taken place. We bend over backwards to avoid missing childhood meningitis. We can do no less for the potentially abused child.

3.10. DIFFERENTIAL DIAGNOSIS

For nonspecific injury, of course, the most difficult differential diagnosis involves distinguishing accidental from nonaccidental trauma. For fractures most specific for abuse, such as metaphyseal fractures or posterior rib fractures, the differential diagnosis is limited. It is true that metaphyseal fractures as described above do occur in children with osteogenesis imperfecta (see below), in which case the child is likely to manifest the other stigmata of osteogenesis imperfecta (Taitz, 1987). Additionally, metaphyseal fractures may occur as a result of difficult vaginal breech extraction and have even been reported resulting from traumatic cesarean section deliveries (Chapman, 1990).

For such suggestive fractures as vertebral compression fractures or avulsion fractures of the spinous processes, differential diagnosis necessarily would involve an injury mimicking a shake injury, such as a severe spinal flexion secondary to a frontal automobile accident while wearing a seat belt without a shoulder restraint. Periosteal separation injuries with periosteal new bone formation can occasionally be confused with sickle-cell disease, osteomyelitis (should be focal), congenital syphilis, hemorrhage secondary to scurvy or hemophilia or neoplasia, including acute leukemia. Appropriate diagnostics generally provide the answer.

Newborn infants, perhaps related to rapid growth or birth trauma, will sometimes exhibit periosteal new bone formation of their long bones, particularly of the lower extremities but also the humerus. This should be symmetrical, should not appear before 1 month of age, should be peaking by 6 months of life and should be gone by a few months thereafter (Caffey and Silverman, 1967; Ozonoff, 1992).

Children with subdural hematomas should have their coagulation functions thoroughly checked to rule out the possibility that the hematoma is a result of a hemorrhagic diathesis.

3.11. DIFFERENTIAL DIAGNOSIS OF MULTIPLE FRACTURES

Perhaps generating the most concern is the possibility that some type of congenital or acquired metabolic bone disease with multiple fractures will be confused with child abuse, with the parents falsely accused.

3.11.1. Osteogenesis Imperfecta

This rare defect in collagen generally causes such typical manifestations that confusion with child abuse is unlikely if a careful history and examination is performed. However, types III and IV are not associated with blue sclera and therefore might very rarely represent a diagnostic challenge. A positive family history, osteoporosis, wormian bones, hearing loss, hyperlaxity, short stature, increased sweating, fragile skin, or dentinogenesis imperfecta usually provide the distinguishing information (Ablin *et al.*, 1990).

It is theoretically possible for one of these conditions, occurring sporadically without a family history, to confuse the examining physician. Taitz (1987) and colleagues estimate that this would occur no more than once in every million births, or about three or four times each year in the United States. During the same period about 300,000 substantiated cases of physical child abuse would be expected to occur. This statistical mismatch does nothing, however, to reduce the anguish of a family investigated for child abuse when their child has, in fact, osteogenesis imperfecta. Errors, if they are unavoidable, must be made in the direction of protecting the child and making the report. However, if confusion is present, the child should be referred to an appropriate center for evaluation.

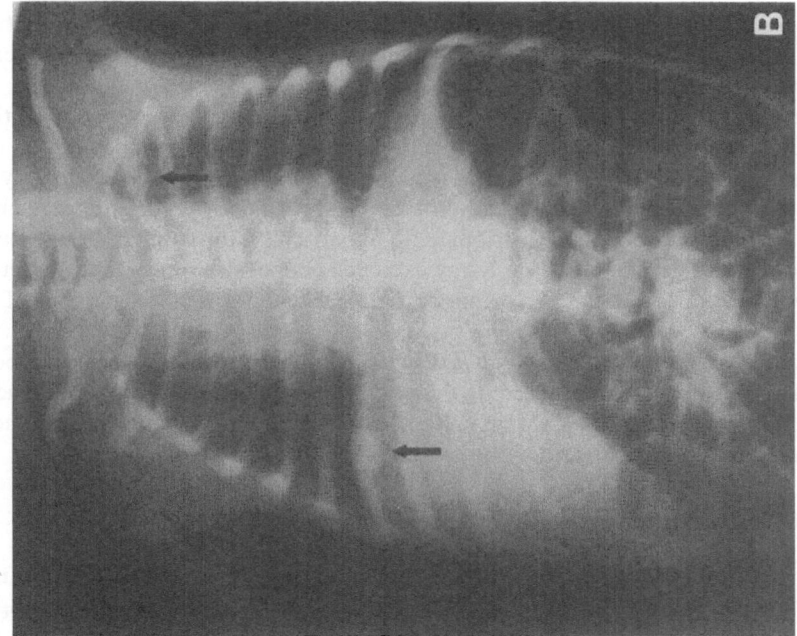

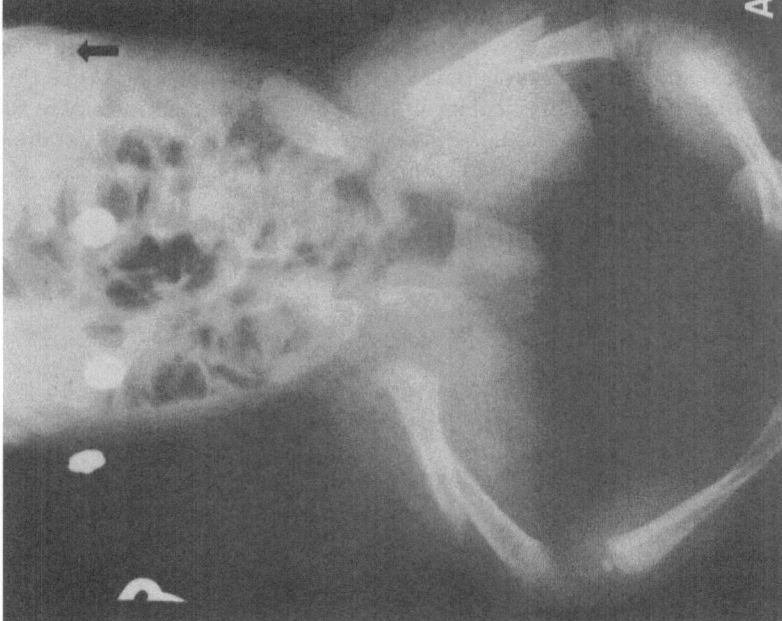

Figure 3.7. (A) Bilateral femur fractures and rib fracture (arrow) in a 2-month-old female who was initially thought to be abused. (B) Review of chest X-ray on day after birth, however, revealed multiple healing rib fractures (arrows), presumably the result of intrauterine fractures. The diagnosis of osteogenesis imperfecta was made on the basis of congenital healing fractures, blue sclera, short stature, and wormian bones.

3.11.2. Copper Deficiency

Copper deficiency is a very rare condition which might theoretically be confused with child abuse. It has achieved some prominence lately and will be discussed because of its forensic implications.

There have been only about 100 cases reported in infants and in only 16 of these were fractures reported. Furthermore, only 5 of these were full-term babies and all were either receiving an abnormal diet or on total parenteral nutrition. Additionally, all children with fractures had obviously abnormal bones, with osteoporosis, retarded bone age, and metaphyseal cupping distributed symmetrically throughout the skeleton. Normal bone age or normal bones on X-ray excludes copper deficiency. Skull fractures have not been described in copper deficiency. Breast feeding is not a nutritional risk factor.

If fractures in preemies, babies on TPN, or malnourished babies with bad bones represent a diagnostic problem regarding the possibility of abuse and copper deficiency is raised as an explanation, look for laboratory features of copper deficiency including neutropenia, anemia, or low serum copper and ceruloplasmin (Chapman, 1987).

3.11.3. Other Explanations for Multiple Fractures

Other possibilities are usually easily excluded on the basis of the child's clinical picture. They include Caffey disease which is a form of focal hyperostosis affecting the mandible and clavicles most frequently. More common previously, it is now virtually unreported. Rickets (see Chapter 4) might be a cause of confusion in children with multiple fractures but should be associated with generalized rachitic change which is recognizable on X-ray, including bowing of lower extremity long bones, osteoporosis, thickened physes, and fraying and cupping of the metaphyses of long bones.

Finally, children with sensory deficits might be unaware of their injuries to such an extent that nonaccidental trauma would be considered. This might occur in children with spina bifida or in the very rare child with congenital insensitivity to pain. A neurologic examination should answer the question.

4

Developmental Orthopedics

4.1. INTRODUCTION

Though common and concerning to family members, none of the problems discussed below are serious. They exist usually as outriding points on a spectrum of normalcy and usually require no specific therapy. In fact, short of surgery, very little therapy is available for any of these conditions and little of what is available has ever been submitted to controlled trial evaluation.

What these conditions do require is lots of education, explanation, and reassurance directed to the parents (and frequently, the grandparents). Happily, they are developmental in the sense that they change, usually for the better with time, if we give them the chance. Because these problems occasionally mimic serious, progressive pathological processes, diagnostic attention must be paid to ferret out and exclude more significant alternative explanations for the child's complaints, or the parent's concerns.

4.2. INTOEING

Three bony explanations exist for intoeing in most children and may occur alone or in combination:

1. Intoeing resulting from incurvation of the forefoot, termed metatarsus adductus or metatarsus varus
2. Intoeing resulting from torsional rotation of the tibia, internal tibial torsion, or
3. Intoeing resulting from internal rotation of the entire lower extremity as a result of increased anterior displacement of the femoral head relative to the femoral shaft, known as femoral anteversion or internal femoral rotation

Each has its own epidemiology and differential diagnosis. All have in common a negative foot progression angle (FPA). The FPA measures the angle of deviation of the foot from the direction of movement of the patient. If the long axis of the foot is parallel to the direction of movement, the FPA is zero. If the patient is intoeing, the FPA is negative.

Though neurologic, muscular, or inflammatory processes may intervene to cause intoeing on occasion, most intoeing is idiopathic in causation with some contribution from intrauterine positioning, sleeping posture, and/or genetic predisposition.

4.2.1. Metatarsus Adductus

Metatarsus adductus, known also as metatarsus varus, represents incurving of the forefoot, easily identified by the "C" curve of the lateral border of the foot. Frequently associated are a transverse plantar crease extending laterally from the apex of the concavity on the medial side of the foot as well as an increase in the space between first and second toes.

This condition is usually noted by parents in infancy and is thought to be related to intrauterine positioning. Certainly it is easy to reproduce the incurved, flexed posture with one forefoot curved over the other. One associated deformation is worth noting, the association between metatarsus adductus and congenital dislocation of the hip (see Section 6.3.3.1). Jacobs (1960) found the incidence of hip dysplasia in metatarsus adductus to be 10%.

Physical examination must be directed to ruling out hip problems and distinguishing metatarsus adductus from more significant congenital foot abnormalities. Even in the

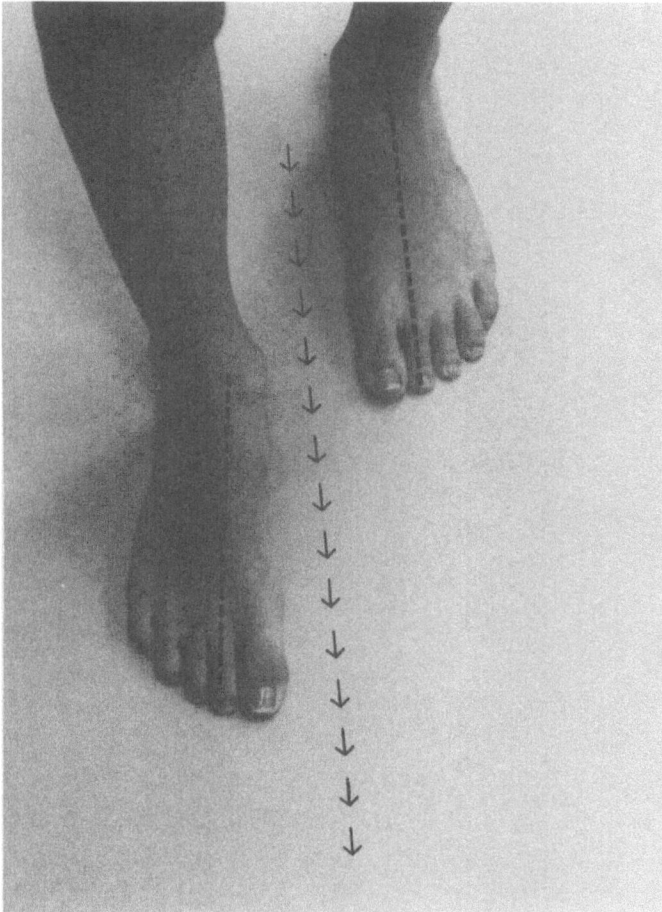

Figure 4.1. The foot progression angle (FPA) is formed by the long axis of the foot and the direction of movement. In this case, 0° on the left and very slightly positive on the right. Children who intoe have a negative FPA.

Table 4.1. Causes of Intoeing

Metatarsus adductus	Other causes
Internal tibial torsion	Cerebral palsy
Femoral anteversion	Residual clubfoot
	Hip dysplasia

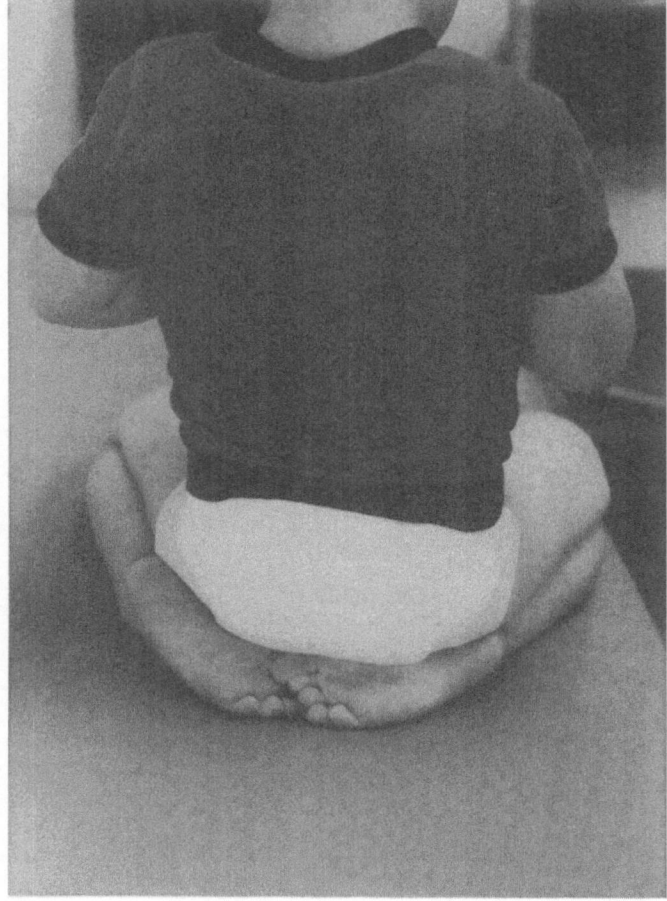

Figure 4.2. Extrauterine posturing, as demonstrated here, may contribute to persistent intoeing

presence of a normal hip exam, radiological or ultrasonographic evaluation should be considered in the child with metatarsus adductus if other "at risk" factors are present, such as twin birth, breech delivery, or positive family history, since the diagnosis of congenital hip dislocation from physical exam alone is sometimes difficult.

Distinguishing rigid metatarsus adductus from talipes equinovarus (TEV, clubfoot; see Chapter 6) is also sometimes difficult. TEV includes three specific foot deformities in concert:

1. Adduction or varus angulation of the forefoot
2. Varus angulation (inversion) at the ankle (actually the subtalar joint), and
3. Equinus posturing with the toes down, the heel up, and the calcaneus difficult to feel

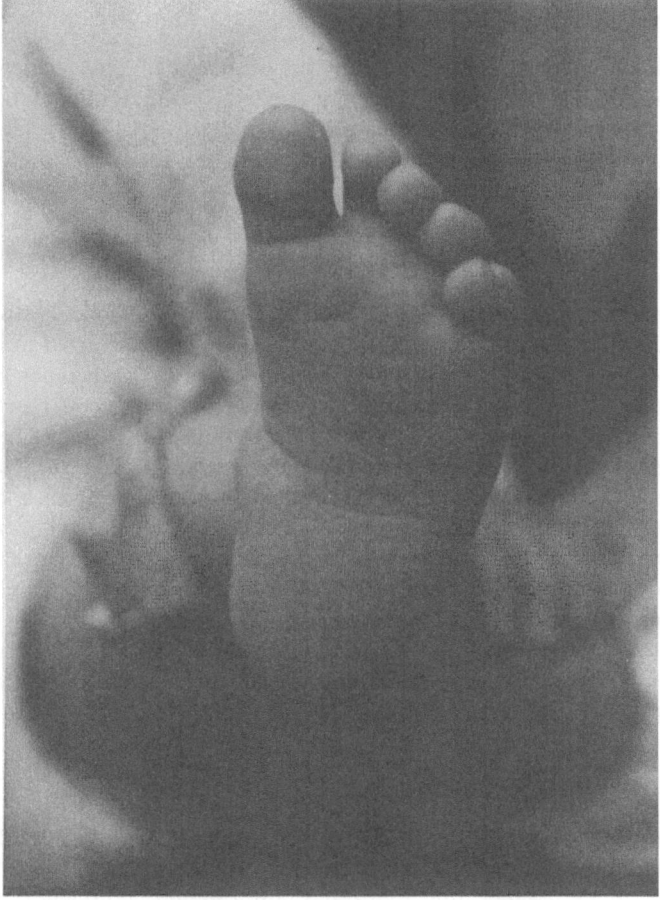

Figure 4 3. Mild metatarsus adductus, note transverse crease, slight increase in space between toe and second digit, and lateral "C" curve

Look at the baby's heel to make certain that the normal, mild valgus angulation (eversion) of the ankle is present with the foot in the neutral position (perpendicular with the tibia). Make sure that normal ankle dorsiflexion is possible. In TEV, the foot is in equinus and full dorsiflexion is not possible.

Since intrauterine deformation is also thought to contribute to the causation of TEV and other foot abnormalities (see Chapter 6), the presence of metatarsus on one side does not exclude the possibility of more significant deformity affecting the contralateral foot. Look closely at both feet and independently come to a decision regarding each.

Treatment of Metatarsus Adductus

Decision-making regarding treatment by the primary care physician versus referral to an orthopedic surgeon for sequential casting depends on the rigidity of the foot and the degree of the deformity. A flexible deformity should be easily correctable to neutral and, in fact, should overcorrect. If correction causes the infant discomfort or if such pressure is required to correct the deformity that the examiner's fingertip is blanched, then the deformity is rigid and severe enough to merit referral. If referral is to occur, it should optimally be done prior to 3 or 4 months to take advantage of the normal flexibility of the young infant.

Flexible metatarsus adductus deformities will usually respond to stretching exercises done at the time of each diaper change. The parent is instructed to hold the heel in one hand and repetitively correct the deformity to neutral ten times each session, holding the foot in the neutral position for 10 seconds at each repetition. If no improvement results over a period of 2 months, straight last shoes might be considered.

The last is the mold on which the shoe is made. A straight last makes a shoe that is symmetrical (the "left" is the same as the "right"). Children's shoe stores sell (with your prescription) tiny "open-toed straight last prewalkers" which will provide a little direction for the growing foot and are sometimes helpful in borderline circumstances when referral doesn't seem necessary but the family continues to be concerned about the lack of improvement with exercises alone. They are, however, expensive. An alternative is to have the family put regular shoes on the wrong foot in an attempt to produce the same effect. However, children's shoes cannot usually be purchased small enough to do much good for the feet of a 3- or 4-month-old.

4.2.2. Internal Tibial Torsion

Internal tibial torsion (ITT) is the term used to describe internal rotation or medially directed torsion of the long axis of the tibia. It occurs more often in toddlers and younger children than in either infants or older children and is thought to be related to intrauterine positioning perhaps aggravated by the tendency of many of these children to "sit on their feet" with their lateral malleolus on the floor and their medial malleolus under their buttocks. There may be a genetic predisposition to this condition as well. Regardless, initial internal tibial torsion makes for greater comfort as the child sits or sleeps as described above which makes for continued rotatory stress on the growth plates resulting in persistent torsion. Parents also complain that the intoeing is worse when the child is fatigued at the end of the day or when wearing heavy shoes. Typically, both legs are affected, though there may be a small difference in the amount of torsion exhibited by each.

Since it is the tibia that is twisted or rotated on its axis, the angle made by the long axes of the foot and thigh (the foot–thigh angle) will be abnormally negative (foot pointing medially). The usual angle is slightly positive (5 to 10°) (Staheli, 1986). Children brought for evaluation of intoeing with ITT usually have foot–thigh angles more negative than $-20°$. Since developmental problems like ITT are most often bilaterally symmetrical, a discrepancy in foot–thigh angles of greater than 10° between

Table 4.2. Physical Findings for Intoeing

Intoeing caused by[a]	Age	Physical findings
Metatarsus adductus	Infancy	Lateral foot border curved
Internal tibial torsion	Toddler	Negative foot–thigh angle
Femoral anteversion	School-aged	Hip internal rotation greater than external

[a]See text

extremities requires consideration that other processes may be contributing to the child's intoeing, such as hip disease or an occult, mild hemiparesis Further evaluation, including hip and lower extremity radiographs, may then be necessary

Therapy for Internal Tibial Torsion

Therapy must primarily be directed toward explaining to the parents that ITT is a self-limited condition that will improve with time They should know, however, that intoeing may continue to some degree throughout childhood **Shoes, twister-cables, or braces have no documented effectiveness.** Keeping the child out of an internally rotated sitting or sleeping posture may be most important and may account for the improvement seen in some children after night bracing is initiated

A less expensive alternative to braces such as the Denis–Browne bar is to ask the parents to punch holes in the medial side of the heels of an old pair of sneakers and tie them together at night so that the child is prevented from sleeping with the legs internally rotated Proven effectiveness here, as with more conventional night bracing, is lacking

4.2.3. Femoral Anteversion

Femoral anteversion (FA, medial femoral rotation) affects mainly school-aged children and is the result of excessive anterior displacement of the femoral head relative to the femoral shaft To be seated securely in the acetabulum, internal rotation of the entire lower extremity will thereby result from this anterior accentuation

The child walks with their kneecaps pointing medially The degree of femoral rotation is almost always symmetrically equal and is reflected in the discrepancy between internal and external rotation at each hip Under normal circumstances, these are usually equal In FA, internal rotation is significantly greater than external rotation (see also Chapter 1)

Therapy for Femoral Anteversion

Unfortunately, little can be done to correct FA short of rotational osteotomy Happily this is usually not necessary either from the point of view of cosmesis or function Children frequently develop compensatory mechanisms, including external tibial torsion, which serve to allow them to point their toes, if not directly ahead, at least almost so As with ITT, shoes and braces have no demonstrable benefit

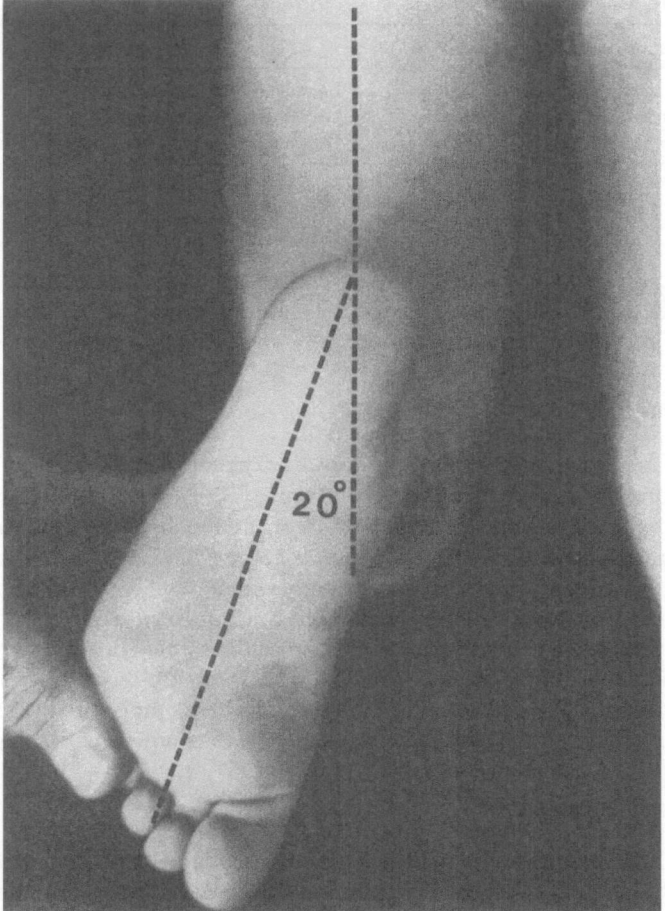

Figure 4.4. Demonstration of foot–thigh angle. In internal tibial torsion, this angle is negative and represents internal (or medial) rotation of the tibia around its long axis.

4.3. OUTTOEING

Parental concern regarding outtoeing surfaces at about the time the infant first begins to bear weight and starts to walk. Perhaps to improve balance, outtoeing is typical at this formative stage and families should be instructed and reassured that their baby won't walk like Charlie Chaplin all of their life, only for the next few months.

Outtoeing resulting from true femoral retroversion (the opposite side of the coin from FA) does occur. Like FA, however, little can be done short of osteotomy. External tibial rotation also occurs occasionally, but is more common as a compensatory mechanism to FA.

4.4. BOWLEG

Bowleg may be a better term than genu varum to describe the legs of these little children because the angular deformity is really not at the knee itself, most of the time. In causation, bowleg can be ascribed to one of three possible mechanisms:

1. Localized problems with linear growth at the knee caused by problems such as Blount disease or a growth plate fracture
2. Generalized defects in bone metabolism and growth, e.g., rickets
3. Neither of the above (physiological bowleg), by far the most common

4.4.1. Physiological Bowleg

We are all, of course, bowed at birth. Gradually we improve so that by 18 to 24 months our legs are straight. We then go through a knock-kneed phase (Shopfner and Coin, 1969). Defining bowing as "physiological" requires that it be symmetrical bilaterally, that it not be severe, that the child be of normal height (see below), and that, most importantly, the bowing improve with time.

To monitor this, and other physiological deformities, a cheap Polaroid-type camera is useful. Stand the child up against the wall with their ankles barely touching and take their picture. Alternatively, measure as accurately as possible the distance between the medial aspect of each knee, with the ankles together (weight-bearing, if possible). Either way, if improvement does not occur within 6 months, further investigation is warranted, including radiographs and chemical measurement of bone metabolism.

If physiological bowleg seems doubtful based on the above, an AP X-ray of the lower extremities (preferably standing) is indicated. The radiologic picture of physiological bowing includes slight lateral bowing of the tibial and femoral shafts with beaking of the medial aspects of both the distal femoral and proximal tibial metaphyses to roughly the same extent. Thickening of the medial wall of the tibia is typical as is slight tapering of the distal femoral and proximal tibial epiphyses to form wedges medially.

4.4.2. Blount Disease (Tibia Vara)

Blount disease is a localized growth disturbance of the medial and posteromedial aspects of the proximal growth plate of the tibia. There are two separate and distinct age peaks. The first is in children between 1 and 3 years (infantile Blount disease) and the second is in preadolescents between 6 and 13 years (juvenile or adolescent Blount disease). Blount disease results in progressive deformity and intraarticular derangement which, if untreated, may result in severely disordered joints in adulthood.

The cause of infantile Blount disease is obscure but often described as related to excessive "loading" of the medial aspect (causing slower growth) and "unloading" of the lateral aspect (causing faster growth) of the proximal tibial growth plate as a result of accentuated physiological bowing (Wenger and Rang, 1993). The problem then becomes cyclical as decreased medial growth contributes to greater and greater degrees of varus

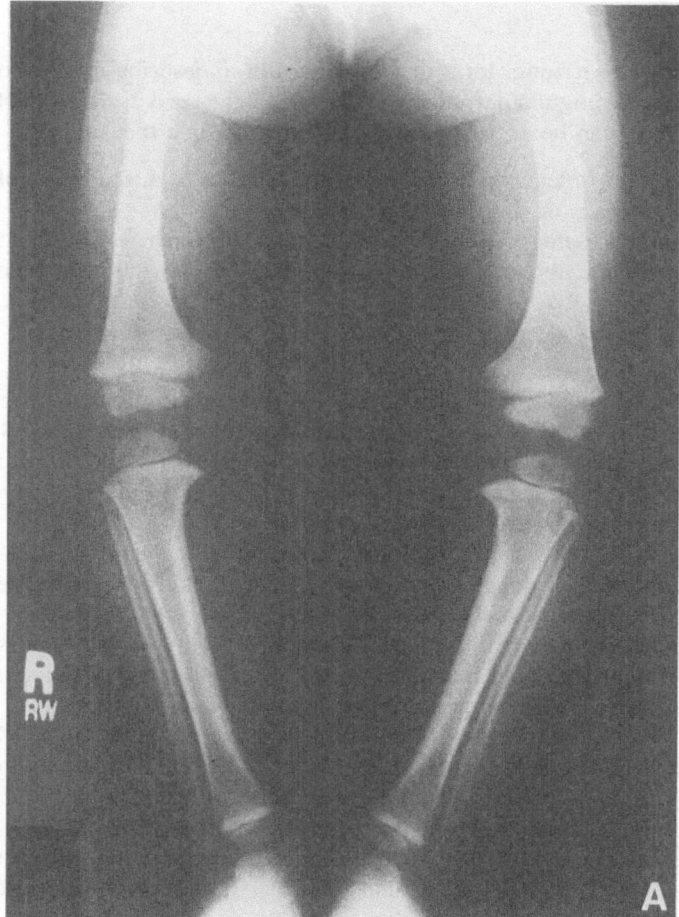

Figure 4.5. (A) Physiologic genu varum in a 21-month-old boy. The "beaking" of the medial aspect of the proximal tibial metaphysis, thickening of the medial tibial cortex, ankle obliquity, and decreased ossification of the medial aspect of the distal femoral epiphysis are all typical. (B) Much improved without therapy after 2 years.

angulation and worsening lateral joint instability. Although black infants and obese infants *may* be at greater risk (Edmonson and Crenshaw, 1980; Langenskiold, 1989), other authors disagree (Smith, 1982). Early walking does not seem to be a risk factor (Smith, 1982). It occurs bilaterally between 50 and 80% of the time (Turek, 1977; Smith, 1982).

Adolescent Blount disease is thought to be most often caused by damage (infection, trauma) to the medial portion of the proximal tibial growth plate, resulting in premature closure and abnormal angular growth (Langenskiold, 1989). It is therefore not surprising that adolescent Blount disease occurs unilaterally 90% of the time (Smith, 1982).

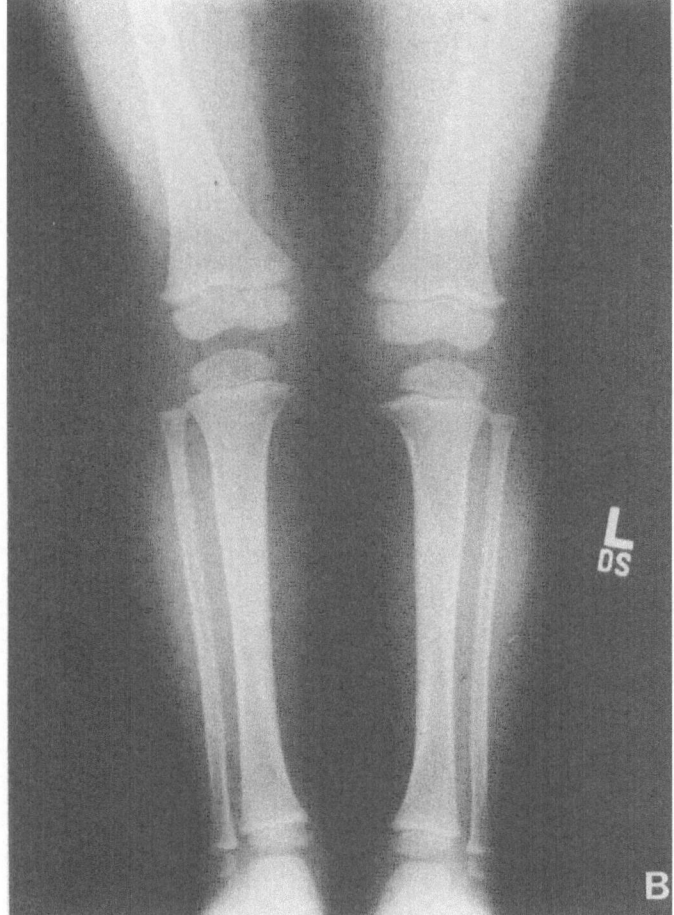

Figure 4.5. (*Continued*)

Radiographs in both types reveal sharp angulation of the proximal tibia with beaking and, eventually, fragmentation of the medial aspect of the metaphysis. "Early" Blount disease in a toddler may be impossible to distinguish from accentuated physiological bowing. Full-fledged radiological changes have not been described in preambulatory children (Langenskiold, 1989).

Table 4.3. Types of Bowleg

Physiological
Caused by local growth disturbance (Blount)
Caused by generalized bone problem (rickets)

**Table 4.4. Characteristics
of Physiological Bowing**

Better with time
Symmetrical
Normal height
Mild or moderate

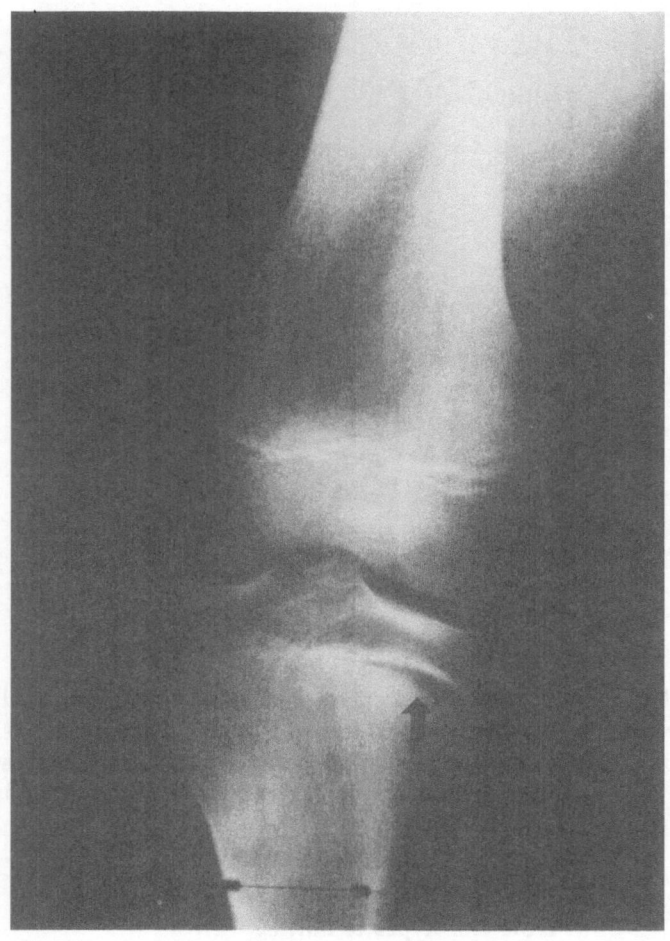

Figure 4.6. Adolescent Blount disease in a 13-year-old boy Note medial widening of proximal tibial physis (arrow)

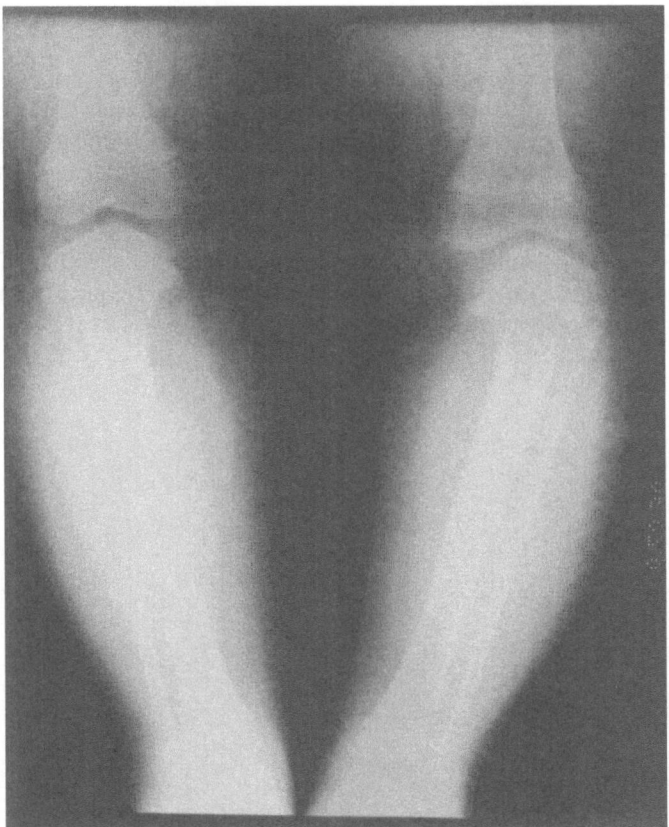

Figure 4.7. Infantile Blount disease in a 5-year-old boy who is very obese. Note bilateral disease, lateral tibial subluxation, disorganization and fragmentation of medial aspects of both tibial metaphyses, genu varum, and poor development of medial aspects of tibial epiphyses.

Treatment of Blount Disease

If begun before age 3, long-leg braces designed to resist varus angulation may be effective if worn regularly while the child is awake and if continued for at least several years. In children for whom braces are not effective and for all children with adolescent Blount disease, osteotomy to realign the angulation and correct the rotation is the treatment of choice. Early surgical intervention when necessary generally improves outcome as it provides the maximal time for longitudinal growth to contribute to correction.

The diagnosis of Blount disease by the primary care practitioner should lead to referral at the time of diagnosis to an orthopedic surgeon experienced in the care of this type of problem.

4.4.3. Other Causes of Bowing

There are a variety of less common but important pathological causes of bowing, all having to do with either defects in mineral metabolism or dysplasias of the epiphysis or metaphysis. They need to be excluded before a label of accentuated physiological bowing can be applied to any child. They have in common three attributes not found in children with physiological bowing.

First, these children are very often short. To know that someone is short, it is necessary to record their height on a growth curve normed for age. It is important to avoid dead reckoning because even experienced observers are frequently wrong if they don't avail themselves of a growth chart.

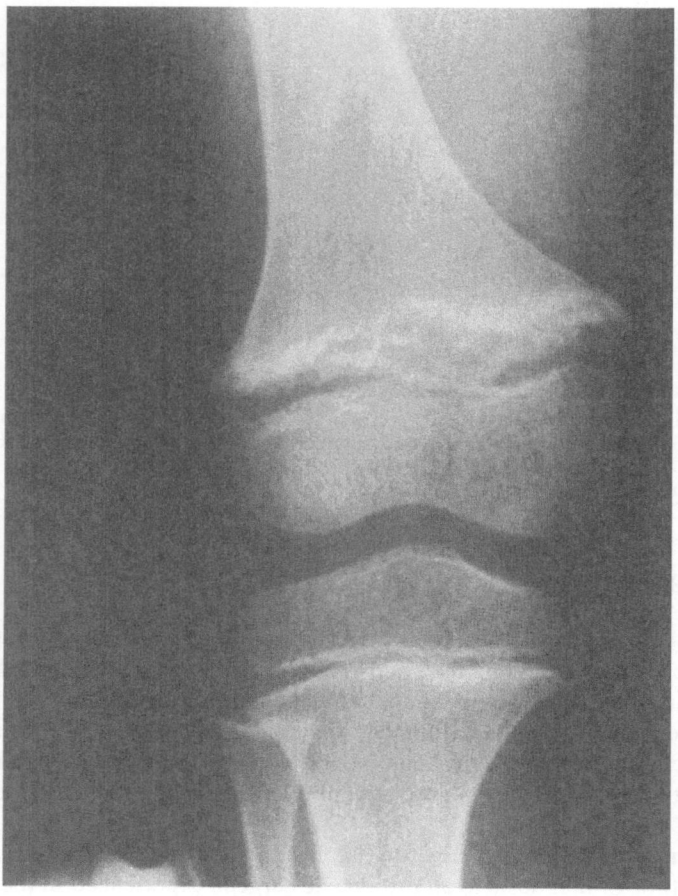

Figure 4.8. Metaphyseal chondrodysplasia (Schmid type) in a 4-year-old girl looks a lot like rickets (see Fig 4 9) Her serum chemistries, however, were all normal

Second, their lower extremity bowing is progressive. Unlike normal children, their bowing doesn't get better from birth but gets worse.

Third, there are often associated and usually obvious bony abnormalities other than the bowing. These include extremity shortening, truncal shortening, clubfoot, short neck, barrel chest, lumbar lordosis, a waddling gait, frontal bossing, nasal bridge depression, and a variety of other structural abnormalities which are usually your's for the looking. The presence of any of these three features mitigates against the diagnosis of physiological bowing and requires further investigation, including radiographs and serum chemistries (see below).

4.4.3.1. Rickets

Derangements in calcium and phosphate metabolism have a major effect on skeletal competency during the very rapid growth of early childhood. Rickets as a general heading can be further subdivided into a group of diseases caused by vitamin D deficiency, a second group related to renal tubular wasting of phosphate, and a third, somewhat miscellaneous group. None are common but all can cause bowing.

Dietary deficiency rickets is rare today since vitamin D is added to milk and infant formula but occurs occasionally as a result of fat malabsorption caused by cystic fibrosis, celiac disease, or chronic liver disease. "Deficiency" rickets also occurs in children on chronic phenytoin or phenobarbital therapy as a result of interference with vitamin D metabolism by these anticonvulsants.

Rickets caused by renal failure (renal osteodystrophy) similarly affects mineral metabolism not only as a result of impaired renal hydroxylation to form active vitamin D but also as a result of secondary hyperparathyroidism. The latter is caused by hypocalcemia due to hyperphosphatemia as a result of a decreasing glomerular filtration rate.

The archetypical phosphate wasting syndrome is familial hypophosphatemia (vitamin D-resistant rickets), an X-linked dominant disease of complex physiology and unknown etiology. The tubular reabsorption of phosphate is impaired as well as the second hydroxylation step for vitamin D. The children present with bowing as soon as they start walking. Phosphate wasting occurs with a variety of other tubular conditions including Fanconi syndrome and type II renal tubular acidosis. Some mesenchymal tumors have also been associated with hypophosphatemia and resulting rickets, though the etiology is obscure.

The third group includes a variety of conditions without any commonality except for the rachitic change they cause. Included are (1) hypophosphatasia, a congenital deficiency of alkaline phosphatase, (2) hyperphosphatasia, the opposite problem, although the results are somewhat similar, and (3) vitamin D-dependent rickets, an even more rare heritable disorder of vitamin D end-organ resistance or failure to effectively form dihyroxyvitamin D, the most active form of the molecule.

Radiologically, rickets is characterized by generalized osteoporosis with coarse trabeculation. Incurvation of weight-bearing long bones, fraying and cupping of metaphyses, and increased width of growth plates are also typical.

Serum alkaline phosphate is elevated (except in hypophosphatasia) and serum phosphorus is low (except in renal osteodystrophy). Serum calcium may be low or

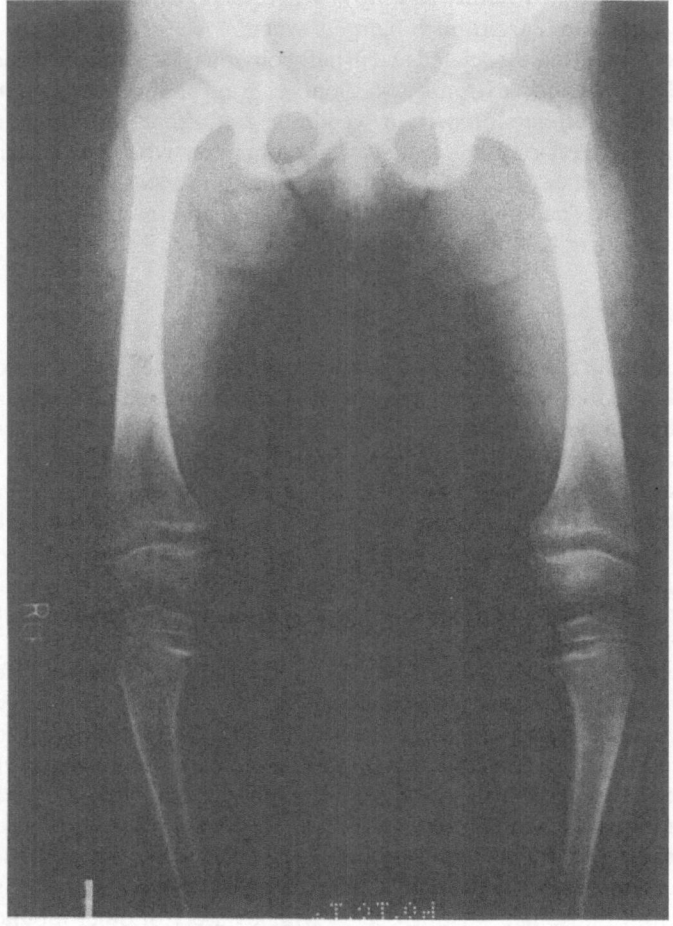

Figure 4.9. Hypophosphatemic rickets in a 5-year-old girl, with typical bowing, widening, fraying, and cupping of metaphyses, and an increase in the width of the growth plate. Rickets looks very much the same, regardless of whether it results from nutritional deficiency or decreased tubular reabsorption of phosphate, as in this case.

normal in deficiency rickets and is usually normal in the phosphate deficiency syndromes. Care should be taken when reviewing serum phosphate levels in children with suspected rickets. Children have higher levels than adults normally. Many laboratories list only adult norms on their laboratory printouts. A serum phosphate level of 3.0 mg/dl might therefore not be noted as abnormal when, in reality, it is low for a child. Rickets associated with renal or hepatic disease will also be associated with the typical chemical derangements associated with these conditions.

4.4.3.2. Bony Dysplasias and Related Conditions

Dysplasias of bone and cartilage include a variety of heritable conditions often resulting in bowing. They include the metaphyseal dysplasias, metaphyseal dysostosis, hypochondroplasia, achondroplasia, pseudoachondroplasia, the epiphyseal (and spondyloepiphyseal) dysplasias, and diaphyseal dysplasia.

As described above they almost always involve progressively worsening deformity with short stature and other associated orthopedic abnormalities.

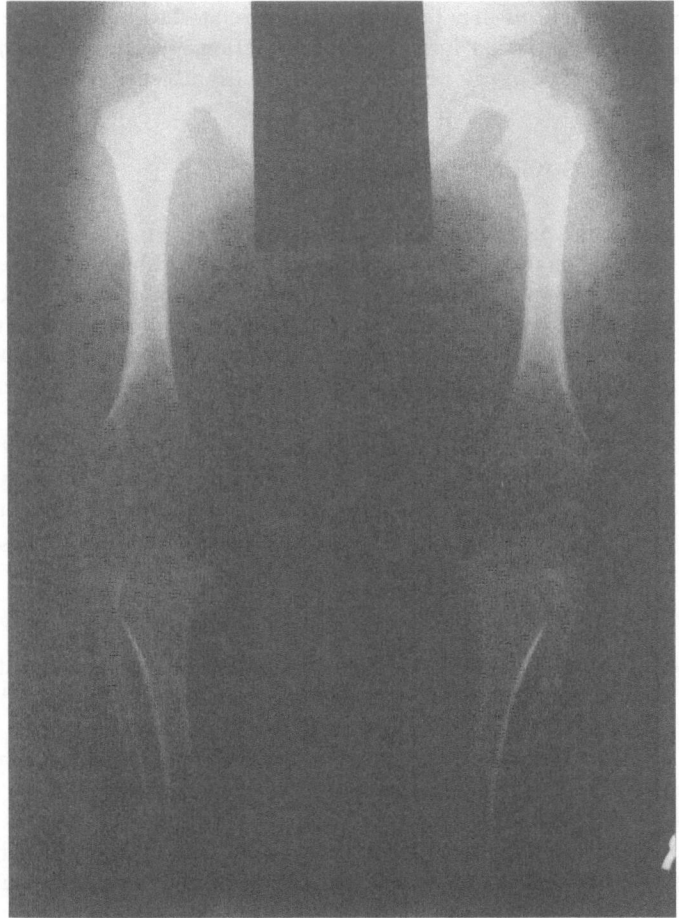

Figure 4.10. Achondroplasia in a 7-year-old girl.

4.4.3.3. Treatment of Other Causes of Genu Varum

Treatment for any of the above involves remediation, if possible, of the metabolic derangements that caused the bowing. Additionally, judicious bracing and/or osteotomy have their place when dealing with progressive deformity.

4.5. BACK KNEES

Back knees or genu recurvatum is most often associated with the same kind of benign hyperlaxity that causes pes planus. Like flexible flat foot deformity, it requires no therapy. It also exists, however, as a manifestation of congenital dislocation of the knee (see Chapter 6), polio, quadriceps contracture, and after intraarticular injury to the knee.

Quadriceps contractures may be congenital or related to injury to the quadriceps muscle, often as a result of an intramuscular injection. Physical therapy and serial casting is tried first with surgery reserved for recalcitrant cases.

4.6. KNOCK-KNEES (GENU VALGUM)

As the normal child progresses from varus angulation (slightly bowed) at the knees to the normal adult valgus angulation (slightly knocked) of about 5°, there appears to be, at least in some children, an accentuation of this valgus which manifests itself at about age 4 years. Many children at that point exhibit up to 10° of valgus at the knees, a situation that can be concerning to the family. Knock-knees are often associated with flat feet or outtoeing, though any causal link is debatable. It may be that ligamentous laxity predisposes to all three.

As with varus angulation, such children should gradually improve with time, should not be short, should not have abnormal upper segment to lower segment ratios (see Chapter 1), and should have bilaterally symmetrical knees. Only after these reservations have been addressed can a child be labeled as having "physiological knock-knees."

4.6.1. Pathological Causes

Traumatic injury to the distal femoral or proximal tibial physis can result in angular abnormalities around the knee as longitudinal growth is restricted around the damaged area of the growth plate. Additionally, by a mechanism not apparent, genu valgum can result as well from a nondisplaced fracture of the proximal tibial metaphysis. Other localized derangements of physical growth can do likewise. They include enchondromatosis and focal fibrous dysplasia.

As with genu varum, the list of generalized growth disturbances resulting in genu valgum is long. It includes such dysplastic processes of bone as diaphyseal dysplasia, some types of epiphyseal dysplasia, Morquio's syndrome (one of the mucopolysaccharidoses), Gaucher disease (one of the lipidoses), osteogenesis imperfecta, diastrophic dwarfism, and metaphyseal dysplasia, among others. Additionally, problems of calcium

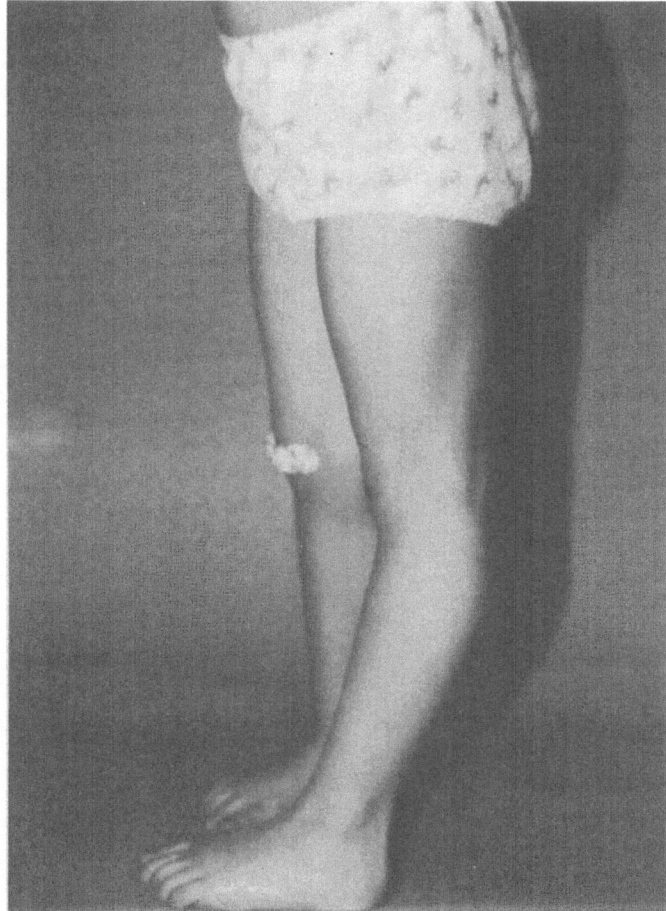

Figure 4.11. Mild knee recurvatum is common in hyperflexible little girls

metabolism, such as rickets (see Section 4.4.3.1), though usually resulting in varus angulation, can also cause genu valgum. If concern exists that the problem is not physiological, radiographs and appropriate chemistries should be obtained. Following the child over time can be accomplished through clinical photographs or by measuring the intermalleolar distance with the child standing and the knees just touching.

4.6.2. Therapy

Knock-knees are more important cosmetically than biomechanically and parents should be reassured. Shoe corrections have not been demonstrated to be of benefit. If severe, bracing may be attempted.

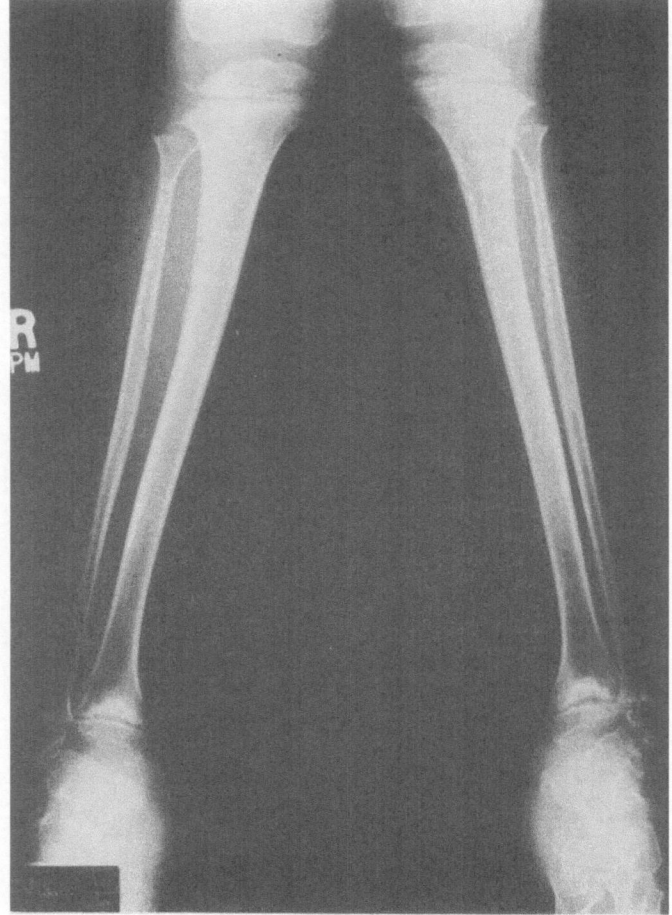

Figure 4.12. Morquio's syndrome, or type IV mucopolysaccharidosis, results in orthopedic problems, including genu valgum, and severe short stature. There is no mental retardation.

4.7. FLAT FEET

Flat feet, pes planus, is loss of the normal longitudinal and transverse arches. It is often associated with valgus angulation (eversion) at the ankle and is then referred to as a planovalgus foot deformity. Many parents of toddlers worry that their child has flat feet because the fat pads over the instep and the child's wide-based gait encourage eversion and make the feet look flatter than they really are. This "pseudo" flat foot deformity should be gone by 2 or 3 years.

There are two varieties of true flat feet: (1) flexible, which is usually benign, and (2) rigid, which is usually not.

4.7.1. Flexible Flat Feet

This is usually related to generalized and demonstrable ligamentous laxity which is often present in other family members. This is true even in the absence of specific, connective tissue abnormalities like Ehlers–Danlos syndrome.

Arches are present when the child is not weight-bearing and "collapse" when the child stands. If he is old enough, have the child walk on his toes. The arch will be obvious to all, including the parents. Flexible flat feet are common enough to be considered normal and are not usually painful. They improve over time as soft tissues tighten, the intrinsic muscles of the foot become stronger, and cartilage ossifies. Treatment is generally not necessary. Parents should be reassured that this is a benign condition and that special shoes are not necessary. Expensive "orthopedic" shoes may keep the feet well-arched while in the shoes but will do nothing to prevent the feet from becoming flat again the moment the child is unshod. They are not corrective. Well-made shoes with a good heel-cup (counter) will keep the child from excessive pronation. Loafers or moccasins without any support at all should be discouraged. High-top gym shoes should be recommended because of the support provided at the ankles and because of the usually good internal arch supports.

Molded shoe inserts to support the arch and keep the heel out of excessive valgus may be warranted under the following conditions: (1) if the child complains of significant pain, (2) if the deformity is severe, or (3) if there is excessive and expensive shoe wear

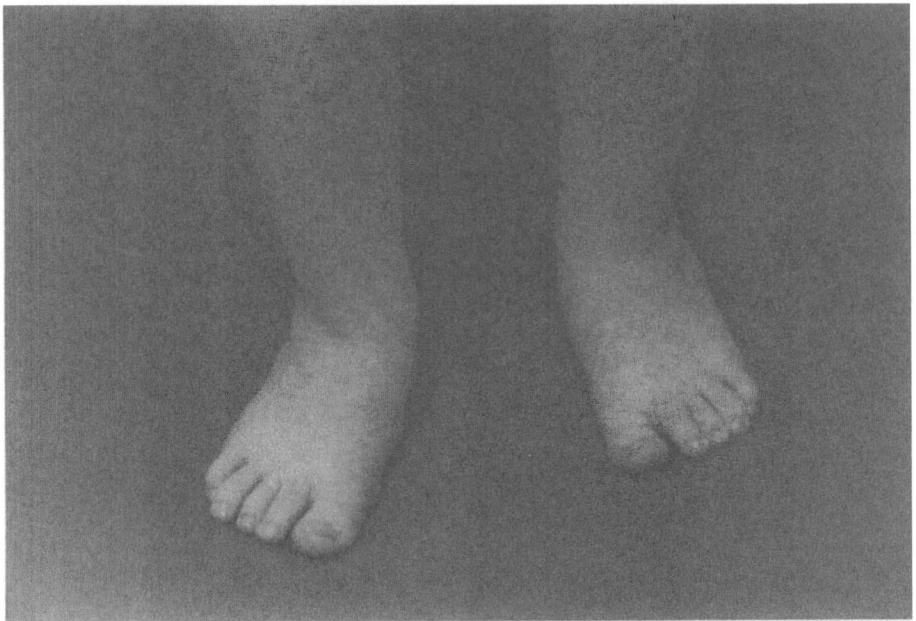

Figure 4.13. Typical flexible flat feet.

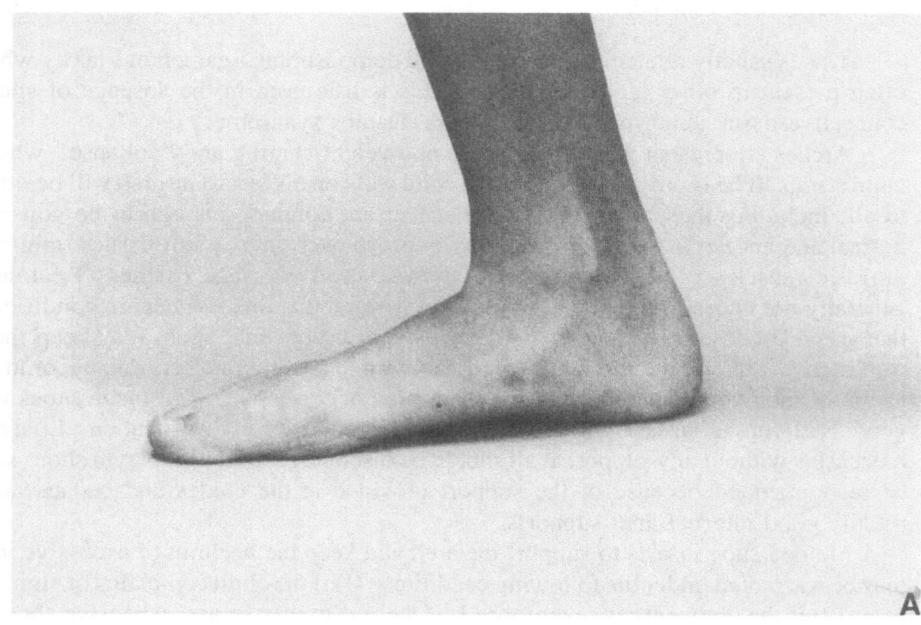

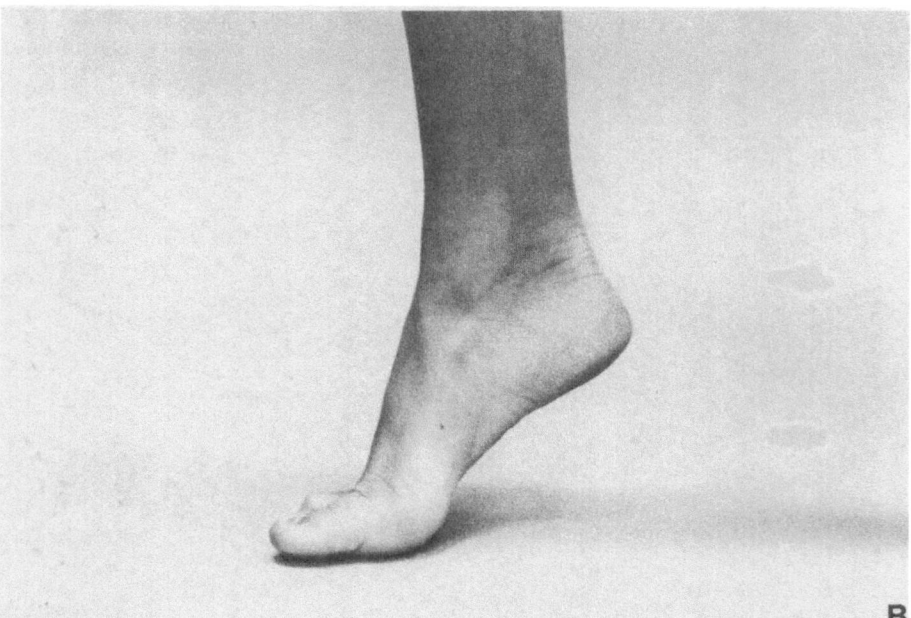

Figure 4 14 Flexible flat feet (A) get better when the patient stands on his toes (B) It s also a good way to reassure parents that their child does have an arch though temporarily absent

affecting the medial heel and sole. Arch-supporting molded shoe inserts can be obtained by writing a prescription to any local brace shop. They are expensive and are often not covered by conventional insurance plans. Parents need to be warned.

4.7.2. Rigid Flat Feet

Rigid flat feet are rigid because they can't be passively manipulated without causing pain. This occurs because of a variety of specific abnormalities. With rigid flat feet, the patient's feet are rigid regardless of weight-bearing or position. When they stand on their toes, if they are able, their feet are still flat. Pain is usually a prominent symptom. Causes of rigid flat feet include the following.

4.7.2.1. Tarsal Coalition

The lack of a mobile joint between any of the tarsal bones is termed a *tarsal coalition*. Though the result of failure of embryonic segmentation, symptoms usually don't develop until ossification is relatively far advanced, usually between 8 and 16 years of age. Radiographs prior to 9 or 10 years of age are likely to be negative until the coalition ossifies. Although any combination of talus, calcaneus, navicular, or cuboid coalition can occur, calcaneonavicular and calcaneotalar are the most common. When present as a primary phenomenon, coalitions are thought to be inherited as an autosomal dominant trait and occur bilaterally about 50% of the time (Edmondson and Crenshaw, 1980). They also can result from chronic inflammation to the joint as might occur with JRA.

On examination, subtalar motion will be markedly reduced and will be painful, particularly with inversion. Painful spasm of the peroneus longus muscle resulting from rigidity of the hindfoot renders the peroneus longus tendon tight and easily palpable posterior to the lateral malleolus. The alternative name for this condition is peroneal spastic flat foot.

Diagnosis can be confirmed radiologically by ordering anteroposterior views (for suspected calcaneocuboid or talonavicular coalitions) or oblique views of the foot (for calcaneonavicular coalitions). Calcaneotalar coalitions are more difficult to see radiologically and frequently require careful tomography or CT.

Confirmation of or concern about a coalition requires referral to an orthopedic surgeon even though surgery is not always necessary. Molded shoe inserts, casting, and anti-inflammatory medications frequently are of some use, depending on the severity of the bridging. If these are not effective, surgery would then be necessary and would involve excision of the coalition and repair of any degenerative change which had occurred.

4.7.2.2. Rigid Flat Feet Caused by Heel Cord Tightening

Heel cord (Achilles tendon) tightening may be idiopathically related to rapid preadolescent growth or to neurologic problems such as cerebral palsy and muscle disease. When appropriate heel strike or placement is restricted by tightening of the heel

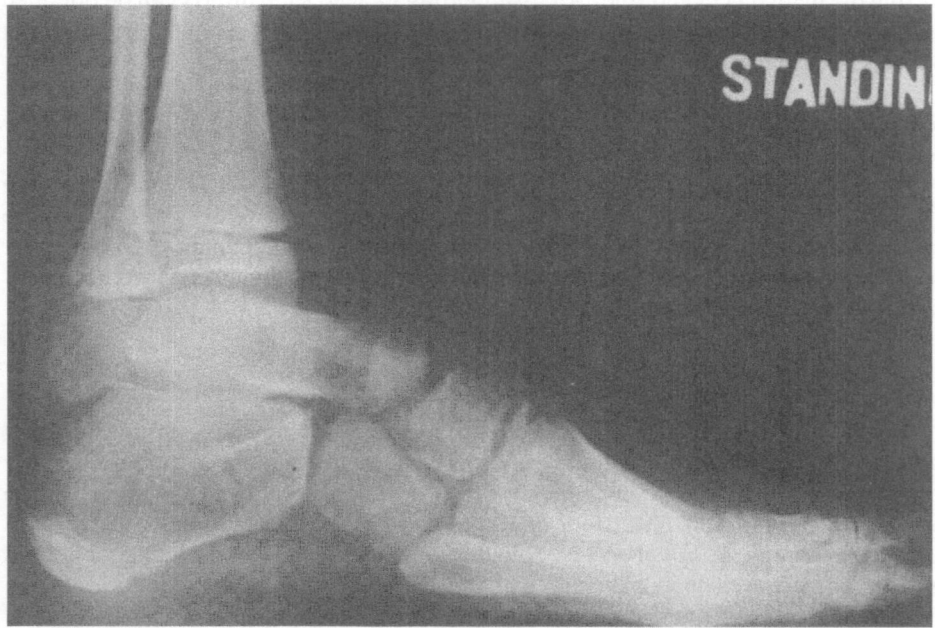

Figure 4.15. Talonavicular coalition in a 7-year-old girl

cord, the midfoot will compensate and "slide" or "break" allowing the heel to make contact with the ground. This compensation can only occur if the midfoot and forefoot is pronated or everted, giving a distinctive planovalgus appearance to the foot. To check for excessive heel cord tightening it is therefore necessary to supinate (invert) the foot, locking the midfoot. Failure to dorsiflex the foot to neutral (perpendicular to the tibia) with the foot in supination is the result of pathological heel cord tightening.

Simple physical therapy to stretch the heel cord is sometimes all that is necessary to treat this condition. If exercises are not effective, bracing with a plastic molded ankle–foot orthosis (AFO) may prove useful if added to the regime. Surgery may be necessary to lengthen the tendon if all else fails. Specific causes, such as Duchenne muscular dystrophy, must, of course, be first excluded by appropriate tests, including muscle enzymes.

4.7.2.3. Accessory Navicular

Pain, often worsened by shoe wear, and fullness over the tarsal navicular is often caused by a small accessory navicular bone with anomalous insertion of the posterior tibial tendon. Resulting spasm leads to pain and a rigid foot. Examination usually reveals tenderness over the navicular with pain on inversion against resistance resulting from maximal contraction of the posterior tibial muscle. Buying shoes to avoid pressure over

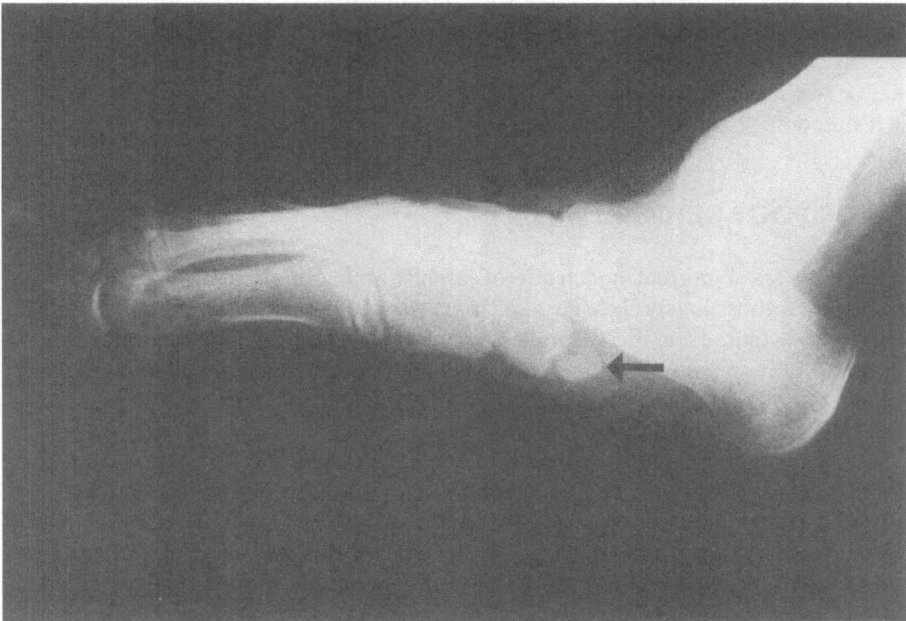

Figure 4.16. Accessory navicular (arrow), when symptomatic, is associated with pain, tenderness, and swelling over the navicular.

the area and providing molded arch inserts to counter muscle spasm are useful in most cases. Surgery may be necessary, and involves removal of the accessory bone and rerouting of the tendon.

Making things a little complex here is the recognition that many feet have accessory navicular bones but are without symptoms and that some children with typical pain and posterior tibial spasm are absolutely normal radiologically.

4.7.2.4. Vertical Talus

This condition, also termed *congenital convex pes valgus*, represents a congenital dislocation of the talonavicular joint such that the talus is aligned in a more vertical position than is usual. The vertically oriented talus pushes the calcaneus more laterally

Table 4.5. Rigid Flat Foot

Tarsal coalition
Heel cord tightening
Accessory navicular
Vertical talus

than is normal and rigidly locks the hindfoot, producing a rocker-bottom appearance. Though present idiopathically in some children, vertical talus is often associated with neurological syndromes such as spina bifida, orthopedic abnormalities such as arthrogryposis, or trisomy of chromosome 13. Early orthopedic referral is likely to result in improved outcome if surgery is deemed necessary.

4.8. CAVUS FOOT DEFORMITIES

Since there is a normal spectrum of arches, most high arches are no more troublesome than most low arches. In fact, most people with high arches are proud of them. However, acquired and increasingly higher arches over time may be a reflection of peripheral nerve or spinal cord abnormalities. This is particularly so when associated with "clawing" of the toes (hyperextension at the metatarsal joints with hyperflexion at the interphalangeal joints).

Certainly a thorough physical exam, particularly looking for abnormalities in strength, sensation (including position and vibratory sense, decreased in Charcot–Marie–Tooth), deep tendon reflexes, atrophy, and tone, is warranted. The presence of a dysraphism causing cavus feet may be suspected by the presence of lumbosacral hemangiomatosis, a pigmentary macule, a hairy patch, or a sinus tract or dimple. Radiography (anterioposterior and lateral of the lumbosacral spine) may demonstrate a bony but occult spina bifida. Magnetic resonance imaging, to investigate the possibility of a spinal cord lesion, or nerve conduction velocities and EMG, for a peripheral neuropathy, may be necessary.

Just as pes planus is associated with valgus deformity at the ankle, pes cavus is associated commonly with varus angulation. Such angulation leads to asymmetrical weight-bearing on the lateral side of the foot, instead of the normal circumstance with weight-bearing spread evenly across the first and fifth metatarsal heads and the heel. Progressive cavus deformity may require orthopedic surgery if persistent pain becomes a problem or to prevent worsening deformity, regardless of cause.

4.9. LEG LENGTH DISCREPANCIES

Regardless of cause, asymmetry of lower extremity lengths causes a variety of secondary difficulties. These include cosmetic appearance, the potential for scoliosis, and an abnormal gait. Depending on the degree of discrepancy, children may walk with a vaulting type of gait, with equinus on the shorter side or with a flexion contracture of the knee on the longer side (see also Chapter 1). Though very often idiopathic, when specific causes of leg length discrepancies (LLD) do occur, they frequently have additional repercussions for the health of the child independent of the LLD itself.

4.9.1. LLD Resulting from Injury

Even fractures which do not affect the growth plate (physis) of long bones may have an impact on longitudinal growth and the effect may be either to shorten or to lengthen. If

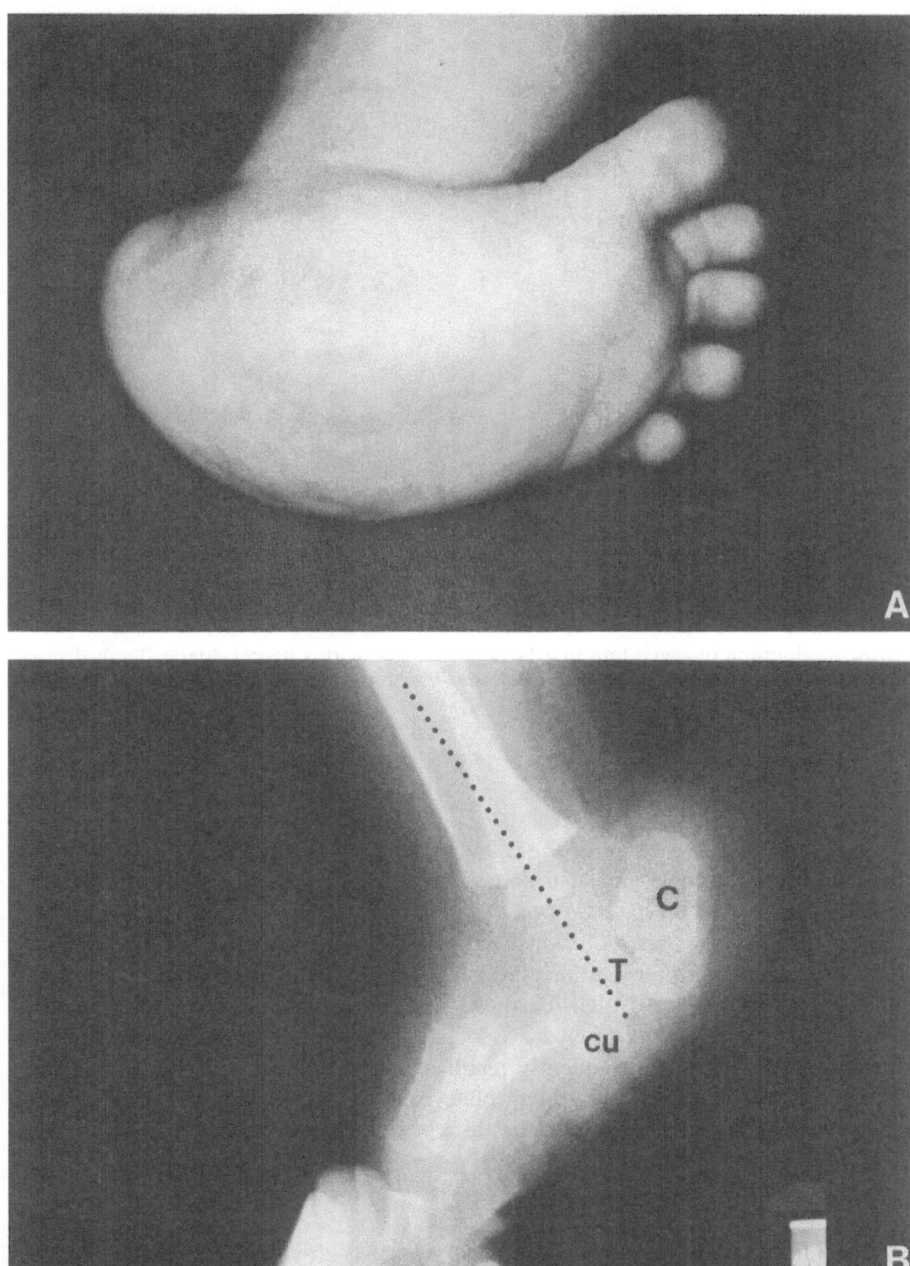

Figure 4.17. (A) Vertical talus, also known as rocker-bottom foot or convex pes valgus, is frequently associated with other congenital defects. (B) On X-ray, note that long axis of talus (T) is parallel to long axis of tibia and that the calcaneus (C) is in severe equinus. The navicular doesn't ossify until about 3 years and so is not seen in this infant's X-ray. cu, cuboid.

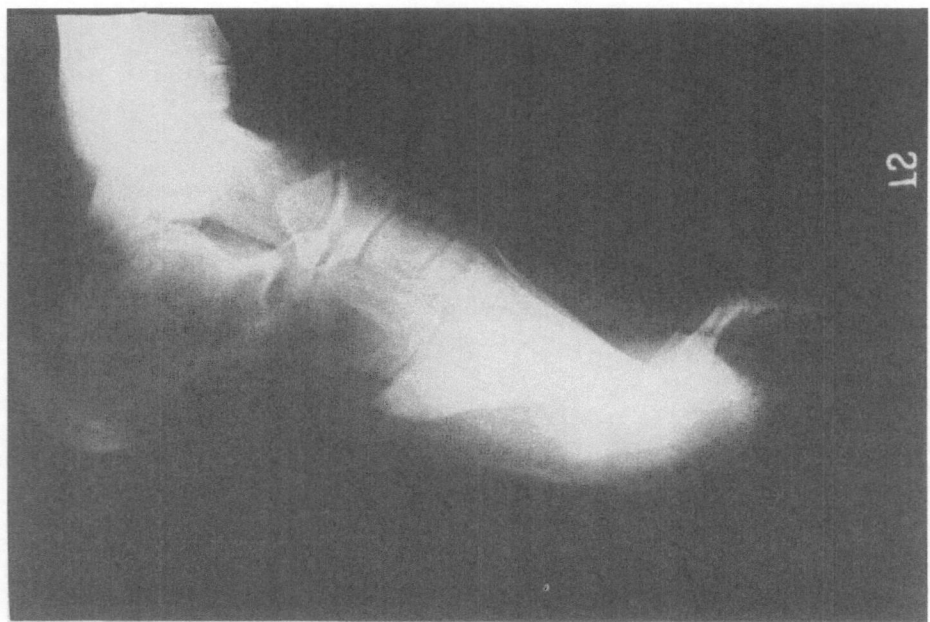

Figure 4.18. Radiograph of cavus foot in a 14-year-old male with Charcot–Marie–Tooth disease. Note hyperextension at metatarsophalangeal joints, flexion at interphalangeal joints (clawfoot deformity), and high arch.

bony deformity results in overlap of the fractured ends, foreshortening may result. On the other hand, the fracture can also somehow stimulate the growth plate, causing overgrowth.

Growth plate injuries are notoriously associated with longitudinal growth problems. It is not necessary for these injuries to be traumatic in the usual sense of the word, however. For example, Legg–Calve–Perthes (aseptic necrosis of the femoral head) or slipped capital femoral epiphysis may be associated with injury to the proximal growth plate of the femur and may subsequently result in severe shortening. Similarly, osteo-myelitis, usually very close to the growth plate, may result in poor growth if damage to the germinal layers of the physis occurs as a result of infection.

4.9.2. Neurotrophic Causes for LLD

An intact nervous system is required for appropriate growth. LLD can be expected when there exists asymmetrical central nervous system or peripheral nerve injury, damage, or malfunction. This might occur as a result of hemiparetic cerebral palsy, for example, or as a result of a unilateral root or peripheral nerve injury such as would occur with polio or after a brachial plexus injury.

4.9.3. Vascular and Inflammatory Causes for LLD

Such vascular abnormalities as arteriovenous malformations or capillary hemangiomatosis result in overgrowth because of increased blood flow to the affected extremity. *Klippel–Trenaunay–Weber* is the term most usually applied to this combination of deep and superficial vascular anomalies together with longitudinal as well as circumferential overgrowth. Look for superficial, often ill-defined, hemangiomata (nevus flammeus or port-wine nevus), increased warmth, or venous varicosities. Listen for bruits resulting from arteriovenous malformations.

Increased blood flow to a joint, and presumably to adjacent epiphyses as well, similarly results in stimulation of longitudinal growth. Asymmetrical arthritis, particularly of the knee, as might occur with pauciarticular juvenile rheumatoid arthritis, frequently results in asymmetrical growth and a LLD. Check for warmth over a joint, swelling, or decreased range of motion.

The opposite is true, as well, when vascular insufficiency restricts growth on the affected side as might occur with linear scleroderma or morphea.

4.9.4. Syndromic Causes for LLD

Several complicated constellations of abnormalities have, as one of their features, a LLD. These include Wiedemann–Beckwith syndrome, Russell–Silver syndrome, McCune–Albright syndrome, and neurofibromatosis, among others.

Wiedemann–Beckwith syndrome includes severe neonatal hypoglycemia, macroglossia, large size, visceromegaly of liver and kidneys, omphalocele, and mild to moderate microcephaly.

Russell–Silver syndrome is characterized by the presence of a small, triangular face, frontal bossing, severe short stature, and, in many cases, asymmetry.

McCune–Albright syndrome includes the association of polyostotic fibrous dysplasia, cutaneous hyperpigmentation (nevus lateralis), and sexual precocity. Occasionally other forms of endocrine disease, including hyperthyroidism or Cushing syndrome, may also be involved.

Neurofibromatosis (von Recklinghausen disease), in addition to cutaneous and central nervous system abnormalities, includes a large number of orthopedic abnormalities, including osseous cysts, bowing and pseudoarthrosis of the tibia, and overgrowth of long bones.

4.9.5. LLD Related to Congenital Malformations

A variety of different kinds of limb deficiencies, such as fibular hemimelia, result in asymmetrical lower extremity growth (see Chapter 6).

4.9.6. Diagnosis of LLD

Documentation of lower extremity asymmetry is the essential first step. This can only be done via direct measurement of each lower extremity from the anterior superior

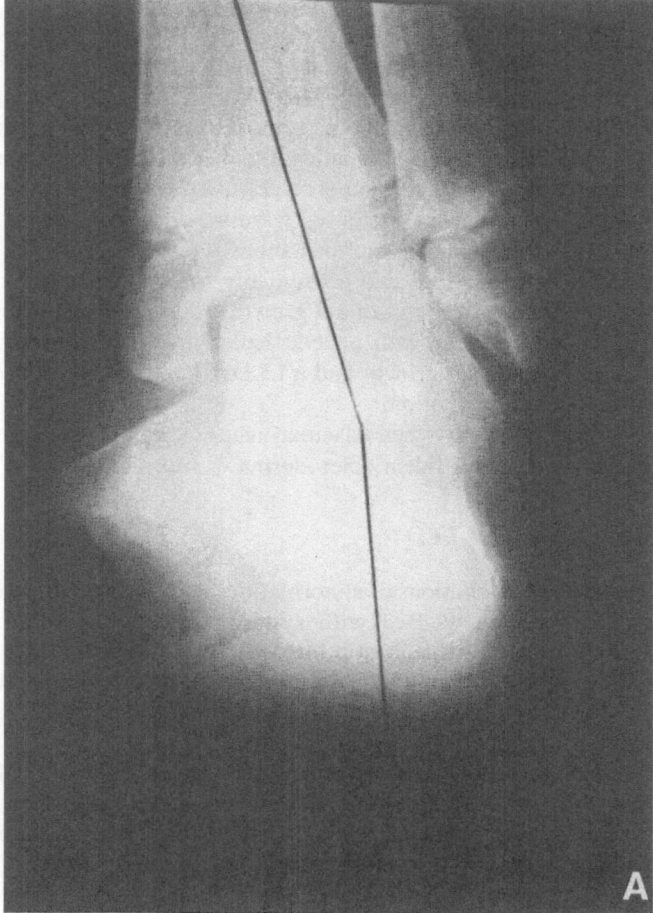

Figure 4.19. (A) AP X-ray of ankle of same patient as Fig. 4.18. Note varus relationship between tibia and calcaneus. Usually, the heel is valgus to the tibia. (B) Clinical photograph of different patient with Charcot–Marie–Tooth showing clawfoot deformities, high arch, and ankle varus.

iliac spine to the medial malleolus of each limb. Measurement from the umbilicus to the malleoli may be inaccurate if there exists an abnormal relationship between the pelvis and the femora or between the pelvis and the lumbar spine. For example, if there is an abduction contracture of the right hip, with compensating adduction on the left, the right lower extremity will be apparently, though not really, longer than the left and will measure longer if the reference point is the umbilicus. A similar process may occur if the pelvis is oblique in relationship to the long axis of the spine, as often happens with scoliosis.

Pelvic obliquity with the patient standing, in other words, is important information

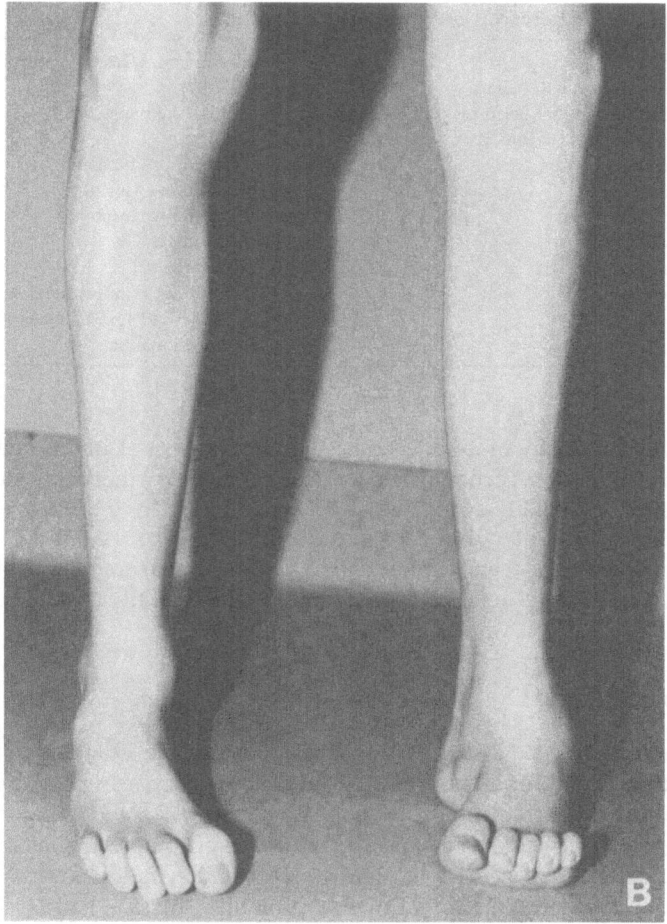

Figure 4.19. (*Continued*)

but is not, by itself, sufficient information on which to base a diagnosis of a LLD. The obliquity may be causing the apparent discrepancy rather than vice versa.

To investigate the possibility of associated difficulties as described above, check for full range of motion at the hip, neurocutaneous abnormalities, hemangiomata, tone, and reflexes. Measure for atrophy and look at the trunk, face, and upper extremity to determine if the lower extremity discrepancy is isolated or is part of a generalized hemihypertrophy syndrome. Check for scoliosis, evidence of trauma, sexual precocity, arthritis, and plot the height and weight carefully.

Radiologic investigation is important, not only to quantitate the discrepancy but to

Table 4.6. Causes of Unequal Leg Length

Fractures	Inflammatory/vascular
Involving growth plate	JRA
Femoral or tibial fractures with overgrowth	Large hemangioma
Other growth plate injury	Syndromes
Aseptic necrosis	Neurofibromatosis
Osteomyelitis	McCune–Albright
Septic arthritis	Hemihypertrophy
Neurotrophic	Exostoses
Hemiparetic CP	Birth defects
Peripheral nerve	Proximal femoral focal deficiency
Polio	Congenital hip dislocation
	Other, idiopathic

investigate the possibility of associated bony abnormalities. Documentation and quantification radiologically is accomplished by a scanogram or orthoroentgenogram. Both of these techniques are readily available in any general radiology department and involve the use of a radiopaque ruler placed under the child's limbs as the X-ray plate is exposed. Direct measurements can then be made and an accurate measurement of the discrepancy, if it exists, can be made. Routine anteroposterior and lateral films should also be ordered as needed.

4.9.7. Therapy for LLD

Referral for orthopedic surgical consultation should be obtained for all discrepancies greater than 2 cm, for all discrepancies which are increasing over time, and for all discrepancies resulting from serious orthopedic conditions, such as growth plate injury.

In general, intervention becomes more and more necessary as the discrepancy approaches 2 cm but depends on the child's height and symptomatology. A shoe lift on the shorter side would be the initial intervention and, for the static discrepancy, may be all that would ever be necessary. Both soles and heels should be included and can be ordered through a brace shop or, oftentimes, through a children's shoe store. The prescribed lift should never attempt to make up the totality of the measured discrepancy; a lift equaling between two-thirds and three-fourths of the discrepancy seems to be tolerated best.

Shoe lifts greater than 4 or 5 cm are often not well tolerated and the problem may then have to be approached surgically. In grown children, osteotomy of the longer extremity or lengthening of the shorter may be warranted.

In the growing child, epiphysiodesis of the longer leg may be considered in order to fuse the growth plate and reduce longitudinal growth by that amount. Alternatively, if short stature is a concern, lengthening of the growing femur or tibia or both might be chosen. Since timing of either of these interventions is critical and the surgery is difficult, children with significant LLDs should always be seen in centers with considerable pediatric orthopedic experience.

4.10. TOE-WALKING

Toe-walking is frequently part of the normal widely based gait of the toddler and will most often take care of itself as the child becomes more secure on his feet. Occasionally, toe-walking will persist and the family will become concerned.

Even if persistent beyond 18 months, toe-walking is most often a benign condition that will resolve on its own. Attention should be paid, however, to the possibility of delayed motor development and tight heel cords. Undiagnosed neurologic difficulties such as mild spastic diplegic cerebral palsy, muscular dystrophy, or spina bifida occulta may be responsible. Even in the absence of demonstrable disease, moreover, tight heel cords may continue to keep the child up on their toes, resulting in continued heel cord tightening, with more toe-walking and so on.

Therapy

In the absence of demonstrable neurologic disease, parents can be taught to stretch the heel cords, three or four times daily with 15 to 20 repetitions at each session. If improvement does not occur over a period of 2 months, casting, bracing, or surgery may be necessary and the child should be referred.

4.11. BUNIONS

Bunion deformity (hallux valgus) is rare in children and most often results from JRA affecting the metatarsophalangeal (MTP) joints.

Bunions begin to make themselves manifest as idiopathic abnormalities during adolescence. They affect males rarely. The term *bunion* is used to describe the painful prominence of the first MTP joint resulting from lateral deviation of the toe distal to the MTP joint. Broadening of the midfoot as well as varus angulation of the first metatarsal ray (metatarsus primus varus) are thought to be etiologically important. The process begins, so the theory goes, with medial deviation of the first metatarsal ray. Shoe wear eventually will then push the first toe laterally, exposing the MTP joint to compressive and irritative forces from shoe pressure.

Increasing deformity leads to decreasing push-off power of the great toe and to increasing pathological loading on the second and third toes. Corns, callosities, and hammertoe deformities occur as a result. Persistent, intractable pain or extreme difficulties with shoeing are indications for surgical repair.

4.12. CHILDREN'S SHOES

There is still the general misconception on the part of many parents that rigid, expensive leather shoes are necessary if their child's feet are to grow properly. Though there is no evidence that such shoes are harmful, there is certainly no reason to recommend them, particularly when rapid foot growth may necessitate three or four

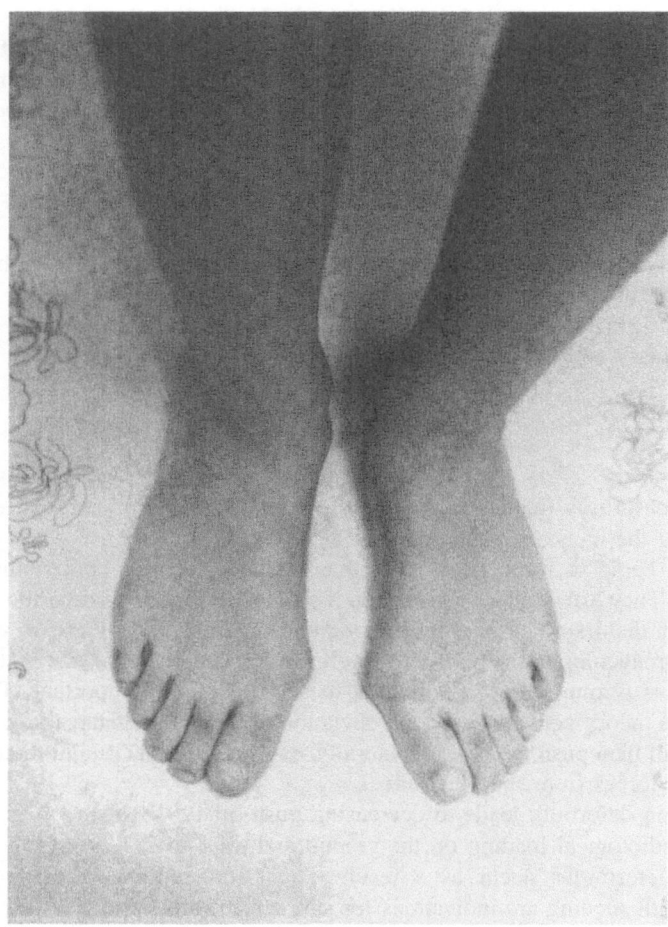

Figure 4.20. Bunion deformities.

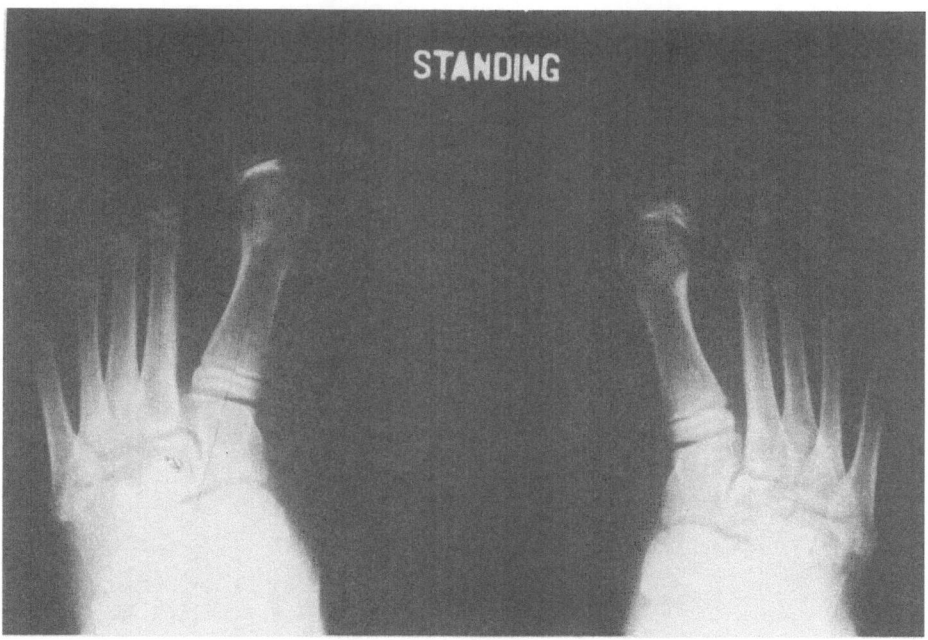

Figure 4.21. X-ray of different patient with bunions, demonstrating hallux valgus and prominence of metatarsophalangeal joints.

different pairs in one year. Simple, inexpensive gym shoes will provide all the warmth and protection from the elements that shoes are supposed to provide.

Similarly, "orthopedic" or "corrective" shoes are generally of no proven benefit in the care of children with most of the normal developmental lower extremity problems described above. There are, however, two shoe corrections that are probably worthwhile.

The first is the use of an open-toed straight last prewalker for stubborn, though not rigid, metatarsus adductus (see above). The second is the use of a special shoe insert for children with severe, painful, though flexible, flat feet. An arch-supporting shoe insert with a shallow heel cup is preferred to an "arch-feature" shoe because the shoe insert can be used interchangeably in a variety of different shoes.

Caring for the Child
with Motor Delay

5.1. INTRODUCTION

This chapter focuses on the child who fails to develop appropriate gross motor skills. In addition to walking, these include rolling over, sitting, pulling up to standing, standing independently, running, walking up stairs, and other functions, deficiencies of which cause parents lots of concern. Expectations regarding motor milestones are listed in Table 5.1. The other areas of childhood development, language, fine motor and social skills, will not be discussed in detail except as they relate to the differential diagnosis of gross motor problems.

Orthopedic considerations have always had an intimate relationship to problems of motor development and still do. Parents often think first of bones as a way to explain their child's developmental problems rather than brain, spinal cord, nerves, and muscles and will bring to your attention some minor normal variant affecting the lower extremities with the expectation that correcting the bowlegs or flat feet will improve the delayed child's ability to walk.

Table 5.1. Major Motor Milestones

Rolls to back from front	3 months
Sits alone unsupported	7 months
Pulls to standing on furniture	10 months
Walks alone	15 months
Runs well	24 months
Up stairs on alternating feet	36 months
Skips	60 months

Additionally, orthopedics as a field has a long and productive history of care for children afflicted with neuromuscular disease. William J. Little, an Englishman working in the mid-19th century, initially associated spasticity with a history of a difficult delivery and asphyxia and pioneered early surgical treatment. For many years cerebral palsy was known as Little's disease.

5.2. SPECIFIC CAUSES OF MOTOR DELAYS

It is useful to order all of the many causes of motor problems in childhood by localizing them to specific levels of the nervous system:

- Brain
- Spinal cord
- Peripheral nervous system, including
    Anterior horn cells
    Peripheral nerves
    Neuromuscular junction
    Muscle

5.2.1. Cerebral Causes

Cerebral causes might be somewhat arbitrarily divided into two large groupings, cerebral palsy and mental retardation, and a smaller group of complex neurodegenerative diseases.

5.2.1.1. Cerebral Palsy

Though an artificial term, *cerebral palsy* (CP) remains a useful one to describe all causes of cerebral damage affecting motor function occurring during prenatal life or around the time of delivery, including asphyxia, trauma, and cerebral infection. CP is a group of problems rather than a single entity. Affected children manifest a spectrum of motor disability from mild defects in coordination and balance to complete lack of ambulation and self-help skills. The implication of the term *cerebral palsy* is that the extent of the encephalopathy is static, though the manifestations are not unchanging

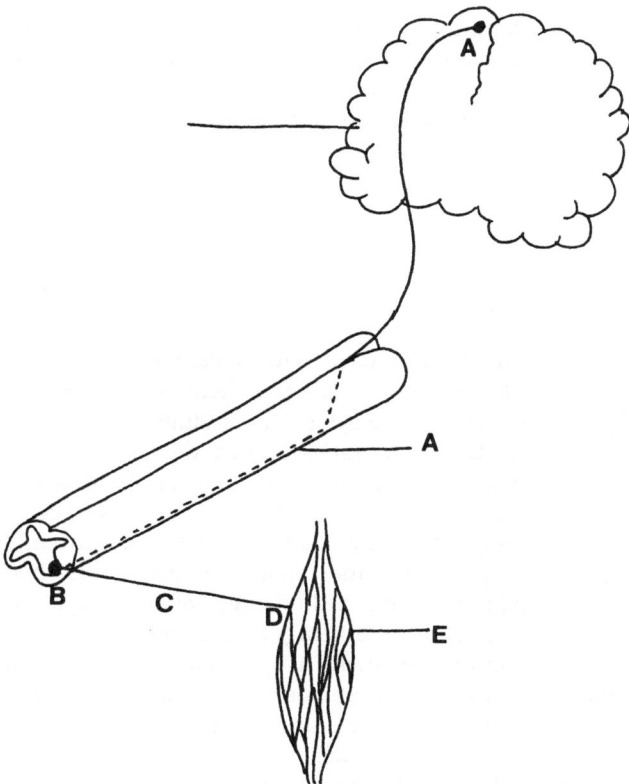

Figure 5.1. Categorizing the presumed level of the nervous system affected in the child with a motor delay provides a structure on which to build an intelligent evaluation. Upper motor lesions include those that affect the brain or the corticospinal tracts (A). Lower motor lesions affect anterior horn cells (B), motor nerves (C), the myoneural junction (D), or the muscle (E).

as the child develops. Children who eventually develop spastic CP, for example, are frequently hypotonic for the first 6 or 10 months of life.

Prevalence rates range from about 2 to 4 per 1000 live births. Recent research has demonstrated that many more children develop CP as a result of prenatal rather than perinatal events. It is often, though by no means invariably, associated with other manifestations of CNS damage such as seizures, strabismus, hyperactivity, hearing loss, and mental retardation.

Though spasticity is most common, children with CP frequently have a mixed picture, spasticity with dystonia or spasticity with chorea, usually with one type of neurologic symptomatology predominating. Ninety percent of children with CP have some spasticity. Athetotic, ataxic, dystonic, and atonic forms are less common.

Spasticity results from corticospinal tract damage resulting in an alteration of the gamma afferent nervous system, rendering the muscle spindles hypersensitive and the muscles hypertonic. Resulting inequalities of muscle balance around each joint lead to characteristic deformities and articular damage. Lack of appropriate ambulation leads to osteoporosis.

The three most common types of spastic CP are:

• Hemiplegia
• Diplegia
• Quadriplegia

5.2.1.2. Hemiplegic Cerebral Palsy

Hemiplegia is not usually associated with apparent problems of pregnancy or delivery and is thought to be often the result of a silent prenatal or perinatal stroke. It manifests itself by mild to moderate delays in motor attainments with walking usually between 18 and 24 months. Both extremities on one side are affected. Children with hemiplegic CP typically walk with equinus posturing of the foot (toe down) and a circumducted gait in which the lower extremity on the affected side is swung widely with a circular motion and slight flexion at the knee. The upper extremity is held flexed at the elbow, wrist, and fingers, with the forearm pronated, the shoulder internally rotated, and the thumb held in the palm. Mild degrees of hemiplegia may only be seen when the child is stressed. In fact, mild hemiplegic CP is sometimes missed until an observant physician (or gym teacher) picks it up when the child is quite old, often at school entry. Abnormally early hand dominance (less than 18 months) is typical and parents may also note decreased movement and fisting on the affected side. Abnormal neurologic control of the affected side will eventually result in circumferential and longitudinal atrophy and a leg length discrepancy.

Though we think of CP as a purely motor disease, children with hemiplegia frequently manifest sensory deficits, most prominently those of stereognosis on the affected side. This sensory loss, together with the motor deficit, causes a significant and persistent functional deficit of the upper extremity. Surgery and splinting for contractures can improve appearance to some degree though significant functional problems often remain.

Children with hemiplegic CP are very likely to have normal intelligence and to function normally in society as adults. Seizures, however, are more common than in other forms of CP and eventually will affect about one-third of all children with hemiplegic CP.

5.2.1.3. Diplegic Cerebral Palsy

Diplegic cerebral palsy causes symmetrical lower extremity spasticity, affecting the upper extremities to a much lesser degree. Associated with prematurity, diplegic CP is thought to be caused by periventricular white matter damage resulting from perfusion abnormalities. The typical pathological lesion, periventricular leukomalacia, is associated with greater damage to the white matter ramifications controlling lower extremity function than upper extremity function, hence the peculiar manifestations of "paraplegia" on a cortical basis. Unlike those with cord lesions, however, children with diplegia will not exhibit a sensory level, an important differential point in the evaluation of the young child with apparent congenital lower extremity weakness and spasticity.

Like children with hemiplegia, children with diplegia usually have a good prognosis for ambulation, usually walking by 48 months. Though mentation is most often normal, children frequently have visual motor handicaps or other types of learning disabilities. Seizures are less likely than in hemiplegic CP.

Lower extremity difficulties include either a crouch gait with hip and knee flexion spasticity or hip flexion with knee hyperextension. Additionally, most children will also manifest internal rotation at the hip with hip adduction spasticity and equinus ankle deformities. Most often, upper extremity involvement manifests itself only by minimal fine motor incoordination.

Therapy is directed toward improving the gait through physical therapy and the judicious use of surgery to correct fixed deformities, most often heel cord release. Selective dorsal rhizotomy is currently being used, mostly as part of investigational protocols, in some centers. Rhizotomy reduces spasticity by interrupting the stretch reflex.

5.2.1.4. Quadriplegic Cerebral Palsy

Quadriplegic cerebral palsy, or "total body involvement," results from diffuse CNS injury caused by asphyxia or some similar diffuse process. Mental retardation, visual and hearing loss, and seizures are therefore more common than in other types of spastic CP and the prognosis for successful ambulation and normal cognitive functioning is not as good. Feeding and nutrition are often problematical and aspiration pneumonia is common. Because community ambulation is less likely, sitting becomes a major focus. Orthopedic surgical care is often oriented toward those procedures that can make the patient more functional in the wheelchair. Scoliosis and hip dislocation are commonly seen.

5.2.1.5. Deformities in Children with Cerebral Palsy

Several specific deformities are associated with spastic CP. These include:

1. **Equinus** deformities of the foot. These may be equinovarus or equinovalgus, depending on the nature of the child's neurologic injury.
2. **Flexion** deformity at the knee as a result of overactivity of the hamstrings and prolonged sitting.
3. **Hip adduction**, particularly in children with diplegia and quadriplegia leading eventually to coxa valga (abnormal straightening of the angle between femoral neck and shaft) and, in many children, to hip subluxation. This may result in pain and worsening deformity.
4. **Internal rotation** of the hips.

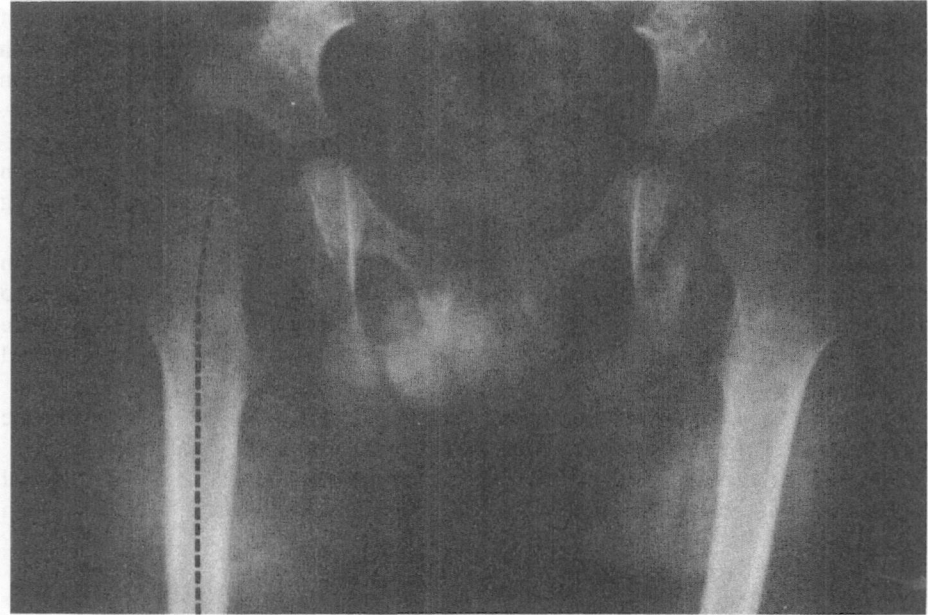

Figure 5.2. Coxa valga in a child with cerebral palsy. Note excessively large angle between femoral neck and shaft. Coxa valga in this context may be the result of unbalanced pull of hip adductors or lack of ambulation or both.

5.2.1.6. Other Types of Cerebral Palsy

Several other, more unusual, types of spastic CP are worth mentioning and include monoplegia, triplegia, and double hemiplegia. Children with double hemiplegia have all four extremities involved but one side much more severely affected than the other. They act more like children with hemiplegia than children with quadriplegia in terms of function and mentation.

Athetosis is the term used to describe slow, irregular, serpiginous involuntary movements. Speech, chewing, and swallowing are frequently also affected. Athetotic CP with bilirubin staining of the basal ganglia from neonatal Rh hemolytic disease is now a rarity. However, athetotic or choreoathetotic CP continues to occur, often associated with quadriparetic spasticity and a particular pathological lesion of the basal ganglia termed *status marmoratus*. Cognitive function is variable but tends to be reasonably well preserved, particularly in those children with less spasticity. Children may appear more affected cognitively than they really are because of their nonvolitional movements and their difficulty with expressive speech. Disability tends to be severe because of the persistent, involuntary movements that afflict these patients.

5.2.1.7. Surgical Treatment in Cerebral Palsy

Surgical treatment in CP is designed to accomplish one of three goals:

1. By lengthening tendons or cutting nerves, surgery can weaken overactive muscles.
2. By transferring tendons, surgery can strengthen weak muscles.
3. By realigning angular deformities, surgery can improve function and appearance.

Goals for each surgery should be well defined prior to the operation and the goal should be explained explicitly both to the family and to the patient.

5.2.1.8. Prognosis in Cerebral Palsy

Prognostically, about 50% of all children with CP will grow up to be community ambulators living independently, about 25% will require total care, and about 25% will be in-between.

5.2.1.9. Mental Retardation

Mental retardation is also known as psychomotor retardation. The motor emphasis is appropriate since children with significant and global developmental problems will often exhibit motor problems that stimulate their families to bring them to the primary care physician for evaluation.

Generally, language function is a more sensitive indicator of cognitive function in preschool children than delays in motor function. However, delays in the area of language acquisition may not be as compelling a problem from the parent's point of view as delays in the acquisition of motor skills. Cognitive deficits which end up being moderate or worse are often associated with motor delays. Mild mental retardation is generally not associated with severe, obvious problems in the area of motor function.

Mental retardation is defined as a measurable deficit in cognition, determined by the effective administration of an appropriate IQ test, associated with deficits in function with the deficits manifesting themselves during the developmental period. In other words, an IQ test result doesn't by itself lead to a label of mental retardation. The person involved must have deficits in daily functional skills as well. Additionally, the deficits must manifest themselves during the first 16 years of life, the developmental period. CNS trauma, stroke, encephalitis, or presenile dementia may leave one dysfunctional but, if they occur after the developmental period, they don't allow for a diagnosis of mental retardation.

People testing within two standard deviations from the mean are normal intellectually. Those testing between two and three standard deviations below the mean are labeled by psychologists as being **mildly retarded** and by educators as **educably mentally handicapped**. They are usually not picked up prior to school, function well after they finish school, work in unskilled or semiskilled positions, and generally marry people who aren't mentally retarded. They eventually develop academic skills to about the third or fourth year level and can read and do all the mathematical calculations most of us ever need to do. They constitute about 90% of all mentally retarded people. Their problems are rarely associated with a specific medical diagnosis.

Moderately retarded people have IQs between three and four standard deviations below the mean and are termed **trainable** by educators. They generally don't develop academic skills beyond survival recognition of important words in their environment, like *exit*, and usually work and live in sheltered circumstances. Their retardation is sometimes associated with a specific medical diagnosis.

Children with **severe and profound** mental retardation can be grouped together and have IQs between four and six standard deviations below the mean. They may have rudimentary language and be ambulatory but all will need institutional-type supervision throughout their life spans. Their conditions are most often associated with specific medical diagnoses.

5.2.1.10. Other Cerebral Causes of Motor Delays

Included here is a group of rare conditions associated predominantly with cerebellar or basal ganglion degeneration including Friedreich ataxia, ataxia–telangiectasia, Refsum syndrome, Wilson disease, Huntington chorea, and dystonia musculorum deformans. Often associated with autosomal recessive inheritance, they present with gait disturbances, ataxia, or a movement disorder. Ataxia–telangiectasia, characterized by ataxia, skin and ocular telangiectases, endocrine abnormalities and immunodeficiency, may present in infancy but the remainder of the conditions present in later childhood or early adolescence and are not usually part of the differential diagnosis of early motoric delay.

5.2.2. Spinal Cord Lesions

A variety of conditions affecting the spinal cord can cause motor delays in early childhood. They include injury to the cord during delivery, a variety of birth defects of the cord, including spina bifida, and acquired diseases of the spinal cord.

5.2.2.1. Birth Injuries to the Spinal Cord

Breech delivery with hyperextension of the neck may result in significant spinal cord injury. Infants affected present with diaphragmatic breathing, respiratory distress, autonomic disturbances, weak cry, a sensory level, and, initially, flaccid extremities. Eventually, spasticity and hyperreflexia become manifest in the lower extremities and, if a high cervical injury, in the upper extremities as well. Many of these infants are thought to have CP because of their spasticity though a careful search for the presence of a sensory level over the neck or upper trunk will reveal the true nature of their injury. Radiologically apparent vertebral fractures in association with such cord trauma are uncommon.

5.2.2.2. Congenital Vertebral Anomalies of the Cervical Spine

A variety of bony birth defects of the cervical spine cause cord dysfunction resulting in motor delays in early childhood. Such children present with signs of a spastic paraplegia or quadriplegia, hyperreflexia, extensor toe responses, neck pain, extremity numbness, sensory deficits, and problems with bowel and bladder function. Included in this group are basilar impression, odontoid separation, and chronic atlanto-axial dislocation.

Basilar impression occurs when the cervical spine invaginates itself into the base of the skull with consequent pressure on the structures around the foramen magnum. It is associated with a variety of other defects of the cervical spine, including the Klippel–Feil sequence. Children with basilar impression, in addition to the above, will complain of headaches and will be noted to have cranial nerve palsies, a short neck, and an elongated skull in the anteroposterior diameter.

Odontoid separation or any cause of instability in the upper cervical area may present with torticollis, intermittent episodes of quadriparesis, progressive quadriparesis related to cord compression, or, unfortunately, death. The intermittent nature of the signs and symptoms makes their diagnosis difficult. Treatment for all of the above is surgical.

5.2.2.3. Familial Spastic Paraplegia

Familial spastic paraplegia is an uncommon condition that may be inherited as either an autosomal recessive or dominant trait. A variety of conditions can be present, including metabolic disturbances, exhibiting progressive spasticity as a result of cortico-spinal tract degeneration. Sensory impairment is uncommon but has been described.

5.2.2.4. Spina Bifida

Spina bifida is a generic term for any defect resulting from failure of normal closure of the posterior neuropore, an event that takes place toward the end of the fourth embryonic week. It includes a spectrum of defects from complete failure of neural tube closure with dysplastic spinal cord tissue exposed (rachischisis or myeloschisis) to spinal cord covered by meninges only (meningomyelocele) to an outpouching of meninges covered by skin but not containing any neural elements (meningocele) to a variety of more mild dysraphic processes involving the lumbosacral spinal cord, including the presence of a lipoma, a dermal sinus, a dermoid cyst, or a thickened philum terminale (spina bifida occulta). These latter are not completely "occulta" since a hemangioma, hairy tuft, deep dimple, or pigmented macule are frequently found in association.

5.2.2.5. Causation in Spina Bifida

Overall, spina bifida occurs once in every 200 to 1000 live births, depending on the population involved. Genetics and environment are both thought to play a role in causation, which remains obscure. Valproic acid taken during pregnancy has been implicated in the causation of spina bifida.

Recently, folate supplementation has been shown to significantly decrease the likelihood of spina bifida. Current recommendations are for all women to take 0.4 mg of folic acid per day (not to exceed 1.0 mg), beginning 28 days prior to conception and throughout gestation. Most adult multivitamin preparations contain 0.4 mg folate and most prenatal vitamin preparations contain 0.8 to 1.0 mg. Women who have already had a baby with a neural tube defect will need more folate. Also, hot tub or sauna use is a risk factor and should be restricted or eliminated.

Recurrence risks for subsequently affected children increase to 4% after the birth of a child with spina bifida though recurrence risk is also dependent to some degree on the baseline risk of spina bifida in the population involved.

5.2.2.6. Presentation of Spina Bifida

Typically the child with spina bifida demonstrates a skin defect in the midlumbar region through which bulges a CSF-filled sac covered by meninges (meningomyelocele). Paralysis of the lower extremities is dependent not only on the height of the lesion but also on its completeness. Intact neural elements below the lesion sometimes give rise to reflex withdrawal activity which can lead to the false hope that true neurologic function extends farther than initially thought. The paralysis tends to be of the flaccid, lower motor neuron type and is associated with loss of sphincter control and hyporeflexia.

Complications include neurogenic bladder, with resulting recurring urinary tract infections, congenital renal anomalies including horseshoe kidney, neurogenic bowel, scoliosis, hydrocephalus which often requires shunting, other CNS malformations, hip dislocation and other lower extremity abnormalities, mental retardation in about 35%, lower extremity sensory loss with ulcerations, precocious puberty, pathological fractures, and strabismus, among others. The continual, multisystem demands that the disease places on child, family, and health care provider are obviously considerable. They represent a major drain on the emotional and financial resources of all.

5.2.2.7. Neurogenic Bladder in Spina Bifida

Clean intermittent catheterization has represented a positive step in the care of the urinary tract problems that these children face. Clean, intermittent catheterization programs can often improve urinary continence, reduce urinary tract pressures, and decrease the frequency of urinary tract infections. Serious, life-threatening allergy to latex, however, has been described and merits caution and strict avoidance of latex products, including latex urinary catheters.

5.2.2.8. Scoliosis

Scoliosis is generally of the paralytic "C" curve type without a compensatory minor curve. This results in more pelvic obliquity than would be expectable if the curve were of the typical "S" type (see also Chapter 9).

5.2.2.9. Hip Dislocation

Dislocation of the hip and other lower extremity deformities result from muscle imbalance. The typical midlumbar meningomyelocele leaves neurologic function intact at L-2 and above. This allows for hip flexion and adduction without the balancing effect of extension and abduction and predisposes to dislocation. Higher lesions which result in all hip muscles being paralyzed and lower lesions which preserve all hip motion

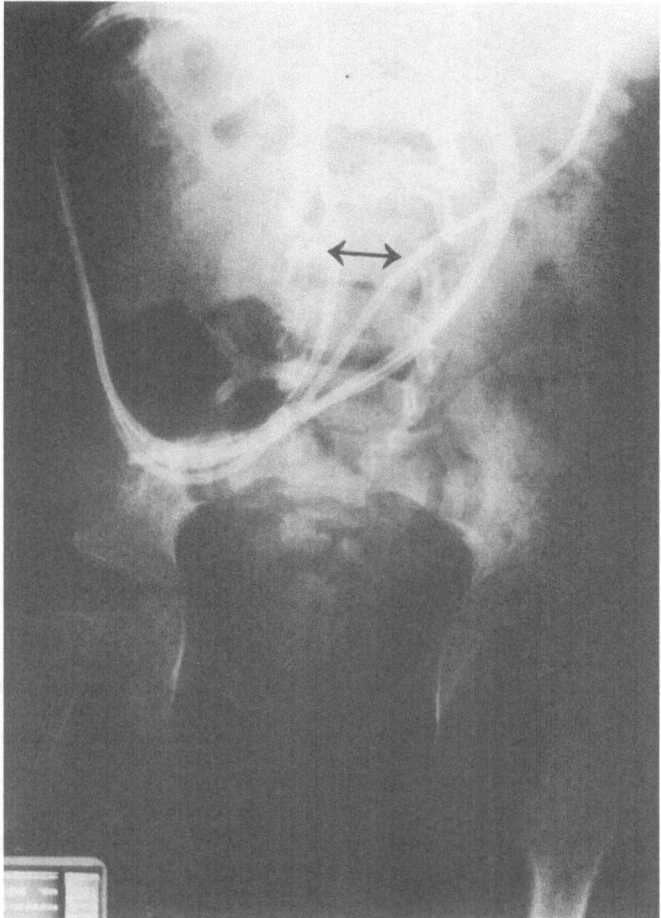

Figure 5.3. Radiological compendium of many of the problems caused by spina bifida. Note ventriculoperitoneal shunt tubing, subluxation of left hip, widening of interpedicular distances of lumbar spine vertebral bodies (arrow), and large amount of fecal material.

generally don't result in dislocation. Other deformities, including talipes equinovarus and calcaneovalgus, may result from abnormal intrauterine positioning caused by prenatal paralysis. Some children may demonstrate arthrogrypotic-like contractures and deformities as well.

5.2.2.10. Spina Bifida Occulta

As all children grow, the distal end of the spinal cord moves in a cephalad direction. Dysplastic elements, including lipomatous masses, dermoid cysts, and midline bony or cartilaginous spicules (diastematomyelia) sometimes tether the cord, putting the remain-

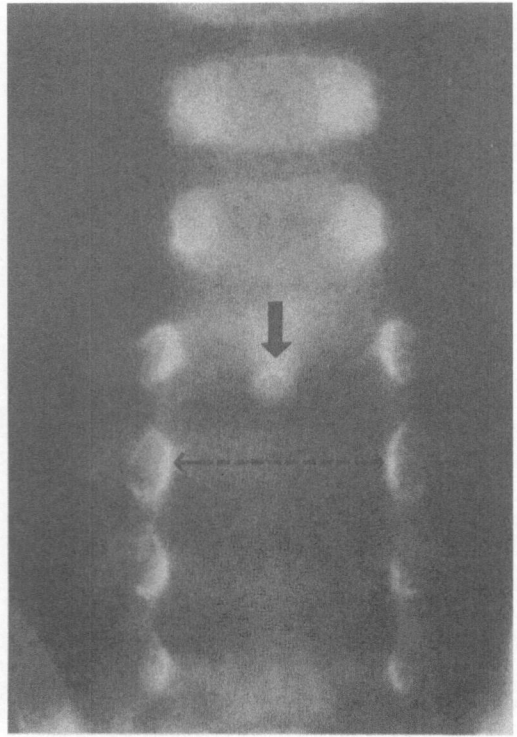

Figure 5.4. Diastematomyelia (arrow) associated with spina bifida. Note widening of interpedicular distances.

ing neural elements on stretch and causing worsening motor or sphincter function. Paradoxically, this may be more apparent clinically in those children with mild disease (spina bifida occulta). Failure to take appropriate diagnostic or therapeutic action may lead to permanent damage even after appropriate surgical intervention. Any change in status of a child with meningomyelocele, including worsening gait, increased frequency of urinary tract infections, change in continence or change in neurologic exam from hyporeflexia to hyperreflexia or hypotonia to hypertonia, merits appropriate evaluation, usually beginning with an MRI of the area.

Additionally, any child without symptoms but with cutaneous stigmata of spina bifida occulta, including hemangiomatosis, hairy patch, deep dimple or pigmentation over the lumbosacral spine, merits evaluation, including an MRI and close neurologic follow-up. Currently controversy exists regarding the need for operative repair of potentially tethering structures in the absence of symptoms, though no one would argue with the need to know that they exist.

5.2.2.11. Prognosis

Prognosis in spina bifida tends to be related to cognitive function as well as the height and completeness of the lesion. Children with a "high" lesion (L-1) may early on ambulate at home and school with crutches and braces from the floor to, and including, the pelvis However, as they become bigger this becomes increasingly difficult and most become wheelchair users exclusively On the other hand, children with low lumbar or sacral lesions should become community ambulators and in fact may be able to walk without orthoses or crutches More and more children, with improved care, are becoming independently functioning adults Since most of the technology involved in the care of people with spina bifida has only been in use for the past 30 years, and some for much less, the eventual prognosis for children born today with spina bifida is unknown but is certainly better than it used to be

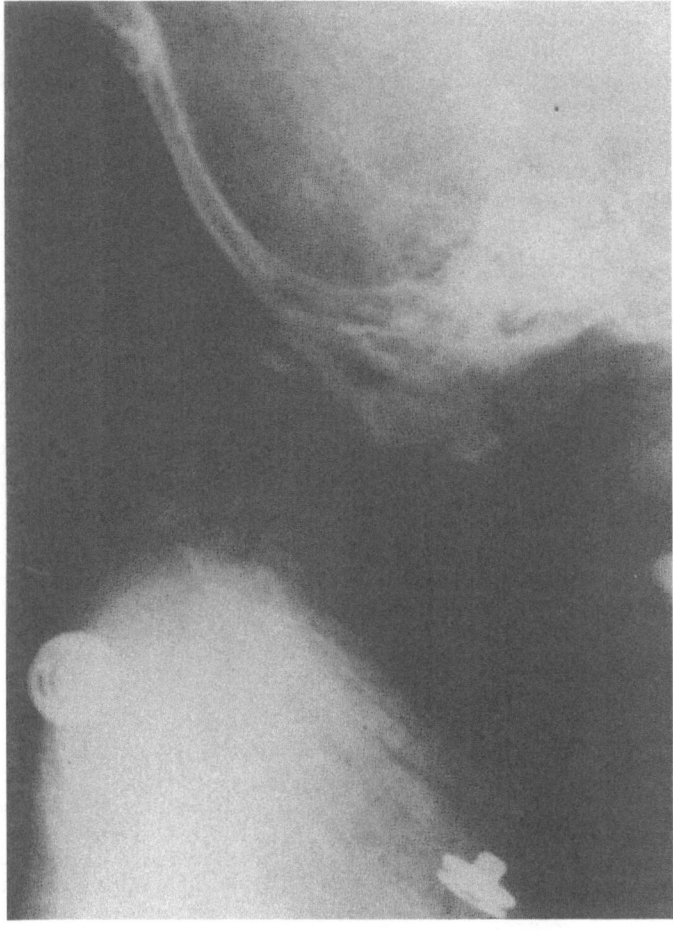

Figure 5 5. Dramatic cervical kyphosis associated with Larsen syndrome Extreme hyperlaxity and multiple joint dislocations characterize this uncommon skeletal dysplasia This young girl exhibited progressive quadriparesis as a result of cord compression

5.2.2.12. Other Cord Lesions

A variety of other cord lesions in children occasionally cause symptoms of spinal cord dysfunction including weakness, tone and deep tendon reflex changes, sensory loss, and loss of sphincter control. They most often either occur in later childhood or present more acutely and are therefore not usually in the differential diagnosis of gross motor delays in infancy or early childhood. They include tumors, syringomyelia, neurenteric cysts, vascular malformations, abscess, transverse myelitis, and such bony anomalies as the Klippel–Feil syndrome.

5.2.3. Anterior Horn Cell Disease

Spinal muscular atrophy (SMA) is the generic term used to describe a group of uncommon disorders characterized by degeneration of anterior horn cells. This results in flaccid weakness with muscular atrophy, fasciculations, and decreased deep tendon reflexes. The motor neurons of cranial nerves can also be involved and result in cranial nerve palsies as well.

Classification of these diseases is based on age at presentation. Group I (Werdnig–Hoffman disease) presents at birth, group II in late infancy, group III by 2 or 3 years, and group IV (Kugelberg–Welander disease) by 3 to 15 years of age.

5.2.3.1. Werdnig–Hoffman Disease

Children with Werdnig–Hoffman disease, the early onset kind of SMA, are always weak by 6 months and sometimes even at birth. Some mothers recall decreased fetal movements compared with their other, unaffected children. They exhibit reduced movements, a feeble cry, decreased deep tendon reflexes, difficulties sucking and swallowing, lingual fasciculations, paradoxical respiration (caused by intercostal weak-

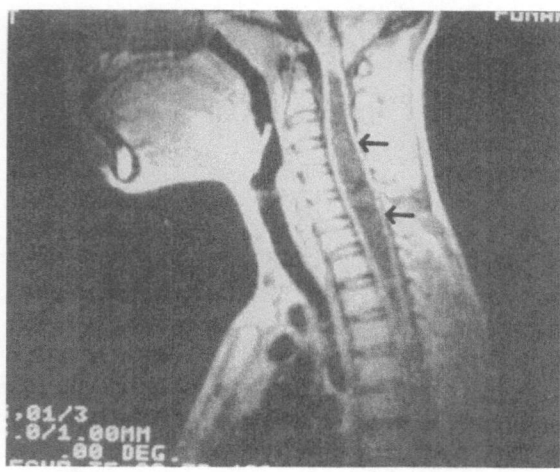

Figure 5.6. Cervical syringomyelia in a 12-year-old male. This manifested itself via decreased sensation in right upper extremity with multiple injuries and persistent cutaneous ulceration. Examination revealed typical hyperreflexia in lower extremities and decreased reflexes in right arm.

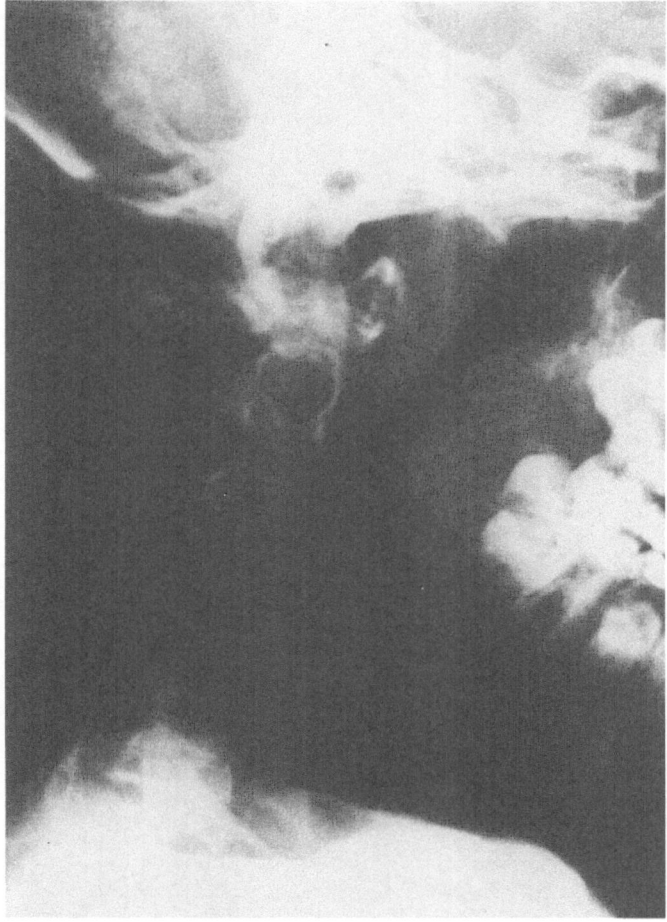

Figure 5.7. Klippel–Feil in a 9-year-old girl. Note abnormal fusion, small size, and irregularities of cervical vertebral bodies.

ness and a functioning diaphragm), and failure to attain normal motor milestones. Sensation is not affected nor are extraocular muscles and the children are alert and responsive. They tend to lie with their arms extended and their legs abducted and flexed at the knees. Werdnig–Hoffman is inherited as an autosomal recessive and occurs once in approximately 20,000 live births. Most children with the early onset form of SMA die of respiratory failure by 12 or 18 months.

5.2.3.2. Late-Onset Spinal Muscular Atrophy

SMA also exists as late-onset forms with presentation between late infancy and adolescence. Symptoms at presentation include decreased coordination, difficulty with

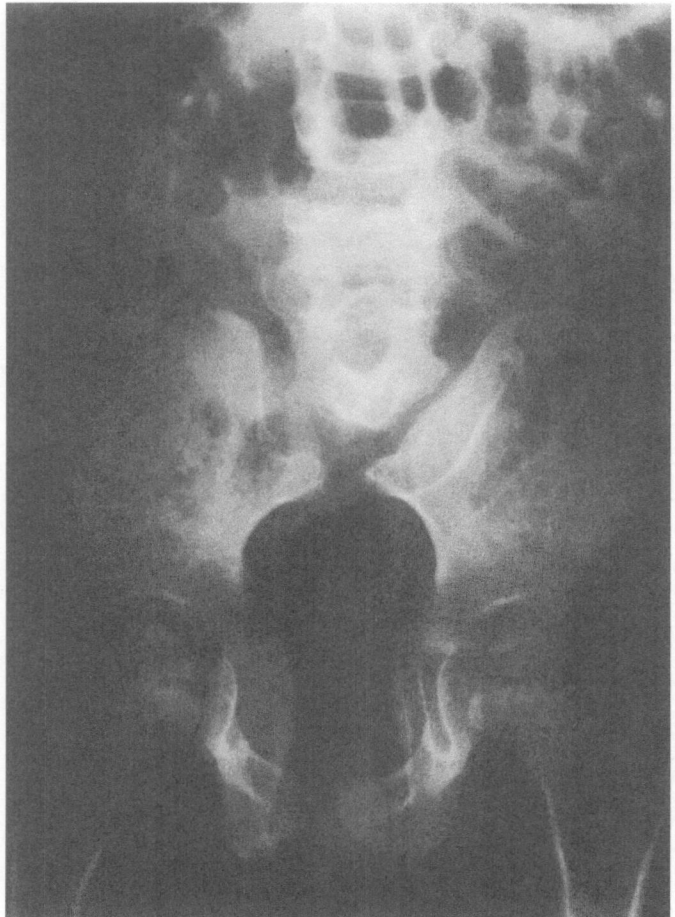

Figure 5.8. Radiograph of a 3-year-old girl with sacral agenesis. Part of the caudal regression syndrome, this anomaly is associated with maternal diabetes. Many of the problems that children with spina bifida have also occur with sacral agenesis, including lower extremity paralysis and a neurogenic bladder.

stairs, and increased falling. Signs of lower motor neuron disease in these patients are more subtle. Weakness tends to be worse proximally than distally and deep tendon reflexes may be normal, at least initially. Chronic and progressive weakness leads to scoliosis and the extensive use of a wheelchair. Survival is variable and depends on severity of disease with survival into adult life expectable in some cases.

Infantile forms of SMA usually do not cause diagnostic difficulties though late-onset forms can sometimes be confused with limb girdle muscular dystrophy or other

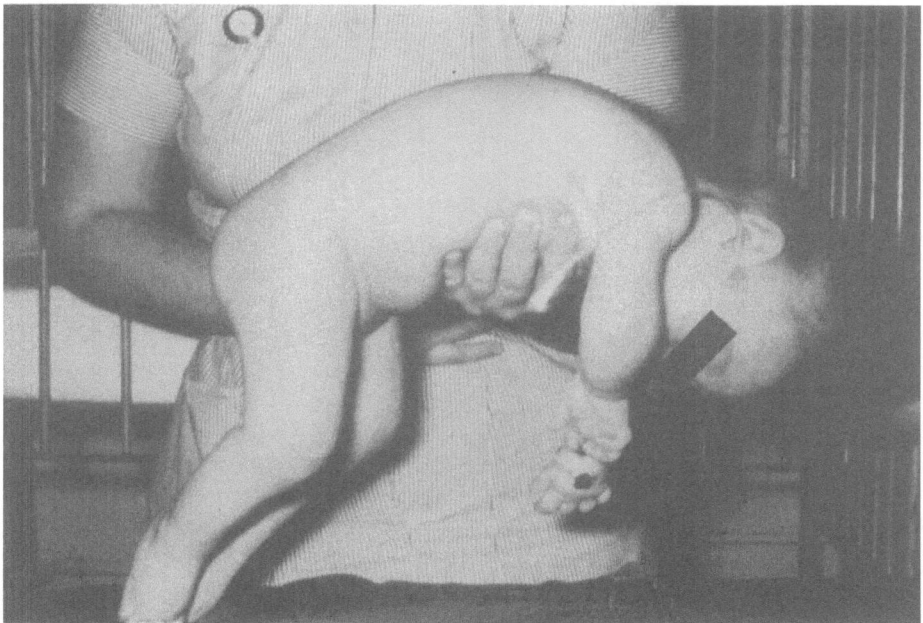

Figure 5.9. Severe hypotonia and weakness typical of infantile spinal muscular atrophy, Werdnig–Hoffman disease.

causes of chronic weakness. Electromyography, nerve conduction studies, and muscle biopsy may be necessary. Muscle biopsy shows patchy denervation atrophy.

5.2.4. Peripheral Neuropathies

A variety of neuropathies, both motor and sensory, can present as motor failure in early childhood. When motor nerves are affected, varying degrees of flaccid weakness, hypotonia, and hyporeflexia result. In general, distal muscle function is more severely affected and proximal motor strength is more well preserved. When sensory fibers are involved, painful paresthesias, loss of sensation, gait unsteadiness, skin ulcers, joint damage (Charcot joints), and loss of fingers or toes may all occur. Orthopedic complications are common and include angulation deformities, scoliosis, and the damaging effects of sensory loss.

Neuropathies may be the result of systemic disease, including diabetes mellitus, uremia, and systemic lupus erythematosus. They may result from deficiencies of vitamins B_1 and B_{12}. A variety of toxic causes for neuropathies exist as well, including heavy metals (lead, mercury, and arsenic) and such medications as isoniazid and nitrofurantoin. Finally, a group of progressive hereditary genetic diseases of unknown causes also are associated with neuropathies. This latter group includes the following:

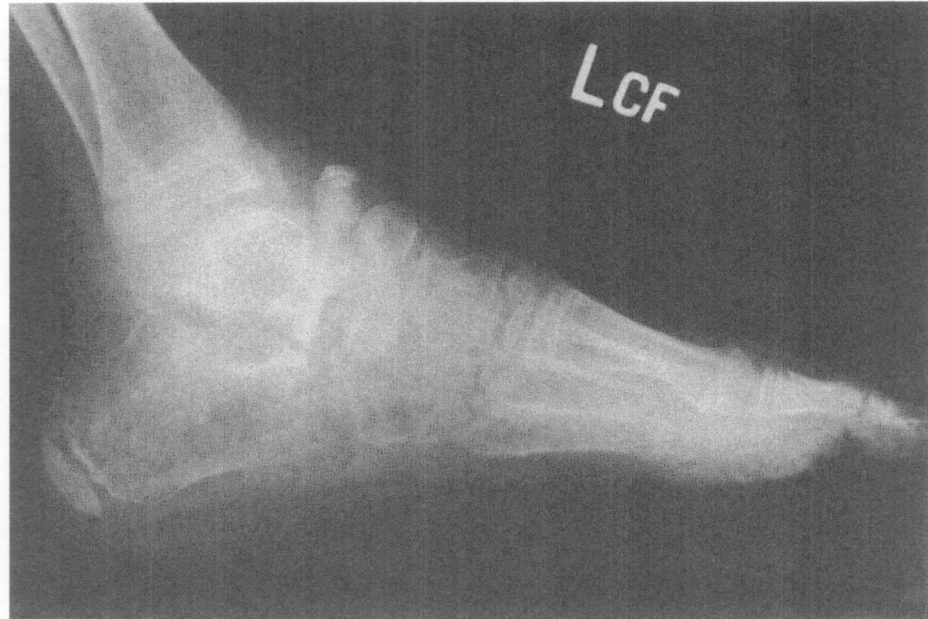

Figure 5.10. Charcot joint in a little girl with sensory problems specific to her joints Sensory perception to touch, pinprick, and temperature change was normal Note destruction and extrusion of talus and deformity of navicular, as well as generalized osteoporosis

- Charcot–Marie–Tooth disease, also known as peroneal muscle atrophy or hereditary motor sensory neuropathy type I (HMSN I), is predominantly a motor neuropathy inherited as an autosomal dominant. It presents in late childhood or adolescence. Slowly progressive, this disease typically causes cavovarus deformities of the feet, distal muscle atrophy, and decreased deep tendon reflexes. Angulation problems of the distal lower extremities and foot drop frequently require bracing or, if severe, ankle fusion.
- Hereditary motor sensory neuropathy type II is a more mild form of disease similar to HMSN I.
- Dejerine–Sottas disease, also known as hypertrophic interstitial neuritis or hereditary motor sensory neuropathy type III, is inherited as an autosomal recessive. It may present early enough that motor delays are apparent from the beginning. Distal sensory loss is common.
- Familial dysautonomia, also known as Riley–Day syndrome, is transmitted as an autosomal recessive gene and occurs almost exclusively in Jewish children. Infants with this syndrome manifest a variety of signs of autonomic and sensory loss including excessive sweating and salivation, urinary incontinence, labile blood pressures, defects in thermoregulation, decreased or absent pain sense, and decreased deep tendon reflexes. Developmental delay on a central basis may be present as well.

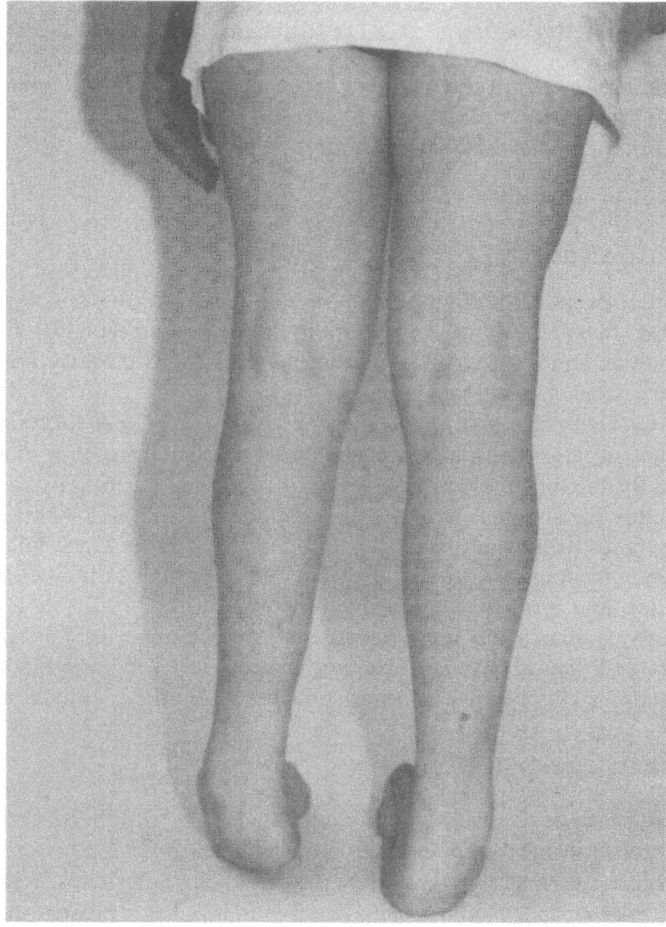

Figure 5.11. Lower extremity deformities in Charcot–Marie–Tooth disease (HSMN I) Note calf atrophy, worse on left, cavus feet, and severe varus angulation of ankles

- Congenital sensory neuropathy and congenital indifference to pain both cause loss of sensation resulting in extremity and cutaneous damage. Anhidrosis and global developmental delays may be present in either. They may be distinguished from each other by the lack of all perception of sensation in the former syndrome with loss of perception of pain only in the latter. Any loss of pain sensation in a joint may predispose to the development of so-called Charcot joints. Repeated trauma and hyperextension of the insensate joint results in recurrent hemarthrosis, loss of structural integrity, and eventual complete joint destruction. Because they do not involve motor nerves, they are not in the differential diagnosis of motor delays.

5.2.5. Diseases of the Neuromuscular Junction

These include several of the childhood myasthenic syndromes, infantile botulism, and tick paralysis.

The myasthenic syndromes of childhood include:

• Transient neonatal myasthenia
• Congenital ("persistent") myasthenia
• Juvenile myasthenia

None figures prominently in the differential diagnosis of motor delays in infancy or early childhood. The first two groups present in the newborn period with respiratory and feeding difficulties and the third presents in late childhood or early adolescence with ptosis, double vision, and bulbar weakness.

Infantile botulism results from intestinal infection with *Clostridium botulinum*. The toxin from this organism impairs acetylcholine release from presynaptic terminals resulting initially in constipation and feeding difficulties. Eventually facial weakness, decreased swallowing and gag, weakness, and hypotonia all make themselves manifest. Pupillary responses to light are typically impaired, a unique sign. Infants between 2 weeks and 6 months are most usually affected. The illness usually lasts several months and tube feeding and artificial ventilation may be required.

Tick paralysis shares the same pathogenetic mechanism of inhibition of acetylcholine release as infantile botulism. Neither is likely to be included in the differential diagnosis of motor delay because of their subacute and unique clinical manifestations.

5.2.6. Muscle Diseases

Intrinsic disease of the muscles in infancy and early childhood can be associated with failed motor milestones and less than normal development. Specific entities likely to present with developmental delay and their clinical characteristics are listed in Tables 5.2 through 5.5. Not every characteristic listed in the tables is present in every patient.

Dystrophies are intrinsic muscle disease which are genetic, progressive, and associated with muscle cell distortion on biopsy. Distinguishing between muscular

Table 5.2. Muscular Dystrophies Presenting in Infancy and Early Childhood

Congenital myotonic dystrophy hypotonia severe early on when mothers affected, myotonia later, autosomal dominant, polyhydramnios, mental retardation, CPK usually normal or slightly up, V-shaped upper lip, distal muscle atrophy, cataracts occur, hypothyroidism, other endocrinopathies

Congenital muscular dystrophy clinically variable, contractures, arthrogryposis, sometimes with mental retardation, cardiomyopathy, usually autosomal recessive, sometimes nonprogressive, CPK elevated, EMG myopathic

Infantile facioscapulohumeral dystrophy early facial weakness, upper extremities worse, particularly triceps, sensorineural hearing loss, CPK elevated, EMG myopathic, autosomal dominant

Infantile polymyositis neck flexors weak, CPK usually up, biopsy shows myositis over time

dystrophies and myopathies is somewhat arbitrary. A detailed description of pediatric muscle disease is beyond our scope here. Appropriate texts should be consulted.

The periodic paralyses associated with defects in potassium metabolism are not discussed because they are not usually in the differential diagnosis of primary motor delay.

Though variable in severity, time of onset, and prognosis, all muscle diseases cause weakness and hypotonia, with weakness more significant proximally than distally (myotonic dystrophy may be an exception). Sensation is intact and muscle fasciculations are usually not present.

5.2.6.1. Muscle Disease in Infancy

Infants presenting in the newborn period frequently demonstrate respiratory and feeding difficulties or facial weakness and occasionally ptosis and decreased extraocular movements. The sequelae of lack of intrauterine movement may sometimes be present as well, such as talipes equinovarus, plagiocephaly, scoliosis, torticollis, and hip dislocation.

5.2.6.2. Muscle Disease in Older Children

In older children, muscle disease may present itself as failure to achieve motor milestones, a waddling gait, difficulty climbing stairs, toe walking, calf hypertrophy, or loss of milestones achieved. Complications include respiratory failure, the usual cause of death, but also include scoliosis, progressive cavovarus deformities of the feet (high arches with inversion), excessive lumbar lordosis, and other orthopedic deformities.

5.3. ASSESSMENT OF THE CHILD WITH MOTOR PROBLEMS

The goal for the primary care provider is not necessarily to make the specific diagnosis when confronted with a child with a motor delay but rather to categorize and

Table 5.3. Myopathies Presenting in Infancy

Central core disease sometimes overlooked early on, no facial weakness, ptosis, ophthalmoplegia, dysphagia, or respiratory problems, very slowly progressive, autosomal dominant, CPK and EMG may be normal, biopsy shows central core

Nemaline myopathy clinically variable, associated with high arched palate, long, dysmorphic facies, prognathism, pectus excavatum or carinatum, autosomal dominant with variable expressivity, normal CPK, EMG myopathic with occasional fibrillation potentials, biopsy shows threadlike rod bodies

Myotubular myopathy. clinically variable, may be severe in males, autosomal dominant, recessive, or sex-linked, normal CPK, EMG myopathic with occasional fibrillation potentials, biopsy shows fibers similar to fetal myotubules

Fiber type disproportion usually severe disease initially, better later, vigorous support warranted, mental retardation in 30%, autosomal dominant with variable expressivity; normal CPK, EMG myopathic, biopsy shows type I predominance

Table 5.4. Metabolic Myopathies

Mitochondrial myopathies: often associated with cardiomyopathy, encephalopathy, lactic acidosis; CPK normal or slightly elevated; EMG normal

Glycogen storage disease: autosomal recessive; cardiomyopathy, muscle cramps, fatigue, and myoglobinuria (type V and type VII); hepatomegaly; hypoglycemia; biopsy shows glycogen accumulation

Carnitine deficiency/lipid myopathy: cardiomyopathy; autosomal recessive; muscle pain and myoglobinuria with exercise; biopsy shows increased lipid

Other myopathies: thyrotoxicosis, hypothyroidism, exogenous or endogenous glucocorticoids, rickets

define the nature of the problem at hand. The best way to do this, still, is with a careful history and physical exam. Appropriate consultation can then be made as necessary.

Specific diseases often cause trouble at more than one level. For example, children with Prader–Willi syndrome are delayed motorically not only because of their mental deficit but also because of their severe hypotonicity. In fact, many children with prenatally caused deficits are at risk for perinatally acquired cerebral damage since they are more likely to be asphyxiated or suffer other kinds of injury during delivery.

Keeping these caveats in mind, it is useful to ask the question: at what level of this child's nervous system is there a problem? Does this child have a cerebral problem, or one that involves the spinal cord, the anterior horn cells, peripheral nerves, myoneural junction, or muscle? Such a process provides us with a structure around which to build an evaluation. To proceed logically requires asking the following questions.

5.3.1. Is There Evidence for Cerebral Disease?

The child's overall development should be studied with an eye to determining if the deficiency in motor skills is part of a global problem or is limited solely to gross motor function. Coexisting cognitive, language, social, or adaptive skills imply a cerebral etiology to the child's motor delays. For example, children with diffuse cortical injury caused by hypoxemia or a syndromic cause for their mental retardation often have associated problems with language acquisition as well as other developmental functions in addition to their motor problems. Their delays are global. Important historical features of diffuse cerebral damage are reviewed in Table 5.6.

Table 5.5. Muscular Dystrophies Presenting in Childhood

Duchenne muscular dystrophy: sex-linked; diagnosis usually early childhood; ambulation usually to adolescence, mean IQ is 80; calf hypertrophy; cardiomyopathy; milder variant presents in adolescence (Becker's); CPK very elevated; EMG myopathic; caused by deficiency in dystrophin

Emery–Dreifuss dystrophy (scapulohumeral dystrophy): sex-linked; no hypertrophy; contractures typical; slowly progressive; normal IQ; cardiomyopathy; CPK mildly increased; EMG myopathic

Limb-girdle dystrophy: autosomal recessive or dominant; sometimes hypertrophy; heterogeneous population, normal IQ; CPK elevated; EMG myopathic

Table 5.6. Historical Features of Cerebral Causes for Motor Delay

Prenatal history TORCH infection, poor fetal growth, drugs or alcohol, X-rays, toxemia, late vaginal bleeding
Perinatal history asphyxia/hypoxemia, seizures, hypoglycemia, prematurity, poor feeding, meningitis, birth trauma, acidosis
Postnatal history. encephalitis or meningitis, head trauma, lead poisoning, developmental regression
Family history· spontaneous abortions, mental retardation, in family or in males only (sex-linked disease), consanguinity

The pattern of the child's development is also important:

- Was early development normal with slowing after an illness, diagnosed or occult? Such a pattern would imply an acute insult, as with viral encephalitis, occurring in a previously normal child.
- Has the child been making progress, albeit slow, from the beginning? This pattern would imply a static deficit related to a CNS birth defect or intrauterine infection.
- Has the child previously attained milestones which they are now losing? Are they not only going more slowly but actually losing ground? This last pattern would imply some form of metabolic or degenerative encephalopathy such as Tay–Sachs disease.

It is true that children with various kinds of progressive peripheral neuromuscular disease, like muscular dystrophy or spinal muscular atrophy (discussed below), also lose milestones. However, with these problems motor functions are primarily affected and language and cognitive skills are not.

5.3.1.1. The Physical Examination in Central Causes for Motor Delay

The physical examination should begin with a period of noninvasive observation, looking at how the child manipulates blocks, how he communicates, how he relates to the examiner and the environment, and how he moves, all best done on the parent's lap. Specifics regarding the physical examination are listed in Table 5.7.

Abnormalities of size may prove important. For example, children with a history of intrauterine infection and fetal growth failure remain small. Children with cerebral

Table 5.7. Physical Findings in Cerebral Causes for Motor Delay

Excessively small or large body size
Microcephaly, macrocephaly, or other cranial contour abnormalities
Minor congenital anomalies like abnormal hair whorls, epicanthic folds, abnormal eye slant, upturned nares, low-set ears, malformed auricle, high-arched palate, thin upper lip, hypoplastic maxillae, short or webbed neck, shield chest, clinodactyly, brachydactyly, arachnodactyly, bilateral simian creases, broad thumbs or great toes, abnormal genitalia, café-au-lait spots, hypopigmented macules, hemangiomata
Neurologic abnormalities like increased or decreased muscle tone, hyperreflexia, no protective reactions, log rolling, persistent Moro reflex, early handedness, chorea
Hearing or visual loss

gigantism (Sotos syndrome) are large. The occipital–frontal head circumference should be measured and note made of excesses in either direction.

Dysmorphic facial and body features may lead to the diagnosis of a specific syndrome. The presence of multiple birth defects leads to the presumption that the brain has been similarly affected by intrauterine developmental anomalies and even in the absence of a specific diagnosis this is important information.

Neurocutaneous abnormalities should be looked for such as café-au-lait spots, hypopigmented macules, or facial hemangiomatosis, raising the question of neuro-fibromatosis, tuberous sclerosis, and Sturge–Weber syndrome, respectively.

Is the child's tone normal? Are the tonal abnormalities worsened by postural change, with increased extensor tone or scissoring during vertical suspension, or extreme floppiness during ventral suspension, with the child draped over the examiner's hand? Some CNS damage is paradoxically associated with hypotonicity rather than spasticity. This may be persistent or, more commonly, there may be a transition during infancy from decreased to increased tone.

Is head control normal? Can the infant rotate the shoulders independently of the pelvis or is there "logrolling" stiffness when the child is rolled over on the exam table, abnormal for infants older than 6 months?

Under ordinary conditions, such automatic reflexes as the Moro reflex (the startle reaction) are gone by the time the infant is 2 months. In the presence of cortical or corticospinal tract damage these reflexes persist.

The automatic reflexes should disappear as the protective reactions emerge. These include several involuntary reactions to body displacement which are not present at birth but develop subsequently and are present thereafter throughout life. Failure to develop these reactions is a reflection of CNS injury. They include protective side-to-side reactions which develop at about 5 to 7 months as a prerequisite to independent sitting. If the child is held in a sitting position on a flat surface and tilted laterally, the child will reach out with the elbow extended as if to protect himself from a fall. A similar reaction is observed in slightly older infants prior to standing and is termed the parachute reaction: if the child is lifted in a prone position and then lowered quickly to the surface of the table head first, they will extend their upper extremities as if to protect themselves from injury.

If the child is ambulatory, what is the gait like? Is it asymmetrical, stiff-legged with circumduction? Is it a crouch gait with excessive hip and knee flexion or internally rotated? Is the child up on their toes?

If the child is mildly affected, gait abnormalities may become more apparent if the child is stressed by running. If the child can't walk, how do they get around? Do they get up on their arms as if to crawl but drag their legs? When they sit, is their back rounded, do they require propping? Most normal children don't develop consistent handedness until they are at least several years old (some not until age 4 or 5 years); the 18-month-old who is firmly and consistently "right-handed" might be so because of left-sided hemiparesis.

Are the deep tendon reflexes normal? Children with corticospinal tract disease will be hyperreflexic, even if hypotonic. Upgoing plantar (Babinski) reflexes may be present to a mild to moderate degree in the normal young infant, sometimes up to walking age. However, they should never be easily elicitable or asymmetrical.

Focal neurologic deficits, spasticity, chorea, or tremor may reflect cerebral palsy, Wilson's disease, or the residua from previous CNS trauma.

Weakness, regardless of cause or associated tone, will eventually lead to fixed muscle contractures. Spasticity can be overcome by a slowly and consistently applied force; fixed contractures can't. Flexion contractures, fixed or otherwise, at the hip are typical when spasticity is present and may not be apparent with the child lying supine on the examination table because of compensatory hyperlordosis of the lumbar spine.

The Thomas test (see also Chapter 1) is one way to check for hip flexion contractures. Flatten the lumbar spine against the table by flexing both hips maximally on the abdomen. Keeping one extremity flexed, extend the other maximally. In children older than 2 years, the extended lower extremity can be placed flat on the table easily; younger children may normally have a few degrees of physiological hip flexion contracture. The angle subtended by the child's thigh and the table represents the hip flexion contracture on that side.

Equinus contractures (toes down) at the ankle are similarly common in a variety of CNS and neuromuscular conditions, including CP and muscular dystrophy. Simply dorsiflexing the foot allows for movement at the midtarsal joints and may underestimate the degree of ankle contracture. To prevent this from happening, invert the foot, thereby locking the midtarsal joint and then dorsiflex. Failure to dorsiflex to neutral reflects an ankle joint contracture, often caused by tightness or spasticity of the calf muscles.

5.3.1.2. Laboratory Evaluation of Central Causes for Motor Delay

There are a large number of laboratory and radiological exams that can be performed on each child with presumed central delay but the chance of success is small unless the tests are performed for specific indications to answer specific questions. Even after thoughtful and thorough assessments, many children with cerebral causes for developmental delays end up without a specific medical label.

A karyotype should be performed on any child with mental retardation with a positive family history of mental retardation or frequent spontaneous abortions. Karyotype on folate-deficient media for fragile sites on the X chromosome should be performed if there is a family history of predominantly male mental retardation. A karyotype should also be performed on any child with mental retardation and multiple congenital anomalies, even if minor.

An MRI scan of the head should be considered for any child with mental retardation and a cranial contour abnormality, including microcephaly and macrocephaly, focal seizures, or if a neurocutaneous syndrome like neurofibromatosis, Sturge–Weber, or tuberous sclerosis is being considered.

Evaluation for congenital hypothyroidism should always be performed in the developmentally delayed infant and young child who manifests either longitudinal growth failure or any of the stigmata of congenital hypothyroidism, including feeding difficulties, somnolence, constipation, umbilical hernia, large tongue, hypothermia,

Table 5.8. Metabolic Causes for Mental Retardation

Galactosemia (check reducing substances in urine) hepatomegaly, seizures, cataracts, vomiting, jaundice
Aminoacidopathies (check urine for qualitative amino acids or urine and serum quantitatively) neonatal
    seizures, acidosis, unusual smell, eczema, microcephaly, blond hair
Wilson disease (check ceruloplasmin and serum copper) chorea, cirrhosis, Kayser–Fleischer ring
Lesch–Nyhan syndrome (check serum uric acid) boys with regression, chorea/athetosis, self-mutilation
Urea cycle abnormalities (check serum ammonia) cyclical vomiting, acidosis
Mucopolysaccharidoses (check urinary mucopolysaccharides) coarse facies, large tongue, corneal clouding,
    skeletal anomalies, umbilical hernia, kyphosis, hearing loss
Gangliosidoses (check enzyme levels in serum, white cells, or skin fibroblasts) regression, coarse facial
    features, organomegaly, cherry red macula, seizures
Metachromatic leukodystrophy (check arylsulfatase activity in urine, serum, white cells, or skin fibroblasts)
    mental and motor deterioration, worsening spasticity, optic atrophy, red macula

extremity edema, enlarged or persistent fontanels, heart murmur, anemia, bradycardia, dry skin, or coarse and scanty hair (see also Chapter 7).

A variety of metabolic tests are available for children whose mental retardation has a biochemical basis. Taken together they are not rare causes of mental retardation. Symptoms include regression rather than progression of developmental milestones, seizures, an odd smell to the urine, movement disorders, coarse facial features, and organomegaly, among many others. See Table 5.8 for a more detailed listing of the indications to test for these metabolic disorders.

5.3.2. Is There Evidence for a Spinal Cord Lesion?

The important historical and physical features of spinal cord problems as they relate to motor delays are recorded in Table 5.9. A high index of suspicion is necessary to avoid labeling these children as having cerebral palsy. A history of breech delivery and the presence of a sensory level should particularly be sought.

5.3.3. Is There Evidence for Peripheral Neuromuscular Disease?

Distinguishing central causes for motor failure from all peripheral neuromuscular ones is usually not difficult. Even when central hypotonia is present, hyperreflexia, decreased mentation, seizures, or other manifestations of central damage are present as well. Similarly, evaluation of the child with motor delay, weakness, and hypotonia

Table 5.9. Spinal Cord Lesions

History breech delivery, intermittent signs and symptoms (craniovertebral anomalies), family history of
    paraplegia, loss of sphincter control
Physical examination sensory level, autonomic disturbances, diaphragmatic breathing, spastic paraplegia,
    DTRs increased, toes up, short neck, decreased neck range of motion, lipoma, sinus, hairy patch,
    hemangioma over lumbosacral spine

Table 5.10. Historical and Physical Features of Peripheral Neuropathies

History diabetes mellitus, uremia, SLE, paresthesias, history of INH or nitrofurantoin, large baby at birth or early handedness (brachial plexus injury), family history of similar problems
Physical findings sensory loss (glove and stocking), Charcot joints or ulcerations, foot drop, distal weakness or atrophy, cavovarus feet, decreased DTRs

resulting from neuromuscular (lower motor neuron) disease can be successful if one keeps in mind the distinguishing characteristics listed in Tables 5.10 to 5.13 and summarized in Table 5.14.

Significant weakness is present in all. Although formal muscle testing on a five-point scale is difficult in infants and the preschool child, a functional approach usually gets at the information necessary. Place the child on the floor. Can they get to standing? Is there a Gower's sign? Do they appropriately resist giving up a proffered toy? Can they get up on all fours? Is muscle atrophy or hypertrophy (pseudohypertrophy) present?

5.3.4. Laboratory Investigation in Peripheral Neuromuscular Disease

It's worth pointing out that children with muscular dystrophy, and boys with Duchenne's in particular, may present with motor delays or clumsiness. As a rule of thumb, all boys presenting with motor delays need a serum CPK level, even in the absence of hypertrophic calf muscles or other specific signs of muscular dystrophy.

When clinical evidence is insufficient to make the diagnosis of a specific neuromuscular disease, serum enzymes (primarily CPK), EMG, nerve conduction studies (NCS), or biopsy are necessary. As recorded in Table 5.14, CPK may be elevated in several different muscle diseases as well as some other peripheral neuromuscular diseases, but variably so, particularly in the slowly progressive muscle diseases. NCS show slow velocities or low amplitudes in diseases of the peripheral nerves but are generally normal in diseases of the muscles.

EMG reveals signs of denervation in diseases of the anterior horn cells and peripheral nerves. As expected, EMG shows "myopathic" changes with muscle diseases, including short-duration, low-amplitude potentials. With myasthenia, EMG shows a characteristic decremental or myasthenic pattern of muscle potentials with repetitive nerve stimulation. Interestingly, infantile botulism shows the opposite pattern, a characteristic incremental response of muscle potential to repetitive stimulation.

Muscle biopsy, if necessary, reveals denervation changes with anterior horn cell disease or peripheral neuropathies. Myopathic change as well as specific histologic

Table 5.11. Historical and Clinical Features of Anterior Horn Cell Disease

History family history of SMA, progressive weakness, difficulty feeding, frequent respiratory infections, decreased movements
Physical findings flaccid quadriparesis, fasciculations of muscle and tongue, markedly decreased or absent DTRs, normal sensation

Table 5.12. Clinical Characteristics of Diseases of the Neuromuscular Junction

History: mother with myasthenia, myasthenic weakness (worse after repetitions), apnea, feeding difficulties, constipation (particularly with botulism)

Physical findings: facial weakness, ptosis, ophthalmoplegia, decreased or absent DTRs, normal sensation, decreased gag reflex, decreased pupillary reaction to light (botulism)

abnormalities (e.g., central core, nemaline) occur with muscle disease. Muscle biopsy in diseases of the neuromuscular junction is generally normal.

5.4. TREATMENT OF THE CHILD WITH MOTOR DELAY

Treatment must be directed not only to the child directly but also to the family. The nature of the intervention will also be affected by community and family resources. Physical therapy is an important consideration in order to teach the child's caretakers how to appropriately care for and handle the child to reduce posturally related spasticity and prevent contractures. Various kinds of braces to control deformities are often used, although the typical "total control" braces which go from the pelvis to the floor are less often employed today than previously. A large number of computerized or electronic devices have become available to help the child with motor delays communicate, including those with visual, printed, and speech outputs, though sometimes the simple manual ones work just as well. Manual and electric wheelchairs continue to improve as do modular designed padded seat inserts. For children with more trouble with balance than weakness, spasticity, or deformity, crutches or walkers have always been useful.

After initial enthusiasm for medications to control spasticity, drugs like Dantrolene, have proven to be a bit of a disappointment though Valium is still found to be effective to take the edge off the spasticity in some children when it is worsened by anxiety.

Surgery, including bony procedures and soft tissue releases, continues to be a mainstay of therapy though debate is constant regarding indications, as well as the details of the procedures themselves. It is imperative in the care of children with CP or neuromuscular disease to find a sympathetic orthopedic surgeon who is experienced in the care of such children.

Neurosurgical procedures for spasticity, like selective dorsal rhizotomy, in which the appropriate sensory nerve roots are incised, are currently being studied and may with time become standard therapy.

Table 5.13. Clinical Characteristics of Muscle Disease

History: waddling gait, difficulty with stairs, chairs, getting off the floor, calf hypertrophy, neonatal hypotonia

Physical findings: proximal weakness, Gower's sign, normal sensation, no fasciculations, mildly decreased DTRs, calf pseudohypertrophy

Table 5.14. Clinical and Laboratory
Comparisons in Neuromuscular Disease

	AHC[a]	PN	NMJ	M
Abnormal sensation	N	Y	N	N
Fasciculations	Y	Y	N	N
Proximal weakness	±	N	Y	Y
Distal weakness	N	Y	N	N
EMG	Den	Den	Myo	Myo
NCS (slowing)	N[b]	Y	N	N
Increased CPK	N	N	N	Var
Biopsy	Den	Den	N	Myo

[a]AHC = anterior horn cell disease, PN = peripheral neuropathy, NMJ = diseases of the neuromuscular junction, M = muscle disease, N = no or absent, Y = yes or present, Den = denervation, Myo = myopathic, Var = variable, EMG = electromyography, NCS = nerve conduction studies, CPK = creatine phosphokinase
[b]Nerve conduction sometimes slow with severe disease

Early intervention programs, including developmental preschools, have become very popular as of late and have, in fact, become a legislated part of the system since the Education for All Handicapped Children Act has been extended to all preschool children in addition to the previously covered school-aged children. Though data documenting effectiveness are scanty, referral to these intervention programs should be considered not only for the therapy, language, and cognitive services that are provided to the child but also for the help provided to the family. These programs provide liaison with other programs, including the public school system. They provide social and psychological support to parents and siblings and the chance to talk with other parents who are also dealing with a child with a disability. They help families to feel that they are not alone, that they have someone in their corner. The therapeutic benefits which may accrue, however, must be evaluated in the light of the cost to the family. These include not only the financial costs but also the disruption of family life that sometimes results from well-meaning but overly enthusiastic use of these services. Parents may be encouraged to forego their responsibilities to other members of their family or to themselves because of the expectation that if twice a week at the center is good, five times a week is better. Keeping parents realistic and yet hopeful is a major responsibility for the physician.

This is particularly so when such special "systems of therapeutic intervention" are being considered. These include sensory integrative therapy, the patterning treatment of Doman–Delacato, the Vojta method, Rolfing, inhibitory casting, and biofeedback, among others. Since most of what physicians and therapists do for children with CP is unproven, at least in the statistical sense, it's appropriate when consulted about such therapies to remain flexible and open-minded. If the costs in time, money, potential complications, and emotions are low, dogmatic condemnation is not useful and may, in fact, antagonize the family who are often desperate to try whatever is recommended.

6

Congenital and Related Defects of the Skeleton

6.1. INTRODUCTION

Congenital defects affecting the skeleton are common, and occur either as single-system defects or as a portion of multiple congenital anomaly syndromes Most often, the cause of such defects is unknown though they are sometimes associated with specific chromosomal, single gene, intrauterine or teratogenic causes Recognizing that the child manifests a previously described constellation of defects is important because of what then may be learned about the prognosis and genetics of the child's condition and what the parents may then be told about the child's future and the family's recurrence risks

Though most of the problems described below are recognizable at birth, and are therefore truly congenital, some are not This latter group includes children who develop structural problems later in childhood to which they are predisposed by their genetic constitution or by other factors They are included in this chapter because it is convenient to do so and seems to make sense

Not every defect is included Though we have attempted to be comprehensive, we have not been able to be encyclopedic We have tried to emphasize those defects important in primary practice

6.2. CAUSAL MECHANISMS

Most birth defects can be categorized etiologically as related to either "manufacturing defects" which are true **malformations**, or "packaging defects" resulting from intrauterine **deformation** or **disruption**.

Malformations result from intrinsic embryologic failure of the developing organism early in gestation. Examples include most limb reduction abnormalities (see below), spina bifida, or congenital heart disease.

Birth defects caused by deformation or disruption result from mechanical factors

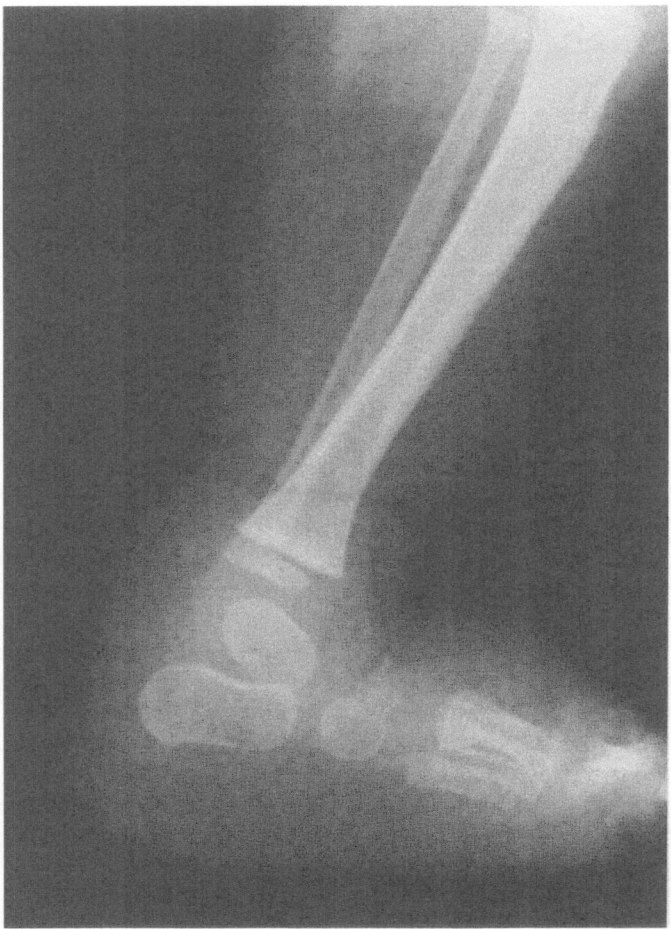

Figure 6.1. Constriction ring around ankle of this 1-year-old boy is a good example of a disruption abnormality, in this case caused by an amniotic band. Abnormal fetal development is not at fault here but destruction of previously normal tissue.

which cause structural distortion (a deformation) or even actual destruction (a disruption) of previously formed elements. Such mechanical factors include oligohydramnios, uterine fibroid tumors, bicornuate uterus, or amniotic bands. Clinical examples include the tibial or femoral bowing common in newborns or congenital amputations resulting from entrapment by constricting amniotic bands.

A third etiologic category, dysplasia, result from abnormal cellular metabolism in one particular tissue type caused by a biochemical defect such as might occur in one of the storage diseases or one of the epiphysial dysplasias. These are too numerous and complex to discuss here. They are handled briefly in Chapters 5 and 7.

6.3. SPECIFIC DEFECTS

Most birth defects affecting the limbs take the form of congenital amputations, more accurately termed **reduction anomalies** or **deficiencies**, which are either **transverse** or **longitudinal**. They may result in loss of the entire limb, the distal part of the limb, or they may be intercalary with distal structures preserved and proximal ones lost. Complete failure of the limb to develop results in amelia and partial failure in hemimelia.

A severe intercalary loss of the proximal and middle part of the extremity with preservation of hands or feet is termed *phocomelia*, the term (from the Greek) referring to alleged resemblance to the flippers of a seal.

The axis of each limb runs longitudinally through the middle digit. By definition, preaxial refers to the radial side of the upper extremities and postaxial to the ulnar side. Longitudinal defects may then be classified as either preaxial or postaxial.

Upper arm or thigh shortening results in what is termed rhizomelic shortening (*rhizo* = root); forearm or leg (calf) shortening in mesomelic (*meso* = middle) shortening; and hands or feet in acromelic (*acro* = point) shortening.

Total transverse deficiency of the hand is called acheiria, of the foot apodia, and of the finger adactylia.

6.3.1. Digits

Limb bud development begins at 4 to 5 weeks of gestation and from the beginning the bud is capped by a thin ridge of apical ectoderm. The apical ridge ectoderm is a prerequisite not only for normal limb development but also for the formation of the digital rays which eventually result in fingers. Embryonic failure can result in one or more of the following anomalies:

1. **Clinodactyly**, which describes curving, usually incurving, of a digit, most often the fifth finger. Curving toward the radius is radial clinodactyly and toward the ulna is ulnar clinodactyly. It often results from hypoplasia of the middle phalanx and though it is associated with a variety of syndromes (Down and Russell–Silver among others), it is most often a minor variant of no particular significance.

2. **Camptodactyly** refers to a congenital flexion deformity of any digit, usually at the proximal interphalangeal joint. Like clinodactyly, it is most often a minor anomaly

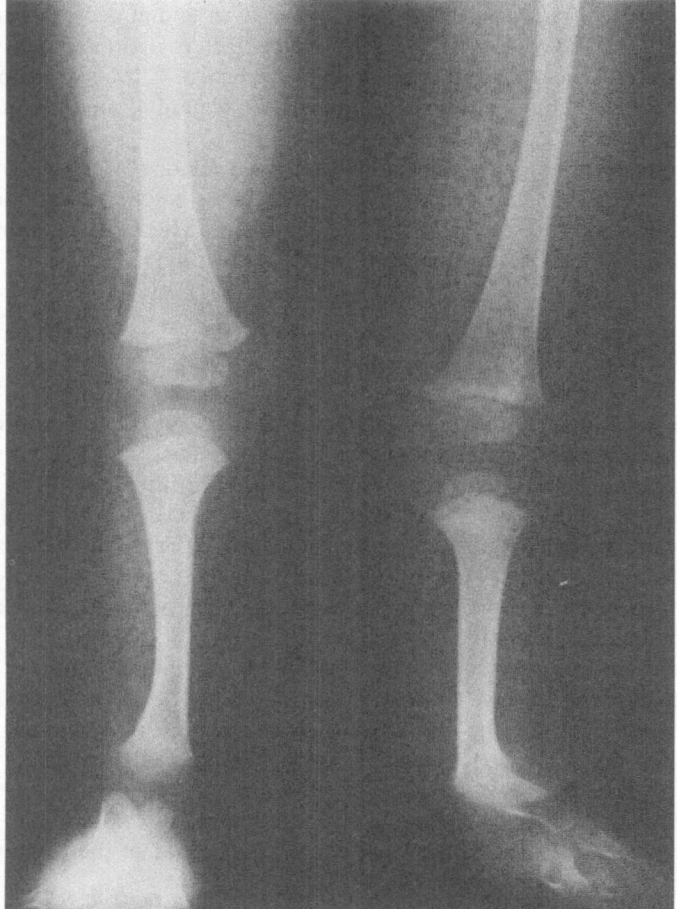

Figure 6.2. Fibular hemimelia, as pictured here, is common and is often associated with other defects of the lower extremities, including distal ray absence, femoral shortening, and tibial bowing

and most often affects the little finger. Other digits may be affected, however, and functional problems may result. Because intrauterine movement is affected, flexion and extension creases at the joint in question are faint or even absent. Camptodactyly may occur as part of dysmorphic syndromes such as Escobar syndrome (multiple pterygia with camptodactyly and syndactyly) or the trismus–camptodactyly syndrome, but can also be inherited independently in an autosomal dominant fashion.

   3. **Syndactyly**, which is fusion of one digit to its neighbor. Though most commonly cutaneous, it may be bony as well. Syndactyly is most often found between the second and third toes and the third and fourth fingers. Cutaneous syndactyly is thought to be caused by embryologic failure of programmed cell death of the mesoderm between the developing digits, leading to persistence of interdigital connections. Bony syndactyly

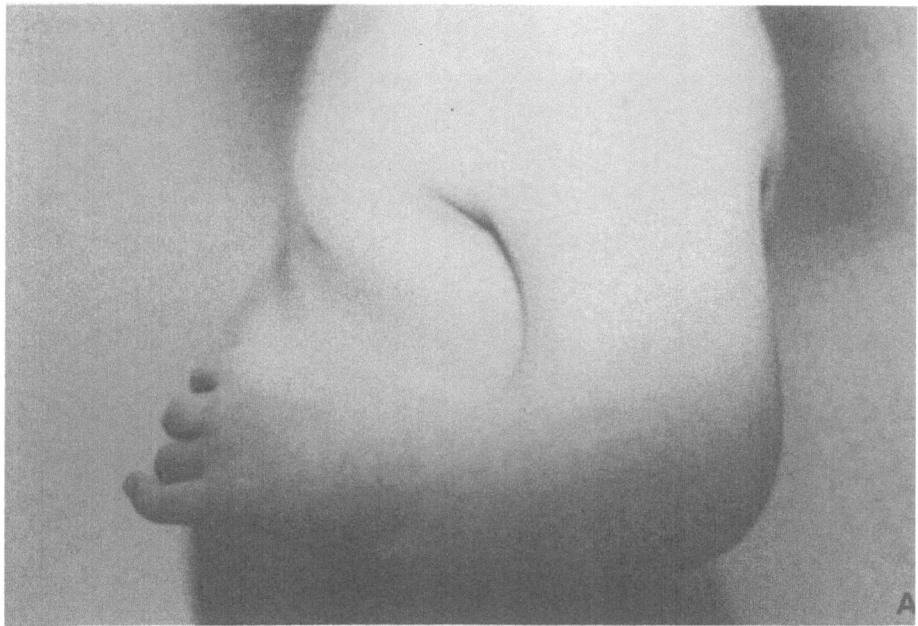

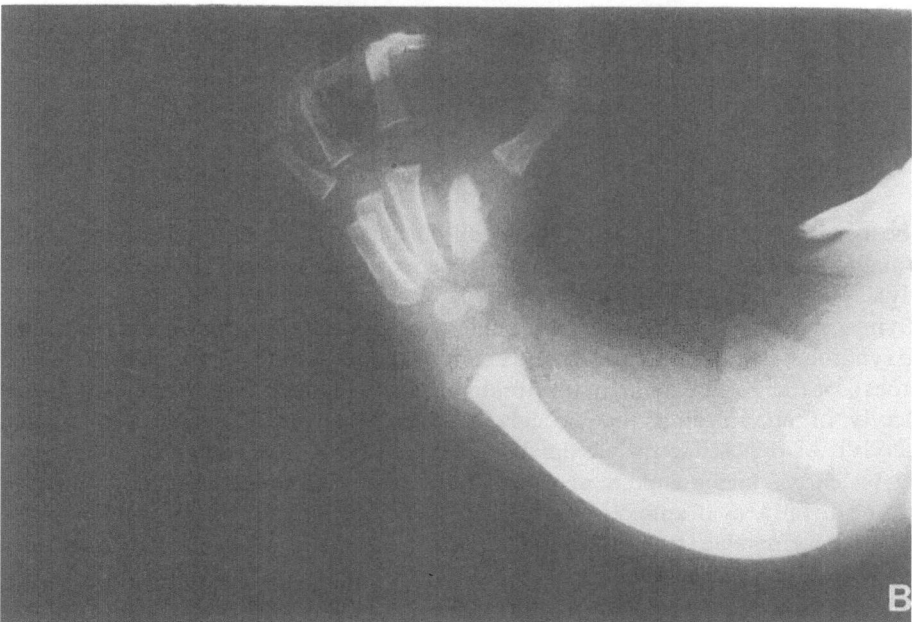

Figure 6.3. (A) Typical appearance of radial hemimelia Also known as radial club hand, this preaxial longitudinal deficiency often involves the thumb as well It is frequently associated with hematologic abnormalities, including thrombocytopenia (TAR syndrome), and pancytopenia (Fanconi syndrome) as well as the syndromic constellation known as the VATER syndrome (vertebral, anal, tracheoesophageal, radial, and renal) and the Holt–Oram (heart–hand) syndrome (B) Radiograph of patient with similar defect Thumb is present but one metacarpal is absent and another metacarpal is short and abnormal

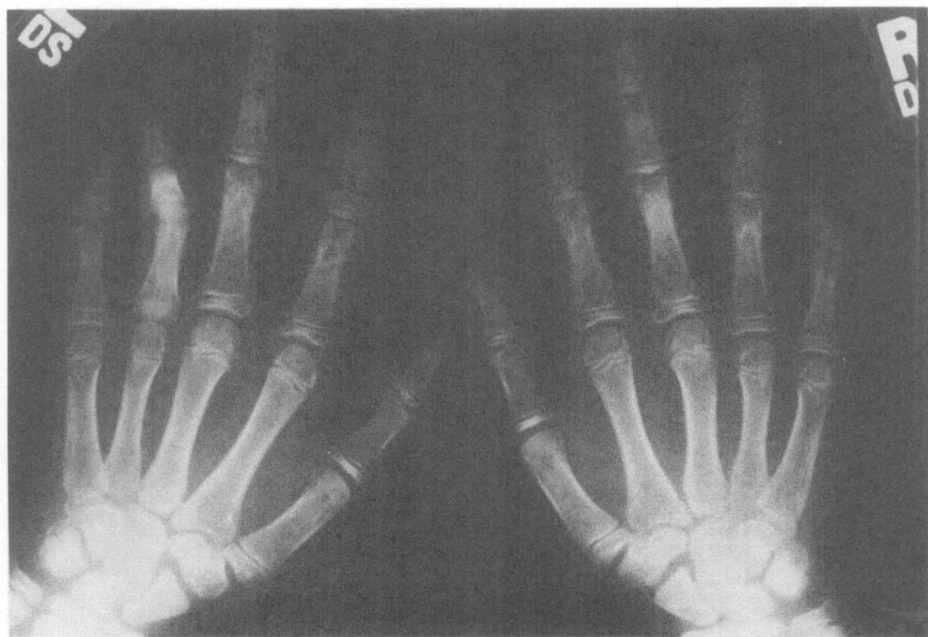

Figure 6.4. Clinodactyly of fifth fingers bilaterally, in this case caused by extreme shortening and growth plate inclination of the middle phalanx. Note also camptodactyly of the fourth digit on the left with a flexion deformity at the proximal interphalangeal joint.

may be caused by excessive cell death with fusion of digital rays, resulting in an abnormally widened digit, sometimes associated with polydactyly as well (polysyndactyly).

Syndactyly may occur as an isolated defect or as part of such syndromes as the de Lange syndrome (second and third toes), the Smith–Lemli–Opitz syndrome (second and third toes), or the Poland anomaly (pectoralis major hypoplasia; see below). Complete syndactyly of all the digits may occur in Apert syndrome (craniosynostosis and syndactyly). As opposed to the proximal syndactyly of true malformations, syndactyly caused by early amnion rupture sequence (amniotic band syndrome) may be more significant distally, as if amniotic tissue had "tied" the tips of digits together. Limb reduction abnormalities, true amputations, cleft palate, and other anomalies are frequently associated (see below).

4. **Symphalangism**, which is bony fusion of phalanges end to end. When symphalangism prevents intrauterine finger movement, there will be no flexion crease at the affected joint. Though occurring as an isolated defect, symphalangism may also be seen as part of a generalized synostosis syndrome with bony fusion at the elbow, wrist, and ankle as well, known as the multiple synostosis syndrome, inherited as an autosomal dominant with variable expressivity. Radiologically, symphalangism may not be present radiologically early on even though functional problems may be apparent.

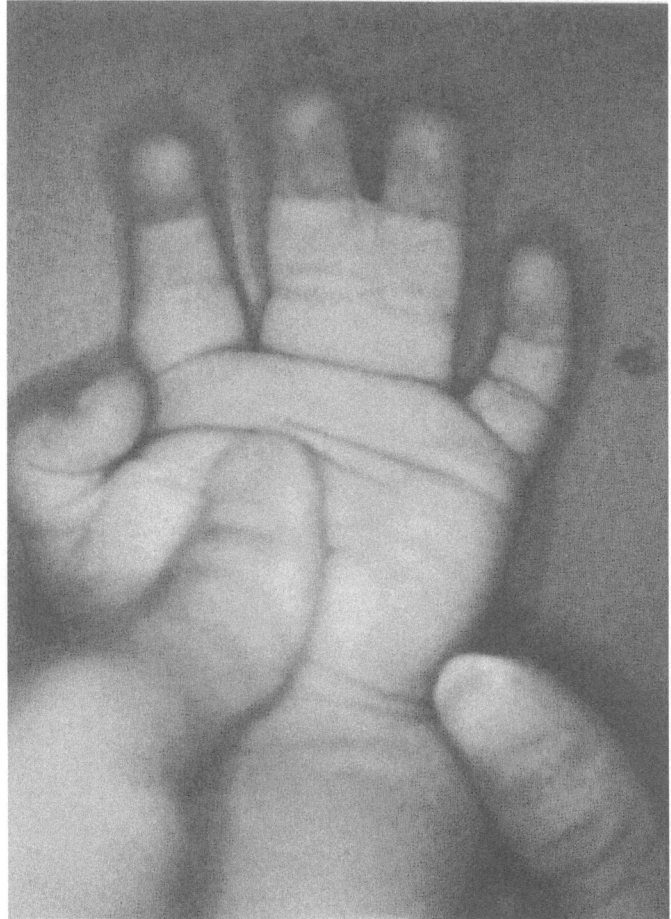

Figure 6.5. Partial syndactyly between the third and fourth digits, the most common location

5. **Polydactyly**, which may range in the severity from an inconsequential nubbin of tissue on the ulnar side of the first phalanx of the fifth finger (postminimus polydactyly) to a well-formed, fully articulated extra digit with its own extra metacarpal. Postaxial polydactyly is more common than preaxial. Usually there is only one extra digit per extremity though occasionally multiple polydactyly may be present, most often as part of a dysmorphic syndrome. The most common form of postaxial polydactyly is an isolated autosomal dominant form which is more common in blacks. Polydactyly occurs with Bardet–Biedl syndrome (retinal pigmentation, obesity, polydactyly), Carpenter syndrome (acrocephaly, polysyndactyly of feet), and Ellis–van Creveld syndrome (acromelic shortening, gingival frenula, heart defects, nail hypoplasia, and polydactyly), among others.

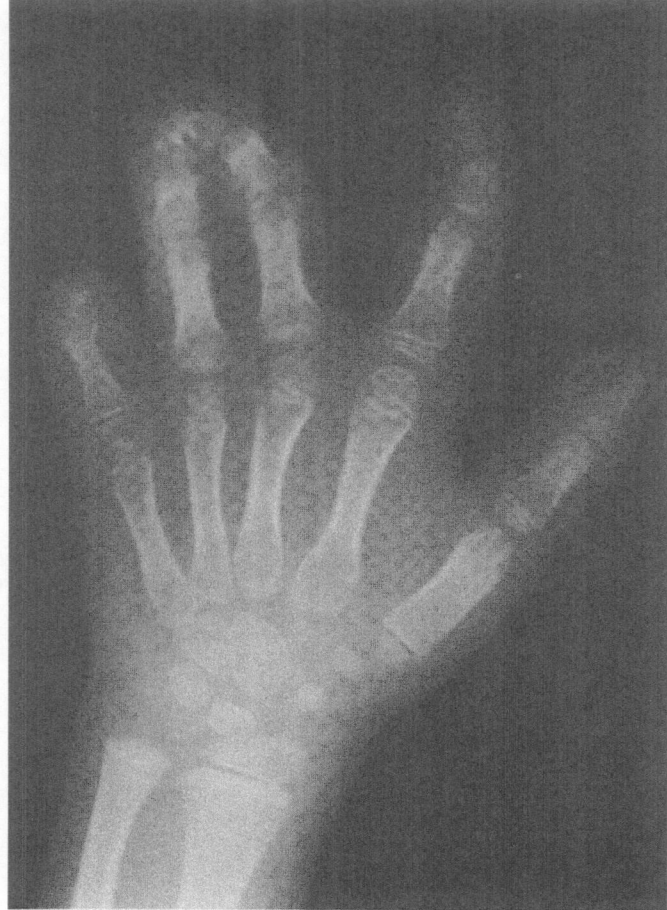

Figure 6.6. Terminal syndactyly, also known as acrosyndactyly, is often associated with amniotic bands. Note also clinodactyly of second digit and camptodactyly, or congenital flexion deformity, of fifth.

    6. **Thumb hypoplasia,** which results from embryologic failure of the apical ridge ectoderm to differentiate appropriately, is often associated with other preaxial reduction anomalies, including radial hypoplasia. Defects range from hypoplasia or "digitalization" of the thumb (the triphalangeal thumb) to complete absence of the thumb and radius. These defects can be associated with hematologic problems and include the TAR syndrome (thrombocytopenia with absent radii), the Aase syndrome (triphalangeal thumb and congenital anemia), Fanconi syndrome (radial hypoplasia, hyperpigmentation, and pancytopenia), and the congenital hypoplastic anemia of Diamond–Blackfan. Other, nonhematologic syndromes involving thumb hypoplasia include the Holt–Oram

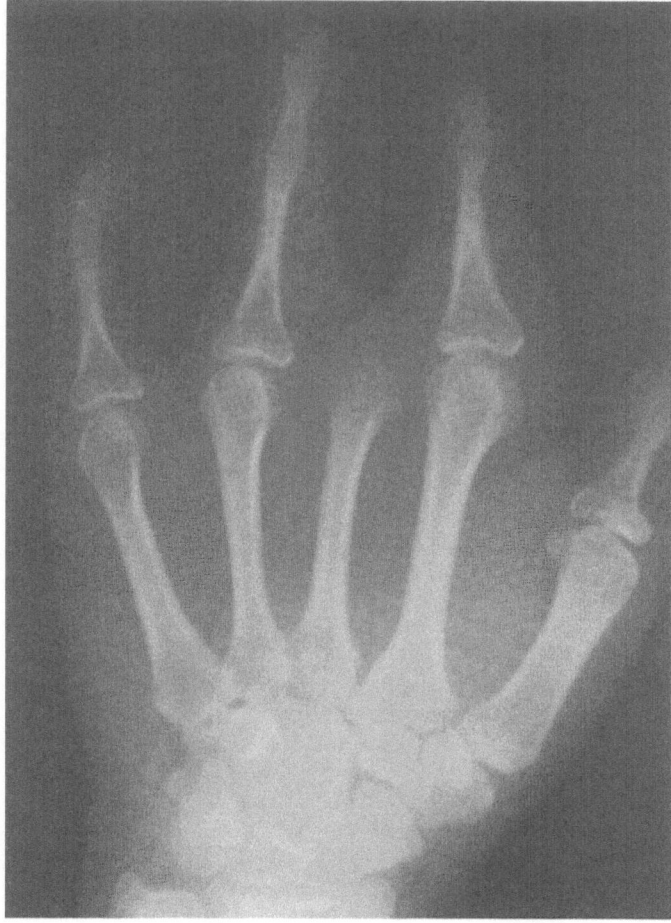

Figure 6.7. Symphalangism is longitudinal fusion of phalanges of the same digit, sometimes associated with tarsal and carpal fusions as well

syndrome (skeletal defects of the upper extremities and congenital heart disease) and the VATER association (*v*ertebral defects, *a*nal atresia, *t*racheo*e*sophageal fistula, *r*adial dysplasia including thumb hypoplasia). Analogous preaxial deficiencies of the lower extremity result in tibial hypoplasia.

7. **Ectrodactyly**, which represents deficiency in the embryologic development of the central digital rays (along the axis), results in a split hand or foot (lobster claw) deformity. Typically, elements of the third digit are missing with the remaining fingers often manifesting other malformations, including camptodactyly, clinodactyly, oligodactyly, or syndactyly. When two or more limbs are involved, autosomal dominant

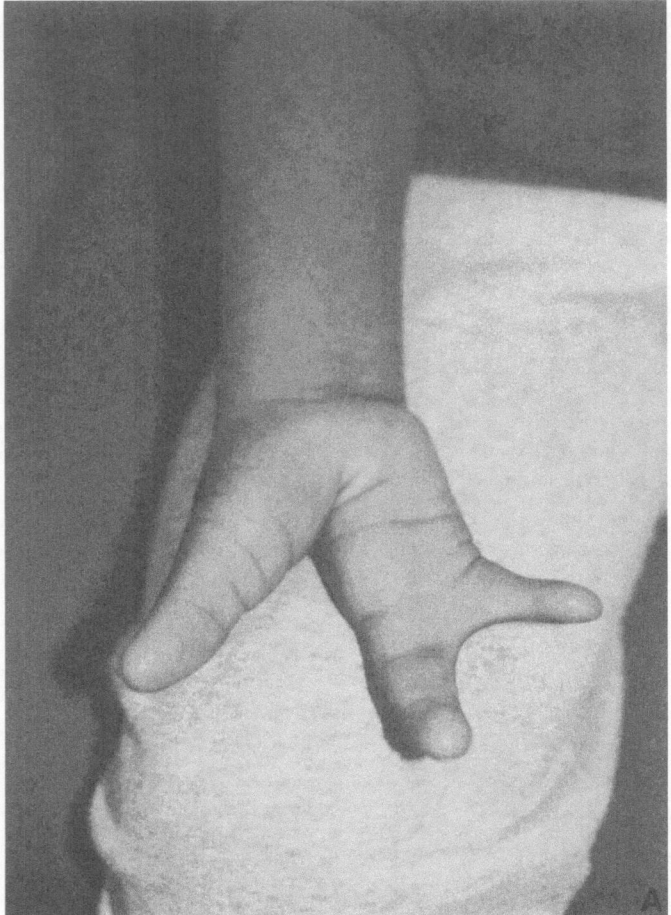

Figure 6.8. (A) Claw-hand or split-hand deformity is sometimes called ectrodactyly. (B) The philosophy of "not what you have but how you use it" is clearly demonstrated here. Surgery is not likely to make this hand more functional than it is already. These defects are often associated with complicated syndactyly, symphalangism, and missing digits.

inheritance is common. Many ectrodactyly–multiple congenital anomaly syndromes have been described.

8. **Arachnodactyly** are long slender fingers, which may be a marker for Marfan syndrome (hyperextensibility, lens subluxation, pectus excavatum, mitral value prolapse, and aortic dilatation), Stickler syndrome (myopia, spondyloepiphyseal dysplasia, hyperextensibility with apparent arachnodactyly), Beals syndrome (joint contractures, crumpled ear, and arachnodactyly) and homocystinuria (lens subluxation, arachnodac-

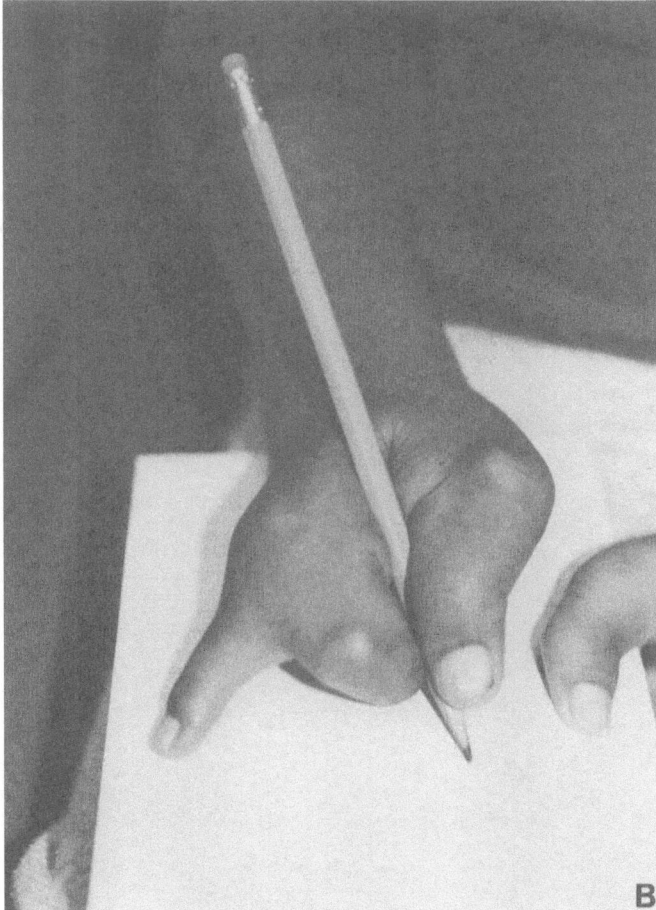

Figure 6.8. (*Continued*)

tyly, and excessive homocystine in urine), among others. Many digits which appear long are not measurably so but rather are normal but thin or belong to tall individuals.

9. Trigger digits which result from abnormalities in function of the flexor tendon in the flexor sheath (rarely extensor tendon), with tethering and, usually, a persistent flexion deformity. About 25% are present at birth and multiple joint involvement is not uncommon. Either narrowing of the sheath or nodules in the tendon are usually found at surgery, which is necessary usually if the child is over 1 year at presentation or if splinting in extension is not effective.

10 "Curly" toes are common and involve varus angulation of one toe, usually under its medial neighbor. These often represent cosmetic or shoe wear problems and

will eventually require flexor tenotomy by the time the child is ready for school. Mildly curly toes might be watched indefinitely if they're not causing anyone trouble.

Other hand defects include a large number of other anomalies that may be useful as markers for a variety of well-defined multiple congenital anomaly syndromes. These include:

1. The broad thumbs and great toes of the Rubinstein–Taybi syndrome (short stature, downward slanting palpebral fissures, mental retardation, and broad thumbs and great toes).

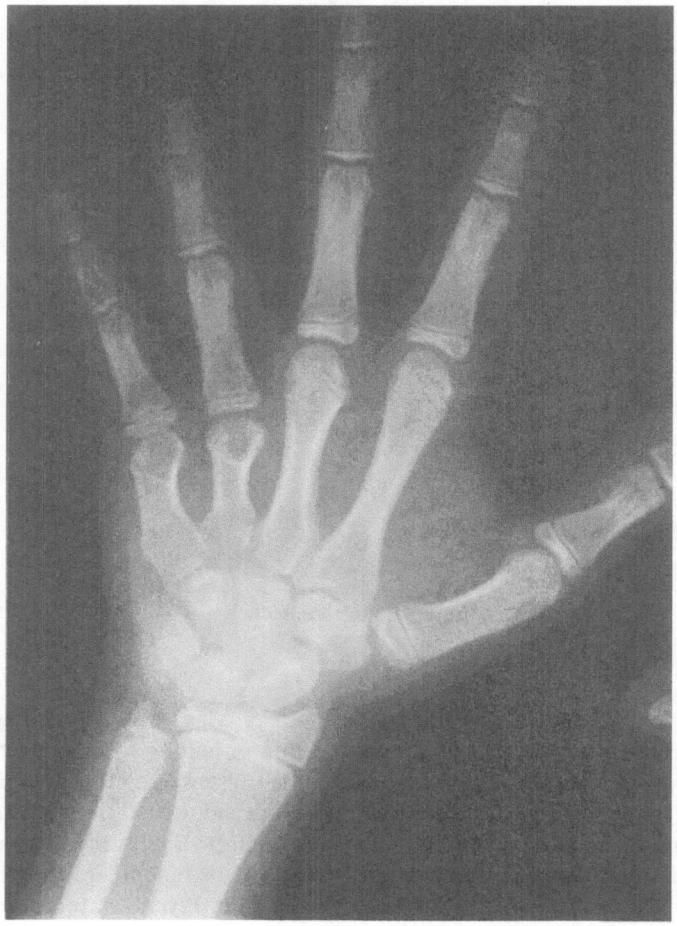

Figure 6.9. Albright syndrome, pseudohypoparathyroidism, is associated with metacarpal shortening, as pictured here, metatarsal shortening, congenital tissue resistance to parathyroid hormone, short stature, mental retardation, and hypocalcemic tetany. It should not be confused with McCune–Albright syndrome, which is polyostotic fibrous dysplasia and precocious puberty.

2. Shortened metacarpals or metatarsals, found in a variety of disorders including Turner syndrome (fourth) and Albright hereditary osteodystrophy (fourth and fifth).

3. Brachydactyly (short fingers), found in Poland syndrome (unilateral deficiency of pectoral major muscle with hand defects; see below), Robinow syndrome (frontal bossing, prominent eyes, hypoplastic genitalia with brachydactyly), and Prader–Willi syndrome (hypotonia, obesity, small hands and feet), among many others.

4. Hypoplastic nails which are found in a large number of syndromes, including fetal hydantoin syndrome, fetal alcohol syndrome (fifth finger), and the nail-patella syndrome (absent patella, hypoplastic nails, and hypoplastic capitellum).

5. A triphalangeal thumb which involves a spectrum of anomalies from an interposed triangular middle phalanx with severe angular deformity (a delta phalanx) to a well-formed fingerlike thumb as part of a five-fingered thumbless hand. It is often inherited as an autosomal dominant trait or may be a part of any of the syndromes associated with preaxial abnormalities including Holt–Oram, TAR, or Aase (see above). Other orthopedic anomalies are common. Treatment is surgical and, in general is performed early on to minimize deformity and maximize function.

6.3.2. Foot and Ankle

6.3.2.1. Metatarsus Adductus

Metatarsus adductus (metatarsus varus) is a common and usually benign deformity discussed in Chapter 4.

6.3.2.2. Talipes Equinovarus

Talipes equinovarus deformity (TEV; classical clubfoot) is comprised of three components: (1) heel inversion or varus with the sole of the foot pointed medially; (2) forefoot or metatarsus adductus; and (3) ankle equinus with the foot in a plantarflexed position. Associated findings include calf atrophy and thinning and redundancy of the skin on the lateral side of the foot. Such markers for occult spinal problems as a lumbar hemangioma or hairy patch should be sought since intrauterine paresis may result in a clubfoot deformity. Similarly, a clubfoot-like deformity which is not present at birth but develops subsequently is always the result of a neurologic abnormality such as might occur with spinal cord tethering caused by spina bifida occulta or diastematomyelia.

TEV occurs between 1 and 2 times per 1000 deliveries, most often in otherwise healthy infants. Fifty percent have bilateral disease and most are male (perhaps 70%). Under ordinary circumstances, the recurrence risk of clubfoot after one affected child is between 2 and 5%. Occasionally, infants will demonstrate other syndromic associations reflecting either decreased uterine capacity or reduced fetal movement, including Freeman–Sheldon syndrome (increased muscle tone with "whistling" facies and club-

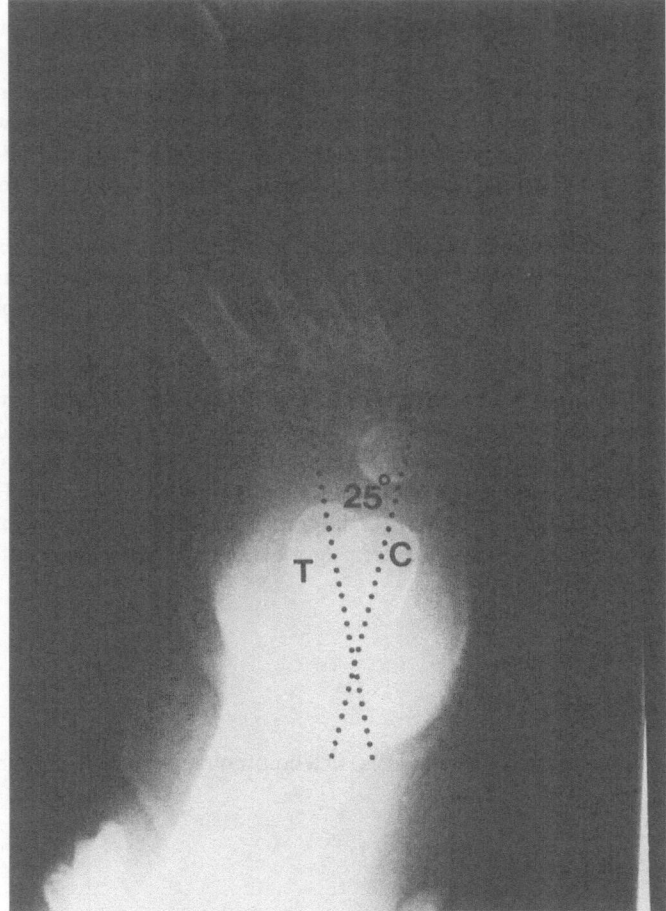

Figure 6.10. Anteroposterior radiograph of young child with metatarsus adductus (MA), also known as metatarsus varus. In MA, the forefoot is abnormal but the relationship between the talus (T) and the calcaneus (C) is normal. That is, the angle formed by the long axes of these two bones (known as Kite's angle) is about 25°. In more severe MA, it is often larger. In true talipes equinovarus (clubfoot), it is always much smaller (see Fig. 6.11B).

foot), arthrogryposis, oligohydramnios, early amnion rupture sequence (amniotic band syndrome), and meningomyelocele. Some maternal illnesses such as myotonic dystrophy increase the risk of the fetus developing clubfoot deformities.

TEV also occurs, presumably as a primary malformation, in diastrophic dysplasia (short tubular bones, joint limitation, hypertrophic auricular cartilage, short stature), Larsen syndrome (multiple joint dislocations, flat facies, clubfoot) and as a result of taking aminopterin or methotrexate early in gestation.

Rigidity of the deformity may be visualized as a spectrum from deformities easily correctable past neutral with minimal effort, to an immobile rigid deformity. Early manipulation and casting takes advantage of the newborn's increased flexibility and is effective in many cases. However, surgery is often required and should not be delayed if it is apparent after 3 to 6 months that casting is not likely to be effective.

Night bracing after surgery is also often necessary using the Denis–Browne bar or a similar splint to prevent a recurrence of varus angulation.

6.3.2.3. *Talipes Calcaneovalgus*

Talipes calcaneovalgus is the "mirror-image" deformity of TEV in which the foot is dorsiflexed, externally rotated, and everted. It occurs usually as a result of intrauterine deformation and is much less severe a deformity than TEV. It usually responds to stretching and waiting though occasionally will require casting if the deformity is persistent or severe or if associated with congenital lower extremity weakness as might occur with a low-lumbar meningomyelocele. Talipes calcaneovalgus is sometimes known as the "other" kind of clubfoot or as "reverse" clubfoot.

6.3.2.4. *Other Foot Abnormalities*

Other congenital foot abnormalities include congenital vertical talus (convex pes valgus) and congenital tarsal coalition. Both of these are discussed in the section on rigid flat feet in Chapter 4.

6.3.3. Other Lower Extremity Defects

6.3.3.1. *Developmental Dysplasia of the Hip*

Developmental dysplasia of the hip (DDH) remains a common and problematic condition. Terminology is confusing and causation is incompletely understood. Previously known as *congenital dislocation* or *dysplasia of the hip* (CDH), the current term emphasizes the fact that some children who eventually manifest dislocation may have a normal examination in early infancy.

DDH includes an entire spectrum of deformity from a shallow acetabulum without hip instability, to excessive femoral head movement within the acetabulum without displacement, to subluxation or loss of contact between the femoral head and the most medial portion of the acetabulum, to dislocation or complete loss of contact between femoral head and acetabulum.

In most cases, a "dislocated" hip discovered in infancy is not persistently and irreducibly dislocated but rather can be felt to dislocate and relocate on physical examination. A small minority of hips are antenatally dislocated completely and are called teratologic dislocations, often associated with other congenital anomalies (as in arthrogryposis) or neuromuscular disease (as in spina bifida).

6.3.3.1a. Epidemiology. Incidences at birth reported by different authors vary considerably, probably related to the broad spectrum of disease, but cluster around the figure

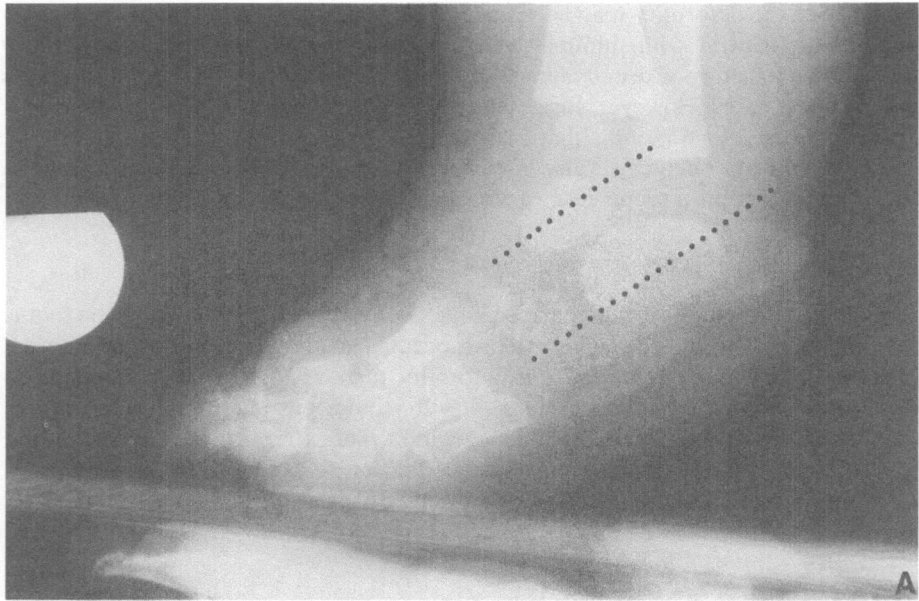

Figure 6.11. (A) Lateral radiograph of a young infant with talipes equinovarus (TEV). Note the "parallelism" between the long axes of the talus and calcaneus. Both are in equinus, even with maximal dorsiflexion attempted. (B) Children with TEV also have metatarsus adductus. Unlike children with simple isolated MA, however, they manifest hindfoot abnormalities as evidenced by the abnormally small angle on this anteroposterior film between the long axes of the talus (T) and the calcaneus (C) (see Fig. 6.10).

of 1 per 1000 live births, with five to ten times more girls affected than boys. Many more affect the left than the right hip and most are unilateral.

6.3.3.1b. Genetics and Environment in DDH.   Environment and genetics each play a role here. Both intrauterine and postnatal positioning have been associated with higher than expectable rates of DDH, including breech position, first born (smaller, more constraining uterus), or anything else that restricts fetal movement. Postnatal factors have been noted, including binding or swaddling the infant in hip adduction and extension as sometimes practiced by native Americans and other ethnic groups.

Genetic influences manifest themselves by the increased recurrence risk of between 2 and 6% after the birth of an affected child and by the 34% concordance for DDH observed in identical twins.

Infants themselves may be biologically predisposed either because of excessive joint laxity or because of a primary defect in acetabular growth and maturation. It has been suggested that more girls than boys are affected because increased intrauterine estrogen levels in girls result in greater joint laxity in the perinatal period. Although some untreated infants with joint instability will improve over time, many affected

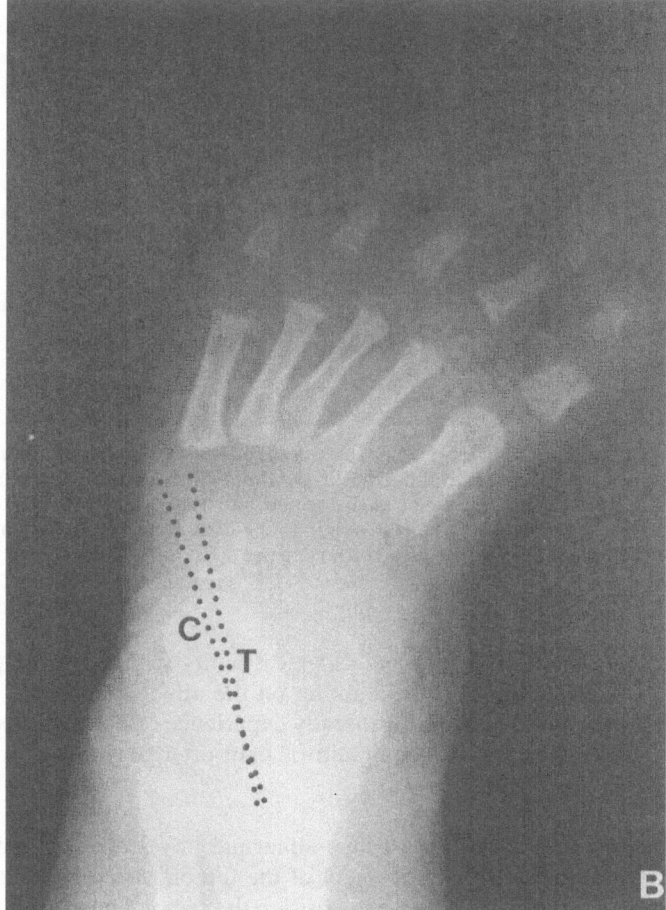

Figure 6.11. (*Continued*)

infants by several months of age will have "tightened up" and will be left with a persistently dislocated hip not easily relocatable.

6.3.3.1c. Presentation. The possibility of DDH should be raised whenever a newborn infant with a history of breech delivery (even if by cesarean section), oligohydramnios, twinning, torticollis, metatarsus adductus, or an affected family member is encountered. The newborn screening examination (see below) is useful but is not always positive in affected infants.

Older infants and young children will present with a shortened extremity, a

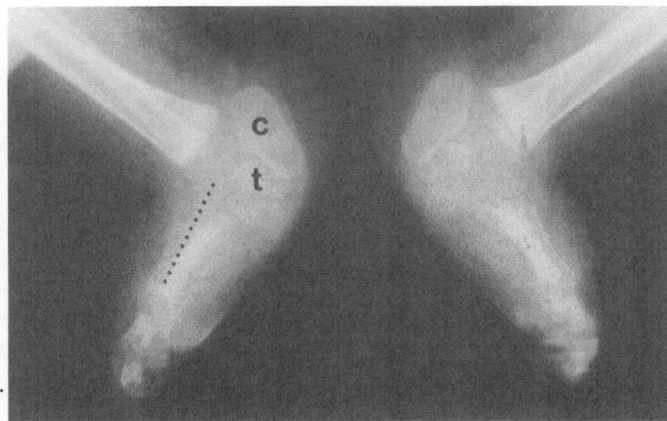

Figure 6.12. Vertical talus in a young infant, also known as rocker-bottom foot or convex pes valgus. Normally the long axis of the talus and the long axis of the first metatarsal (dotted line) are the same. With a vertical talus, the talonavicular joint is dislocated and the talus (t) is oriented vertically, pushing the calcaneus (c) laterally. This results in a rigid foot which cannot be walked on. Sometimes associated with spina bifida, trisomy 18, or arthrogryposis.

waddling gait, excessive lordosis ("swayback"), difficulty with diapering (because of reduced abduction), or intoeing and toe-walking on the affected side.

Affected infants and children don't generally experience discomfort though adolescents with a missed dislocation will complain of pain after they begin to experience degenerative changes in the hip.

6.3.3.1d. Examination. All of the various abnormal physical findings in the newborn period are based on either the movement of the femoral head into and out of the acetabulum or, if persistently dislocated, the position the femoral head eventually takes, superior, posterior, and lateral to the acetabulum.

Because this is a developmental process, one or two good examinations in the neonatal period are not adequate to detect late-occurring dysplasia. Examinations should be performed periodically until the child is walking well. None of the manipulations require much force and, in fact, excessive force makes things more difficult with the infant more likely to cry and damage more likely done to the cartilaginous femoral head.

Table 6.1. Risk Factors in Developmental Dysplasia of the Hip

Family history	Oligohydramnios or other uterine constraints
Breech position (even if cesarean section)	Hyperlaxity
First born	Neuromuscular disease such as spina bifida
Female	Metatarsus adductus
Torticollis	

The infant should be warm and happy. You'll never get any kind of accurate exam on a crying baby—better to come back later. Do one hip at a time so you can concentrate on the hip in hand and do the exam on a flat surface. If you can't do a good exam in the cramped, plastic bassinets popular in many hospitals, take the infant out of the bassinet for the exam.

Look for associated deformations, most particularly torticollis, which is highly associated with DDH. Other associations include metatarsus adductus, and arthrogryposis.

If the hip is dislocated when examined, gentle abduction with the hip in flexion, lifting up on the greater trochanter, will generally result in reduction, associated with a palpable (more than audible) "clunk" or "thunk" as the femoral head slips over the posterior rim of the acetabulum during midabduction. This is the Ortolani maneuver.

The newly relocated hip is then dislocatable by doing the opposite: adducting the hip in flexion and pushing gently down with the thumb. If dislocatable, the examiner will feel the femoral head slip out of the acetabulum with a "clunk" or "thunk" and the sensation of movement. This is the Barlow maneuver.

A similar though less dramatic exam will result from femoral heads which are subluxable rather than dislocatable. Even if not subluxable, some hips are unstable if the examiner finds that the femoral head can be "pistoned" in and out of the acetabulum, demonstrating increased laxity.

High-pitched clicking noises which occur during the exam are probably of no significance if they are unassociated with a sensation of movement. They presumably result from tendons slipping over bony prominences or bursae. Complete reassurance is

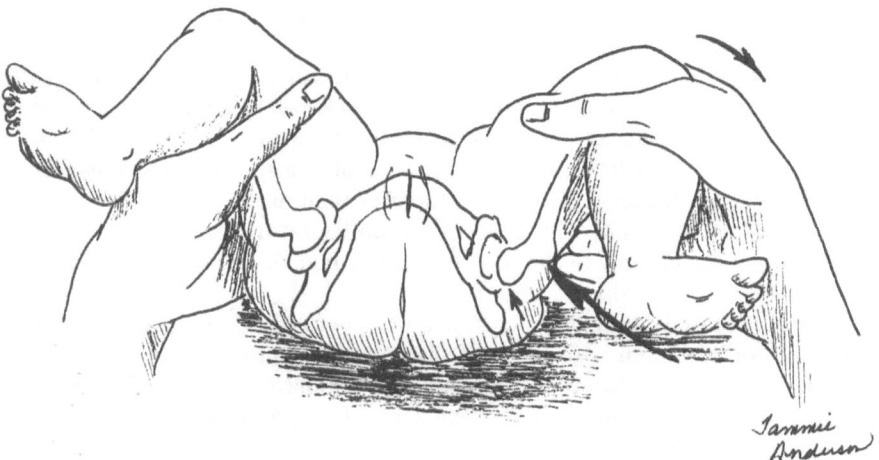

Figure 6.13. Ortolani's test. Marino Ortolani described his test for hip dislocation in 1937. The presumption has always been that Italy figures prominently in the history of infant hip disease (Galeazzi, Ortolani) because Italian women typically swaddled their infants, producing a position (adduction and extension) conducive to subluxation. With gentle abduction and lifting, a reducible hip will produce a "clunk" as it passes over the posterior rim into the acetabulum.

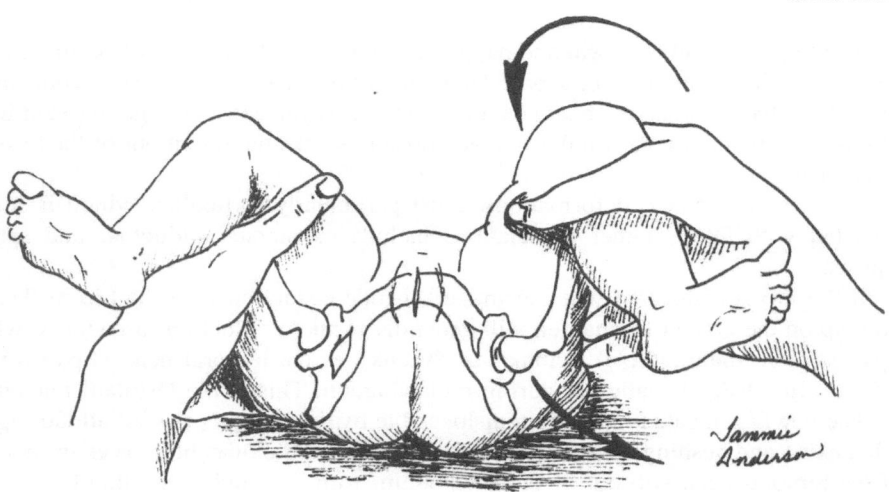

Figure 6.14. Barlow's test is the opposite side to the coin. If a hip is dislocatable, adduction and downward pressure will cause the femoral head to subluxate over the posterior rim of the acetabulum and a "clunk" will be felt.

probably not possible, however, because the presence of a click in one study was associated with a higher than expectable rate of dysplasia. Evaluation and follow-up is warranted if other historical risk factors are present (see below).

If the femoral head is persistently dislocated, the femur may appear short since the dislocation is usually superior. This can be seen by comparing the relative heights of the knees with the hips and knees flexed, the Galeazzi sign.

Abduction, which should be 60° in a newborn, might be reduced on the affected side and extra or asymmetrical thigh folds may also be seen. An imaginary line drawn from the greater trochanter through the anterior, superior iliac spine should point to the umbilicus. If the hip is dislocated, the line will point to a spot inferior to the umbilicus since the greater trochanter will be more superior than usual.

If ambulatory, the child with a persistent unilateral dislocation will walk with a Trendelenburg gait, leaning to the affected side when in stance phase. Toe-walking on the affected side may also be observed.

Bilateral disease is more difficult to diagnose because of the lack of a comparison side. Ambulatory children with bilateral disease will exhibit an accentuated lordotic posture. Children of any age with bilateral disease will have an increased space between their thighs with the perineum easily seen when lying with their knees together, an abnormal situation. They frequently will walk with a waddling "ducklike" gait which parents may find endearing until they discover its significance.

6.3.3.1e.   Radiography in DDH.   The value of radiography is somewhat limited by the fact that femoral head ossification does not begin until about 6 months. Despite this, however, X-rays are useful in diagnosis and follow-up if proper attention is paid to

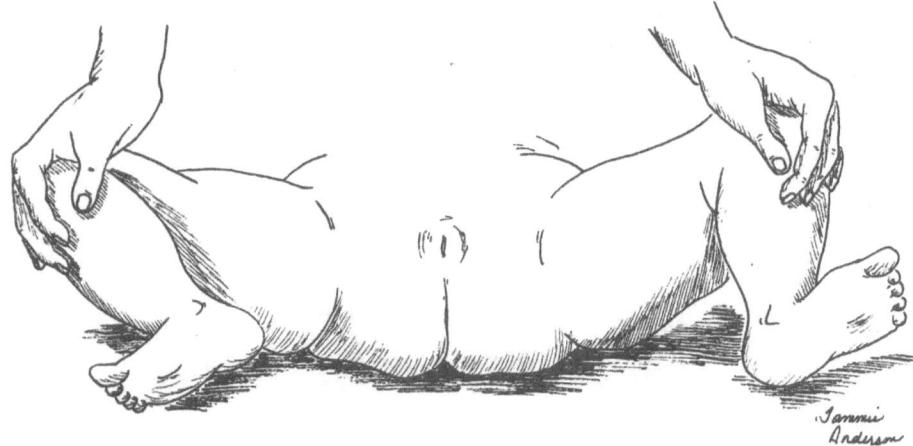

Figure 6.15. Decreased abduction, as demonstrated here on the left, is an important sign of hip pathology. This is particularly so in infants whose dislocation is not reducible and who will therefore not have a positive Ortolani or Barlow test.

obtaining a true, nonrotated anteroposterior film with the infant's hips adducted and slightly flexed. The beak of the proximal medial metaphysis of the femur should normally lie within the inferior medial quadrant formed by drawing a horizontal line through the triradiate cartilage (Hilgenreiner's line) and two vertical lines (Perkins's lines) through the lateral border of each acetabulum.

Shenton's line may be "broken" if the smooth arc normally formed by the medial border of the femoral metaphysis and the inferior border of the pubic ramus is interrupted by lateral and superior displacement which occurs with dislocation. After ossification of the femoral head has begun, delayed ossification will be noted on the affected side. With a dysplastic hip the affected acetabulum may appear shallow and/or the femur laterally displaced. With the hips abducted to 45°, the femoral neck should point to the triradiate cartilage under normal circumstances.

Having said this, one should never rely on radiography for early (neonatal) diagnosis. Radiography should be considered as accessory and confirmatory in the early diagnosis of DDH.

Radiography is more useful in following children in treatment or in the evaluation of untreated children over the age of 6 months who are at risk. Even children with a normal hip examination should have a single anteroposterior view of the pelvis at 6 or 7 months (after femoral head ossification) if they have a history of congenital muscular torticollis or frank breech delivery. Both are highly associated with DDH with about 20% of children having DDH in each condition.

Additionally, radiography at 6 months should be strongly considered for children with normal exams if there is more than one of the following: other kinds of breech delivery, a family history of DDH, metatarsus adductus, a hip click or any other questionable exam in the past even though they had normal X-rays at that time, excessive

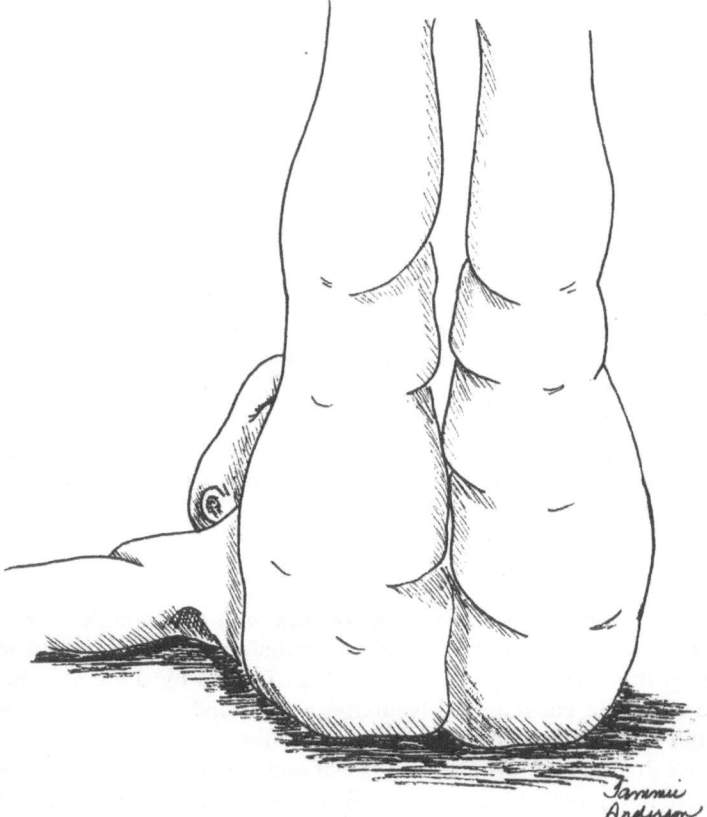

Figure 6.16. Because most dislocations are superior, the femoral length on the affected side will be shorter and the flexion folds may then be asymmetrical. Sometimes the minor folds of fat along the inner thighs will not match up, even without hip disease. The most important folds to check are the ones behind the knees and the ones at the top of the thigh, right inferior to the gluteus muscles. These should normally correspond pretty much exactly to each other.

⟶

Figure 6.17. (A) Left-sided developmental dysplasia of the hip (DDH). DDH is difficult to diagnose radiologically prior to femoral head ossification (about 6–7 months). By dividing each hip into four quadrants with a horizontal line through the triradiate cartilage zones (Hilgenreiner's line, H above), and two vertical lines dropped perpendicularly from the lateral margin of each acetabulum (Perkin's lines, P above), an inference can be reached. The medial beak (arrow) of the metaphysis or the ossification center of the proximal epiphysis, if it has developed, should be in the medial, inferior quadrant on each side. Additionally, a line drawn along the medial aspect of the femoral metaphysis should smoothly continue and underline the inferior border of the superior ramus of the pubis (Shenton's line, S above). Note also shallower acetabulum on affected side. (B) On the frog-leg lateral film, a line drawn along the femoral neck should bisect the triradiate cartilage

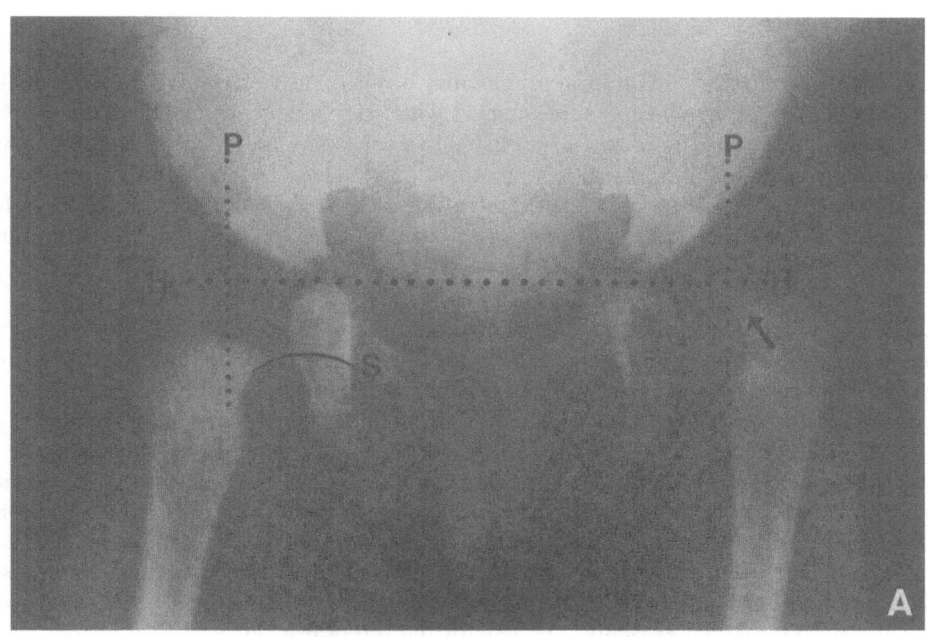

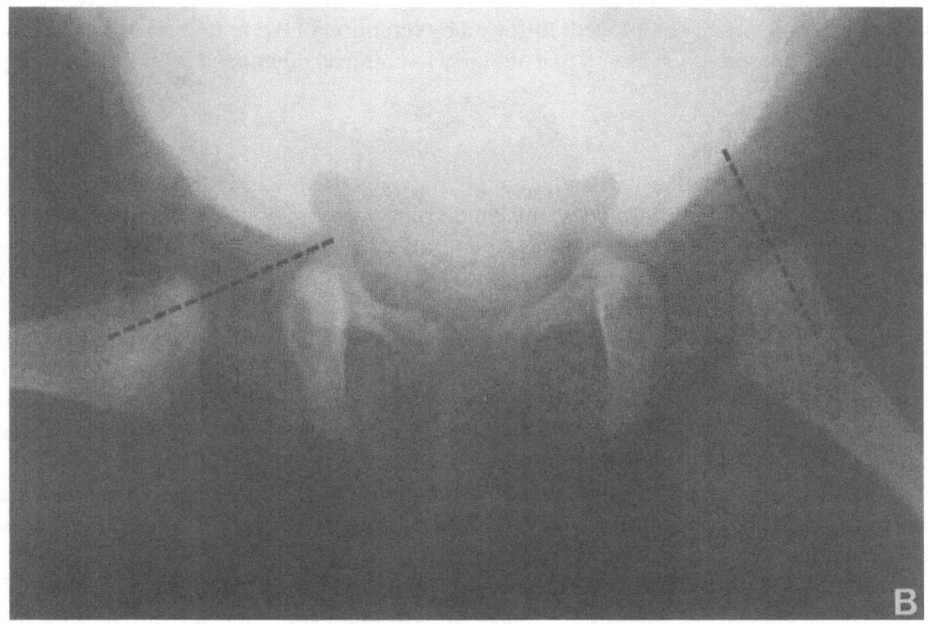

hyperlaxity, oligohydramnios, congenital neuromuscular disease, or if they are a firstborn female.

6.3.3.1f. Ultrasound.   Ultrasonography may be useful as well but is dependent on the skill of the ultrasonographer. In some centers with particular expertise, ultrasonography has been found to be more sensitive than physical examination in screening for hip dysplasia. Competent ultrasound examinations may be an alternative to radiography in at-risk infants with normal physical examinations. The role of ultrasonography both for screening and for diagnosis is evolving and is likely to increase in the future as more experience is obtained.

6.3.3.1g. Treatment of DDH.   The goal of treatment is placement of the femoral head into the acetabulum. Earlier treatment is not only easier but more effective. For this reason, when in doubt, err on the side of treatment. The Pavlick harness is the abduction apparatus used most often in the United States for children diagnosed before 6 months of age. It holds the hips in about 100° of flexion but allows for some movement. It is generally worn 24 hours a day, at least initially. Extreme abduction in the splint is not necessary and may be dangerous. Active adduction to neutral by the infants should be possible. After several months, the splint is slowly weaned, assuming appropriate reduction. Follow-up radiographs should be obtained after placement in the harness, after femoral head ossification has begun and after ambulation begins. Complications are uncommon but include avascular necrosis of the femoral head.

For children diagnosed after 6 months, skin traction and closed reduction under anesthesia are generally employed, followed by retention of the reduction in a cast. Open reduction is sometimes necessary, particularly in children diagnosed after 2 years of age.

6.3.3.2. Coxa Vara

Coxa vara is an abnormally small angle between the femoral shaft and the femoral neck. Under normal circumstances, this angle ranges from about 150° in infancy to 120° in adulthood. Children with coxa vara frequently exhibit shaft–neck angles close to or even less than 90°. Coxa vara can be categorized conveniently as congenital, acquired, or developmental.

Congenital coxa vara is most often found as either a portion of a localized birth defect affecting the proximal femur (see Section 6.3.3.3) or resulting from a generalized osseous dysplasia like rickets, osteogenesis imperfecta, spondyloepiphyseal dysplasia, or cleidocranial dysostosis (absent clavicles, delayed closure of cranial sutures and fontanels, and delayed tooth eruption).

Acquired coxa vara is the result of local injury to the femoral neck or proximal femoral growth plate as might result from trauma, localized infection, or aseptic necrosis of the femoral head (Legg–Calve–Perthes disease).

Developmental or infantile coxa vara is thought to be related to failure of the medial or inferior aspect of the proximal femoral growth plate to ossify, leading to structural weakness and fatigue, increasing varus, and worsening verticality of the growth plate. This leads to secondary small slips of the epiphysis on the metaphysis.

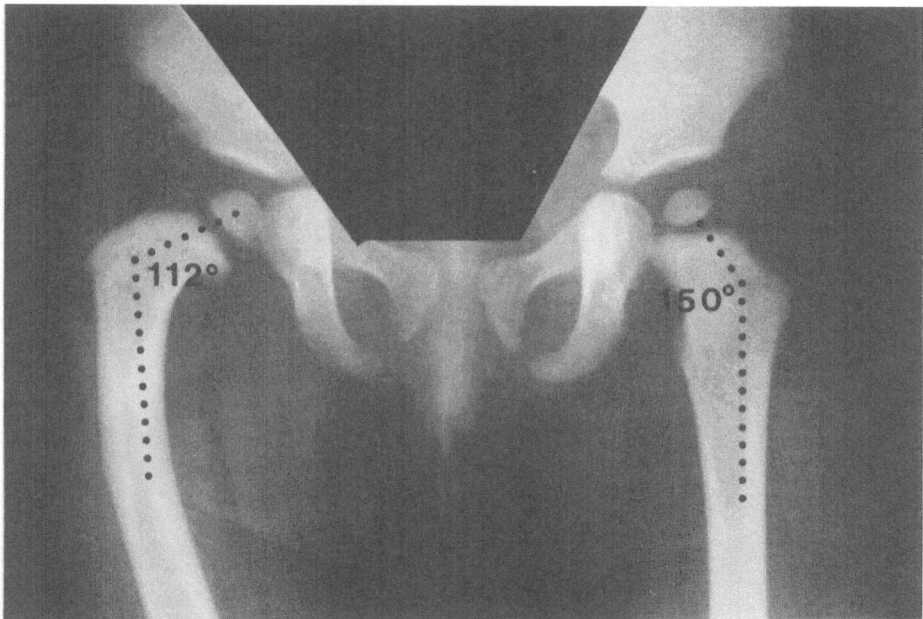

Figure 6.18. Right-sided coxa vara in a 2-year-old girl. Coxa vara is generally defined as being present when the shaft–neck angle is less than 120°. The 120° figure is taken from the normal angle for adults. In fact, children have higher angles (more valgus) at birth and throughout childhood, as is evidenced by the normal 150° shaft–neck angle here on the patient's left.

Coxa vara is rare, occurring once in every 25,000 births, and is without sexual predominance. Left and right are equally represented and between 25 and 50% have bilateral disease. Familial cases have been reported. Children present after 2 and before 6 years with a painless limp, if unilateral, or a waddling gait, if bilateral. Children with coxa vara present similarly to children with DDH diagnosed late.

Physical examination will reveal a modest leg-length discrepancy, a positive Trendelenburg sign, a flexion contracture, and reduced hip range of motion. Radiography performed at birth or in early infancy on patients who subsequently acquire developmental coxa vara is normal. Nonoperative therapy is not useful and most orthopedic surgeons prefer a valgus producing osteotomy of the proximal femoral shaft.

6.3.3.3. Proximal Femoral Focal Deficiency

Proximal femoral focal deficiency (PFFD) is an intercalary limb deficiency (proximal problems with normal distal extremity) characterized by varying degrees of absence or hypoplasia of the proximal femur and acetabulum, often associated with fibrous connections (pseudarthroses) between proximal and distal femoral segments. Other limb

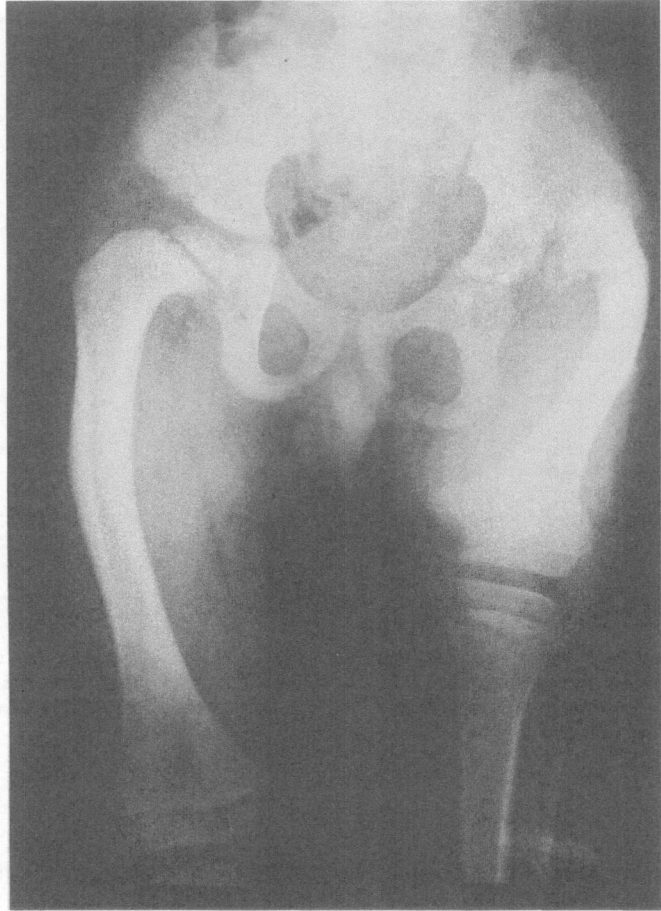

Figure 6.19. Proximal femoral focal deficiency (PFFD) on the left in a 5-year-old boy. PFFD is an intercalary defect which can cause severe leg-length discrepancies. It frequently occurs with other lower extremity defects, including fibular and tibial shortening. Note abnormal bowing and coxa vara on right. Note dysplastic, very shallow acetabulum on the left.

deficiencies are common in children with PFFD, most prominently fibular hemimelia (see below).

Children with PFFD present with short femoral segments which taper sharply to the knee. The hip is held in flexion, abduction, and external rotation. Fifteen percent have bilateral involvement which is usually severe. A variety of clinical staging systems have been developed which rely on the characteristics described above as parameters. Treatment with surgery and the fitting of various prostheses attempt to deal with the shortening, joint instability, weakness, and malrotation inherent in the deformities. The specific cause of PFFD is unknown though it has been described in association with caudal regression in infants of diabetic mothers and in the femoral hypoplasia/unusual facies syndrome.

6.3.3.4. Discoid Meniscus

A discoid meniscus is an abnormally thickened meniscus which lacks the central concavity of the normal meniscus. Its cause is embryologically obscure and it may in fact be a degenerative change rather than a primary malformation. The typical presenting symptomatology of a painful, snapping, locking knee which doesn't fully extend is the result of abnormal meniscal mobility resulting from poor attachment to the tibial plateau, particularly posteriorly. It is often bilateral and only very rarely does it affect the medial meniscus. Although it may present as early as 5 or 6 years, a discoid meniscus typically presents in early to midadolescence. Boys are more often affected than girls. Many children with this condition are asymptomatic.

Diagnosis should be suspected in any child with a typical history and physical findings. A snap or palpable lurch may be felt during passive flexion and extension as the tibia moves abruptly beneath the femur. Lateral joint line tenderness may be present as well as an effusion, particularly so if a meniscal tear has occurred. Radiography may reveal lateral joint space widening though usually the diagnosis is confirmed arthrographically or by MRI rather than by radiography. Treatment often starts with immobilization, with repair or partial meniscectomy reserved for children with persistent symptoms. Complete removal of the meniscus may result in later degenerative changes.

6.3.3.5. Bipartite Patella

A bipartite patella develops when the normal fusion of two patellar ossification centers doesn't occur. Repeated trauma to the cartilaginous connection between the two ossicles causes pain and requires operative therapy if conservative measures of immobilization fail. Patients without symptoms require no therapy.

6.3.3.6. Patellar Dislocation

Congenital patellar dislocation implies a laterally displaced and irreducible patella tethered by soft tissues to the lateral femoral condyle. It is almost always associated with a fixed flexion deformity at the knee. Valgus angulation at the knee is also seen on occasion. If delayed ossification makes the patella difficult to see radiologically, ultrasound may be useful. This defect may appear independently or as part of such generalized problems as arthrogryposis, the nail–patella syndrome, connective tissue disorders, or diastrophic dysplasia. Treatment is surgical release.

Patellas that intermittently dislocate are classified as either habitual or recurrent dislocations. The former group includes children in midchildhood with either a tight iliotibial band or a quadriceps contracture or both, which cause the patella to dislocate laterally during flexion. Holding the patella in the midline prevents flexion. Treatment is surgical release.

Recurrent lateral patellar dislocations occur most often among adolescents and don't happen as predictably as habitual dislocations. Factors predisposing to dislocation include genu valgum, hyperlaxity, medial quadriceps (vastus medialis) weakness or atrophy, lateral condylar hypoplasia, patellar alta, and rotatory problems, particularly if the femur tends toward medial and the tibia toward lateral rotation. Many of these factors are also seen in adolescent females with the patellofemoral pain syndrome (see Section 2.5.14).

Examination, in addition to the above, often demonstrates tenderness on patellar compression and a positive "apprehension" test. When the examiner moves the patella laterally and gently flexes the knee, the patient will sense impending dislocation and will become apprehensive and agitated.

Treatment involves rehabilitation of the medial portion of the quadriceps in order to balance the tendency toward lateral pulling. Straight leg raising with the knee fully extended or knee extension exercises against increasing resistance beginning with the knee in 20° of flexion, are often effective, building up slowly to 50 repetitions daily. Extension exercises beginning with the knee in greater flexion than 20° should be avoided. Doing so results in increased load on the patellofemoral joint resulting in increased patellar compression, joint wear, and pain. Surgery, often involving a lateral release and tendon transfer, may be considered if muscle strengthening is not effective.

6.3.3.7. Popliteal (Baker) Cyst

Baker cysts are small, benign, fluid-filled cysts of the popliteal space which are either outpouchings of the knee joint capsule or bursae between the semimembranosus and gastrocnemius tendons. Some authors reserve the term *Baker cyst* for the latter meaning only. They are usually discovered incidentally by the child or the parents and can present at any time in childhood but are found more often in boys. They are usually unilateral. On examination they are nontender and soft and they transilluminate.

Any chronic increase in intracapsular pressure or synovial fluid production, as in JRA, will predispose to the development of outpouchings of the synovial capsule of the knee. Under most circumstances, however, they occur idiopathically and almost always resolve. Recurrences frequently occur after surgery which is indicated only if the child has considerable symptoms or if the diagnosis is in doubt. The standard semimembranosus cyst rarely needs surgery and is a self-limited problem.

6.3.3.8. Congenital Tibial Bowing

Congenital tibial bowing may be associated with severe difficulties, depending on the direction of the bowing. Lateral bowing is common, usually bilateral and benign, and tends to improve with time (see Chapter 4). Prognosis is less good when associated with specific pathological processes, including Blount's disease, rickets, or epiphyseal injury.

Both anterior and posterior tibial bowing are associated with significant extremity shortening and equinus or calcaneus deformities, respectively.

Anterolateral bowing of the tibia is a much more serious problem because of its

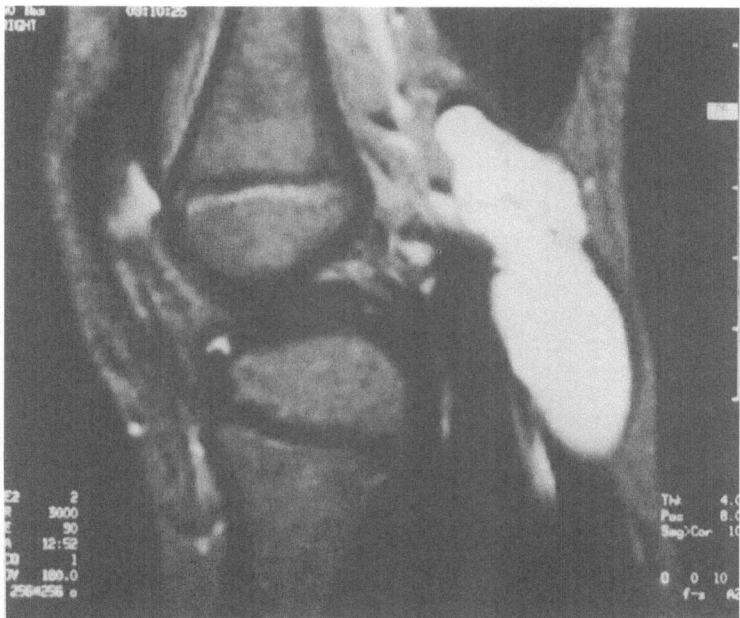

Figure 6.20. Baker cyst demonstrated on a T-2 weighted MRI in this 5-year-old boy. An MRI is not necessary to make the diagnosis, but demonstrates the anatomy well.

association with fracture at the site of the bowing and resistance to healing (pseudarthrosis). At least half of such children have neurofibromatosis (see below) though the exact pathological process involved remains obscure. No neurofibromata are found at the site. What is found is disorganized bone and fibrous tissue. Such pseudarthroses are resistant to bone grafting and, about half the time, amputation is the only solution. Fibular anomalies, including pseudarthrosis, are commonly associated with tibial bowing, though fibular bowing/pseudarthrosis does occur as an isolated phenomenon.

In addition to neurofibromatosis, tibial bowing is extremely common in children with bone dysplasias associated with disproportionate dwarfism.

Children with anterolateral tibial bowing at birth are at significant risk for subsequent fracture and pseudarthrosis and should be treated with a knee–ankle–foot orthosis in an effort to prevent this from occurring.

6.3.3.9. Congenital Knee Dislocation

Congenital hyperextension and dislocation of the knee is an uncommon defect and represents a spectrum of abnormalities. As with hip dysplasia there is a female predominance and many of these children are born in the breech position, often with associated clubfoot deformities or hip dislocation. In some children, predisposing conditions are apparent, and may include excessive ligamentous laxity, arthrogryposis,

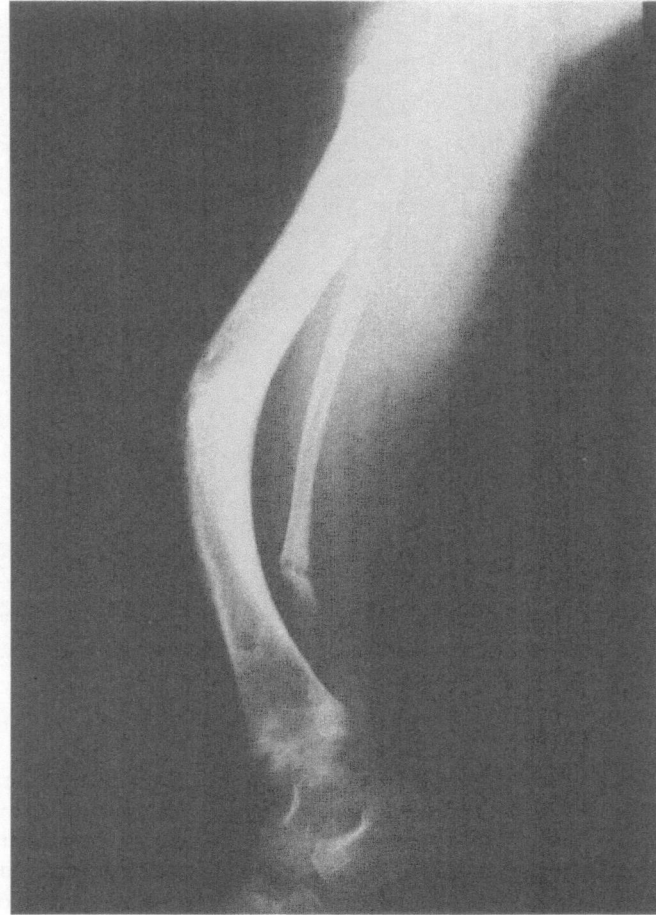

Figure 6.21. Anterior bowing of both tibia and fibula in a 4-year-old girl with neurofibromatosis. Fracture of a bow like this is likely to lead to nonunion (pseudarthrosis) which is difficult to treat.

or spina bifida. Acquired forms can be seen resulting from injury to the quadriceps muscle, as might occur with an intramuscular injection, with subsequent fibrosis and contracture.

Congenitally affected children are born with their knees hyperextended, sometimes with the feet fitting comfortably under the chin and an anterior transverse crease across the knee. The tibia is anteriorly displaced relative to the femur and the femoral condyles are prominent posteriorly. The rectus femoris may be shortened and ipsilateral developmental dislocation of the hip may be present.

Treatment is initially conservative and includes manipulation and casting. Surgical release may be necessary if conservative approaches fail.

6.3.4. Upper Extremity Defects

6.3.4.1. Upper Extremity Synostoses

Taken as a group, abnormal bony fusions or synostoses affecting the upper extremities are not uncommon and include the syndactyly and symphalangism deformities described above. In addition, carpal synostoses are occasionally discovered through usually not because of any functional problem.

Congenital synostoses of the radius and ulna occur proximally only and result in functional impairment because of ensuing difficulties with pronation and supination. Many are bilateral. If supination is severely impaired, even compensatory shoulder rotation will not allow for enough supination to keep coins in an open palm, a significant functional problem. Synostoses of the radius and ulna are sometimes accompanied by radial head dislocation, synostosis with the humerus, or severe atrophy of the brachioradialis muscle. Other bony deformities may be associated, including camptodactyly and syndactyly, and should be searched for. X-rays early on may be misleading as the cartilaginous connection may not yet be ossified. Treatment is surgical with the understanding that return of true supination/pronation is unlikely. Surgery can correct

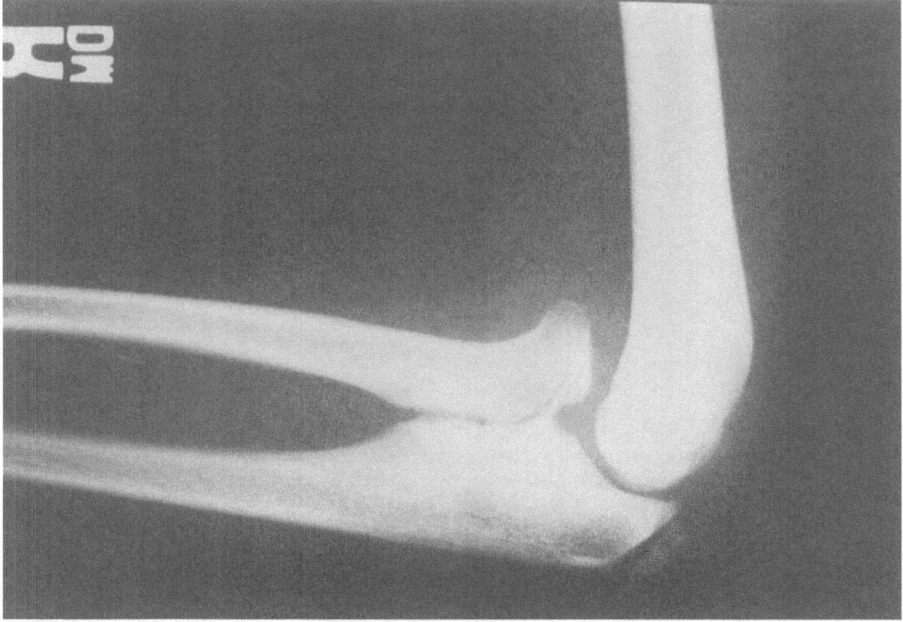

Figure 6.22. Synostosis of the radius and ulna in a 12-year-old boy. This existed as an isolated defect in this patient though radioulnar synostosis has been associated with other birth defects of the upper extremities and with the fetal alcohol syndrome and Nievergelt syndrome (radioulnar synostosis, coalitions of the tarsal and carpal bones, radial head dislocation, and tibial abnormalities)

dysfunctional position by substituting a more functional, albeit still fused, forearm position such that supination can be achieved through compensatory shoulder motion.

6.3.4.2. Congenital Radial Head Dislocation

Congenital radial head dislocation can be anterior, posterior, or lateral and can occur in isolation or as part of a constellation of upper extremity anomalies. It is often bilateral. The capitellum is small and the proximal radius dysplastic. Syndromic associations include that of Nievergelt (carpal and tarsal coalition, radioulnar synostosis, and radial head dislocation), the nail–patella syndrome (hypoplastic nails and patella, iliac spurs, and radial head dislocation), and the Ehlers–Danlos syndrome (skin and joint hyperextensibility).

Children often present in midchildhood with deformity and decreased range of motion.

Occasionally acquired radial head dislocation, if chronic, can be confused with the congenital variety. In the former, the capitellum and the radial head will appear normal radiologically, the dislocation will be unilateral, and associated bony defects will be lacking as will a family history.

Congenital radial head dislocation is not usually painful in childhood. If pain is a problem, surgery to remove the radial head is usually successful in reducing discomfort though not in improving range of motion.

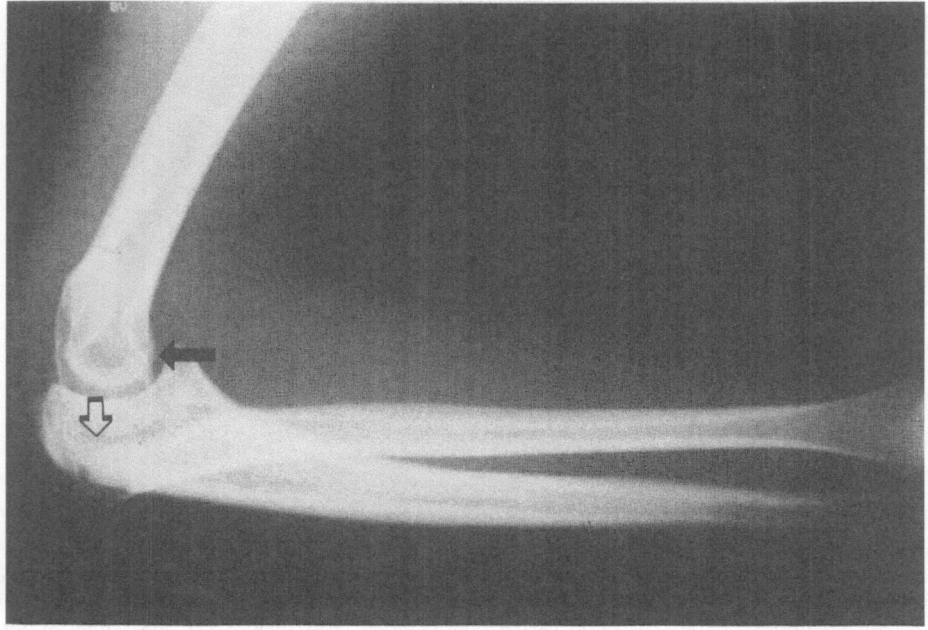

Figure 6.23. Congenital radial head dislocation (open arrow). The radius should be pointing at the capitellum (arrow).

6.3.4.3. Sprengel Deformity

Congenital undescended scapula (Sprengel deformity) is manifest by elevation and medial rotation of the inferior pole of the scapula. Sprengel deformity is the result of embryologic maldescent of the scapula though the exact pathologic mechanism is unknown. Inheritance is not well established since most cases occur sporadically.

Most affected children are asymptomatic with decreased shoulder abduction apparent on physical exam. It is the most common congenital abnormality of the shoulder and, though usually unilateral, can be bilateral in 14% of cases. Elevation of the scapula may be up to about 10 cm, contributing to webbing of the neck, with the scapula itself frequently hypoplastic. Most children with Sprengel's deformity have some other birth defect, including cervical vertebral fusion (Klippel–Feil syndrome), congenital scoliosis, rib abnormalities, cervical spina bifida or diastematomyelia, cleft palate, congenital heart disease, or renal anomalies. Associated abnormal bony or soft-tissue connections between the scapula and spine are termed omovertebral bones and are common. Associated musculature, including the trapezius, serratus anterior, rhomboids, pectoralis major, and levator scapula, may also be hypoplastic or absent.

Treatment is surgical and is more for appearance than for any improvement in function. Renal and cardiac defects must be searched for.

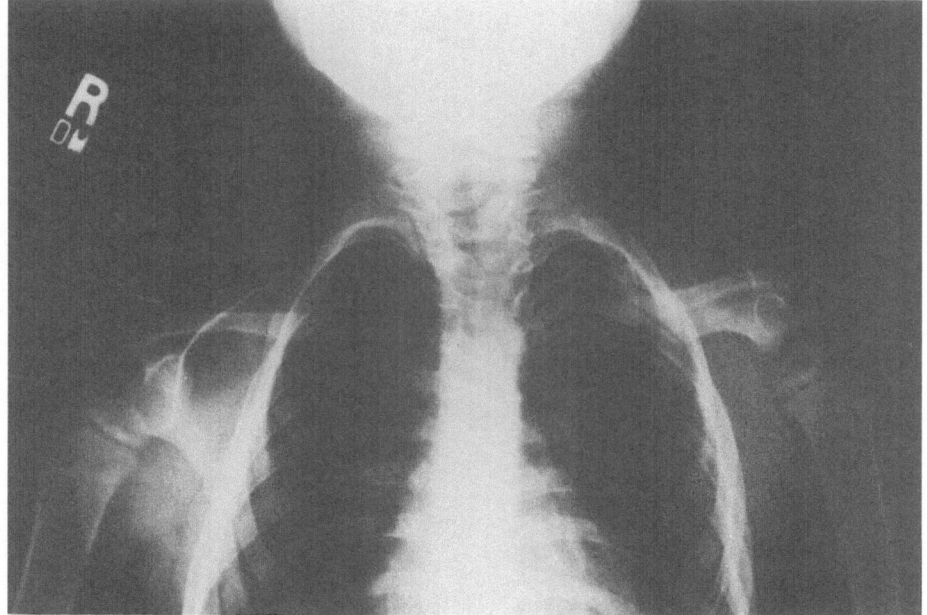

Figure 6.24. Sprengel deformity on the left in a 4-year-old girl. Also known as congenital unde-scended scapula, this deformity occurs more often in girls and is highly associated with other bony birth defects, particularly involving the spine. Note high-riding and rotated scapula on left, cervical hemivertebra, and rib abnormalities.

6.3.4.4. Poland Anomaly

Poland anomaly is unilateral pectoralis major hypoplasia, often with associated abnormalities of the ipsilateral hand. The cause is unknown and generally occurs sporadically although two sibships have been described. It occurs once in about 20,000 births, is more common in boys, and more often occurs on the right side. The defects are variable and include mild hypoplasia to complete absence of the pectoralis major muscle and nipple with variable syndactyly, camptodactyly, brachydactyly, or other abnormalities of the hand and, occasionally, the forearm. Ribs on the affected side may be hypoplastic or absent and the scapula may be elevated. Breast tissue may be completely absent on the affected side with consequent poor breast development during puberty.

6.3.4.5. Congenital Pseudarthrosis of the Clavicle

Congenital pseudarthrosis represents an anomaly in which the medial and lateral ends of the clavicle are not connected. It is almost always on the right and is thought to result from embryologic impingement on developing structures by a superiorly displaced subclavian artery. If you see one on the left, think dextrocardia. Cosmetic, rather

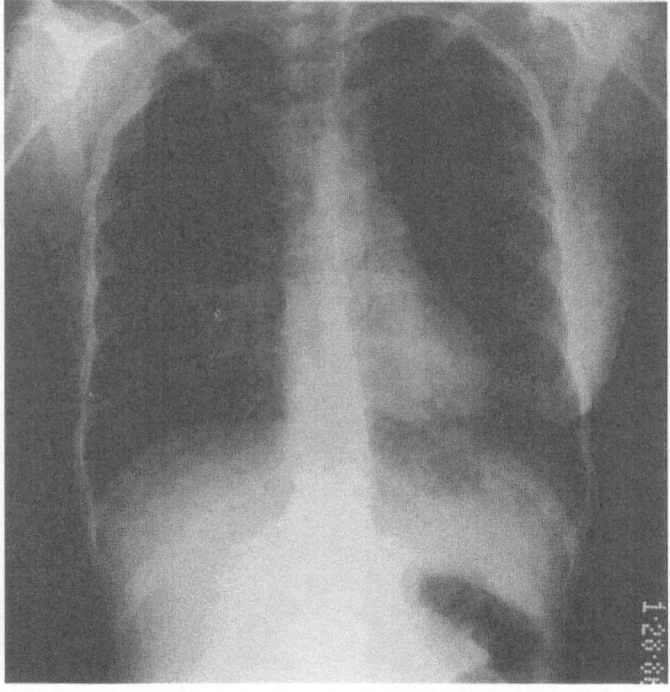

Figure 6.25. Poland syndrome on the right in this adolescent female; also known as the pectoral aplasia dysdactyly syndrome. Note increased lucency of right lung field and absent right breast.

than functional, problems result and manifest themselves by truncal asymmetry and fullness of the neck on the affected side. Cervical ribs and congenital coxa vara may occasionally be associated. Early bone grafting with plate fixation must be performed early (between 3 and 6 years) to reduce asymmetrical shoulder growth and neck line. Neonatal fractures of the clavicle and cleidocranial dysplasia can mimic congenital pseudarthrosis.

6.3.4.6. Madelung Deformity

This is an uncommon deformity of the forearm caused by an abnormality in the growth of the distal radial epiphysis with resulting shortening and bowing of the radius and carpal dislocation. The distal end of the radius and ulna override the wrist bones, producing an inverted fork appearance at the juncture of the wrist and hand. Though radiographic changes may be apparent early in childhood, clinical manifestations of deformity and restricted range of motion do not become apparent until preadolescence.

Most often the cause is unknown. It may be transmitted as an autosomal dominant disorder (dyschondrosteosis of Leri and Weill) and is often associated with other osseous abnormalities including cervical ribs and scoliosis and with other syndromes such as Turner syndrome.

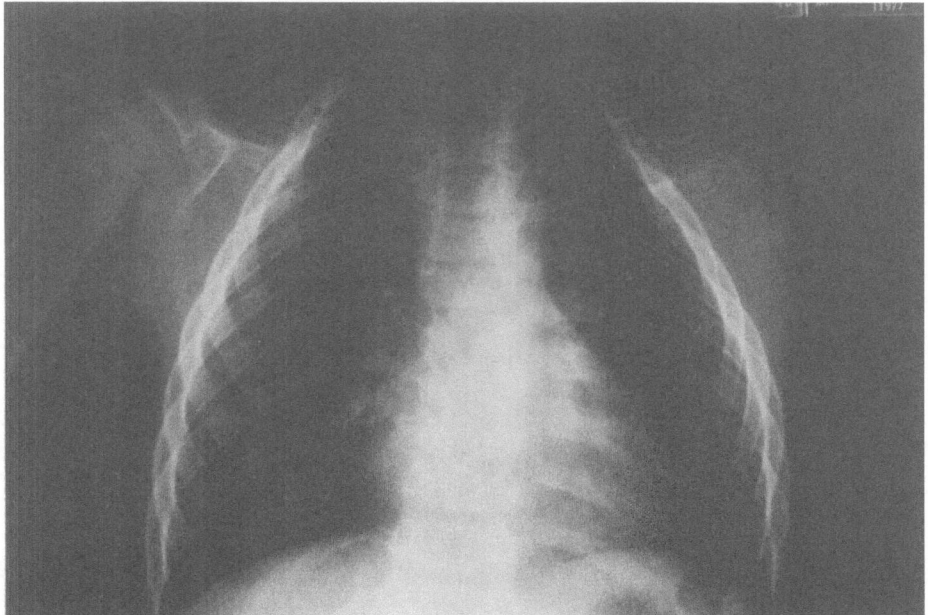

Figure 6.26. Cleidocranial dysplasia is a generalized dysplasia affecting membranous bone formation, including hypoplasia and ossification delays of the clavicles, pelvic bones, skull, and scapulae. Ligamentous laxity and dental abnormalities are often commonly associated. Note absence of clavicles.

6.3.5. Generalized Skeletal Defects

6.3.5.1. Arthrogryposis

Arthrogryposis refers to a group of diseases all of which are characterized by immobile joints at birth (actually, the term *arthrogryposis* means curved joints). When present in its most common, generalized form, it is also known as amyoplasia congenita or arthrogryposis multiplex congenita. It occurs at a rate of about 1 per 3000 live births. A variety of other diseases in which arthrogrypotic joints are a feature are generally excluded from this categorization since a more specific etiologic label can be applied.

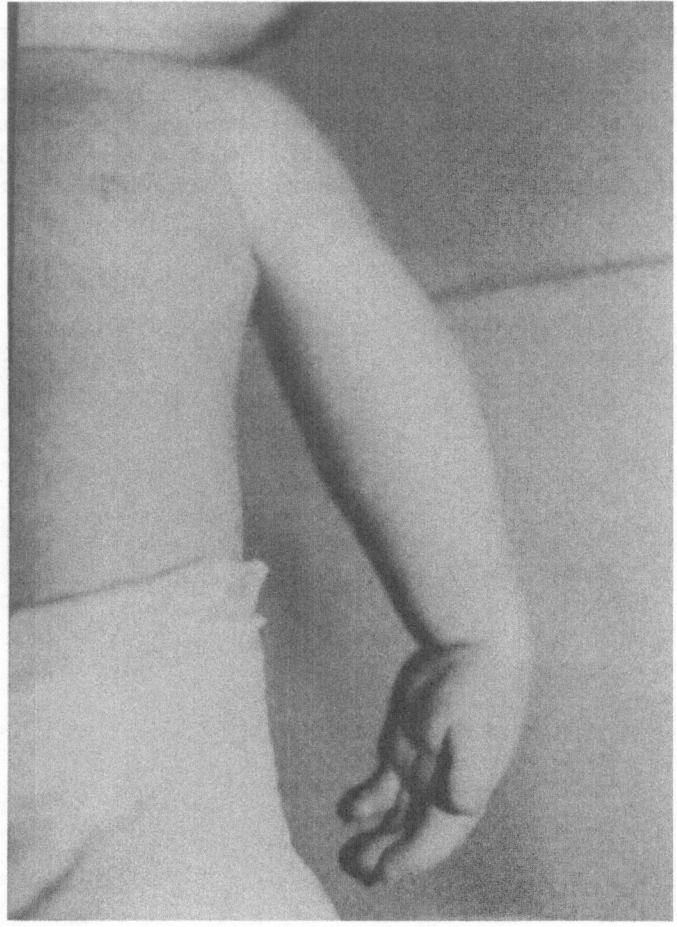

Figure 6.27. Typical "tubelike" arm of a child with arthrogryposis. Note the lack of elbow flexion crease.

These include Potter syndrome, meningomyelocele, diastrophic dwarfism, and congenital muscular dystrophy, to name but a few.

Etiologically, arthrogryposis usually occurs sporadically and probably includes a variety of fetal neurologic or myopathic processes which lead to decreased fetal movement, muscle atrophy, and tight soft-tissue contractures around each affected joint. The joints themselves are radiologically and pathologically normal. A neurogenic basis for arthrogryposis has been demonstrated by finding spinal cord atrophy and decreased number of anterior horn cells in some affected children.

Muscles or muscle fibers tend to be affected in an unpredictable but segmental fashion with one muscle demonstrating dramatic atrophy and fibrous replacement and another, close by, virtually normal. Clinically, infants with arthrogryposis are born with smooth, tubelike extremities, lacking flexion creases. They exhibit rigid joints with marked muscle atrophy, clubfoot deformities, dislocated hips, elbows locked in extension, wrists in flexion, and shoulders internally rotated. Webbing across flexion deformities (pterygia) is common as are dimples over extremity joints. Knee position tends to be somewhat variable. Four-limb involvement is most common, two-limb involvement is next most common, and isolated unilateral disease occurs least often. A history of breech delivery is frequent.

Intelligence and sensory function are most often normal. Other congenital anomalies occurring in some, but by no means all children, include micrognathia, cleft palate, low-set ears, short neck, congenital heart disease, high-arched palate, hypoplastic lungs, hernias, midline capillary hemangiomas, and cryptorchidism.

Other orthopedic associations include scoliosis, scapular maldescent (Sprengel deformity), and thin, immobile, and atrophic fingers. Dysphagia and swallowing problems may lead to aspiration, and chronic pulmonary problems.

Different from generalized arthrogryposis is a somewhat more stereotypical disease affecting hands and feet only. Termed the *distal arthrogryposis syndrome*, these children manifest tightly clenched fists with overlapping fingers (the trisomy 18 position), clubfoot abnormalities, and an autosomally dominant mode of inheritance. Treatment includes physical therapy and splinting as well as soft tissue releases and tendon transfers. Early referral to a pediatric orthopedic surgeon is important.

6.3.5.2. Early Amnion Disruption Sequence

The early amnion disruption sequence is known by a variety of other names, including *Streeter amniotic band syndrome*. It represents the result of fetal deformation or disruption rather than true malformation. Included are a broad range of transverse distal amputations, with no two affected children exactly the same. The middle three digits of the upper extremities are most commonly involved, exhibiting a range of defects from soft-tissue indentation to complete amputation. If the distal portion of the digit or extremity is present, lymphedema may be severe and neurologic compromise may be present as well. Other associated defects include terminal syndactyly, brachydactyly, symphalangism, clubfoot, cleft palate, abdominal wall closure problems, and cranial defects such as encephaloceles. As one might expect, involvement is usually

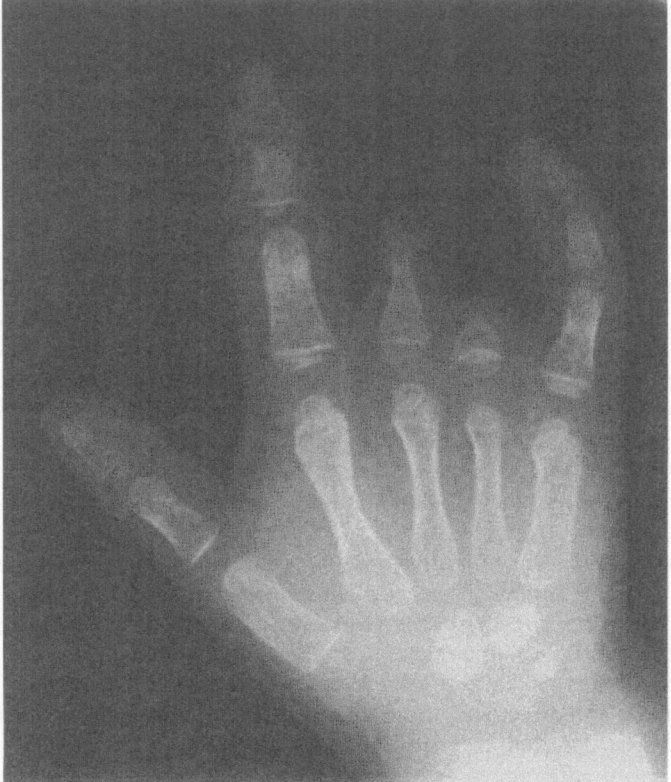

Figure 6.28. Typical congenital transverse amputations of middle digits associated with the early amnion disruption sequence (Streeter band or amniotic band syndrome).

asymmetrical. Incidence has been variably reported as ranging from 1 per 15,000 births to 1 in 2000.

Etiologically, these defects are generally thought to be related to early amniotic membrane rupture with amniotic tissue causing constriction or pressure on developing body parts or with sheets of amnion interfering with palatal or cranial development. Additionally, deformities may also result from fetal growth in a constrained space following the loss of the normal amniotic space. The reason for amniotic disruption is unknown although it is not a genetic condition and risk of recurrence is considered negligible.

Treatment is directed to the release of constricting bands, syndactyly repair, web-space lengthening, and other surgical remedies. Ultrasonic prenatal diagnosis is possible.

6.3.5.3. Neurofibromatosis

Neurofibromatosis, also called von Recklinghausen's disease, is the most common single-gene genetic disorder found in humans (1 in 3000) and is inherited as an autosomal dominant. Though many of its features result from abnormalities of neural crest cells, other manifestations of the disease are the result of dysplasia of embryonic mesoderm. The new mutation rate is high (25–50%) although some patients thought to represent new mutation in actuality have a minimally affected undiagnosed parent. Although penetrance is high (99%), expression is very variable, from scattered cutaneous lesions of no clinical significance to extremely deforming and sometimes fatal abnormalities. Features include multiple café-au-lait spots which are thought to be significant if more than five are present (or six, according to some authors), measuring more than 5 mm in diameter (or 1.5 cm, according to others). Also found are subcutaneous neurofibromas which may be lumpy, pedunculated, vascular, or plexiform as well as axillary freckling.

Somewhat fewer than half of patients with neurofibromatosis have recognizable manifestations of their disease within the first 2 months of life. Two-thirds of patients exhibit at least multiple café-au-lait spots by 1 year.

There are two distinct forms of neurofibromatosis, peripheral (NF-1) and central (NF-2). NF-1 occurs once in about 3000 live births and is characterized by café-au-lait macules and subcutaneous neurofibromas. NF-2 occurs much less frequently, about 1 in 50,000 live births. The NF-1 gene is on chromosome 17, the NF-2 gene on chromosome 22.

Affected children often have large heads (30%), and may have attentional deficit disorder, learning disabilities (40%), or mental retardation (5%). Pigmented hamartomatous nodules of the iris (Lisch nodules) are common. The tendency to develop tumors including acoustic neuromas, brain tumors, and optic gliomas, as well as nonlymphocytic leukemia, Wilms's tumor, and other visceral neoplasia has been well described.

After diagnosis, close follow-up is obviously important. Headache, rapidly growing head circumference, seizures, vomiting, or cranial nerve findings, including decreased vision or hearing, should prompt a search for central nervous system tumors.

Orthopedic manifestations are common and include scoliosis, pseudarthrosis of the tibia (and other long bones), rib fusion, dislocation of radius and ulna, local bony overgrowth (which is sometimes very disfiguring), bone cysts and other forms of osseous dysplasia, and hemihypertrophy.

The spine is abnormal in half of all patients. Though scoliosis is the most common abnormality, others include a peculiar scalloping of the vertebral bodies, cervical spine abnormalities, and spondylolisthesis. The cause of scoliosis in these patients is unknown. It is classically a sharply angulated thoracic curve which may be noted in early childhood and sometimes results in paraplegia as a result of cord entrapment. More typical "idiopathic" curves also occur at least as frequently as the more classical variety. Some of the children with cervical spine disease will present with dysphagia, torticollis, or a neck mass, and spine films are recommended for all children with NF who are to have spinal surgery or traction.

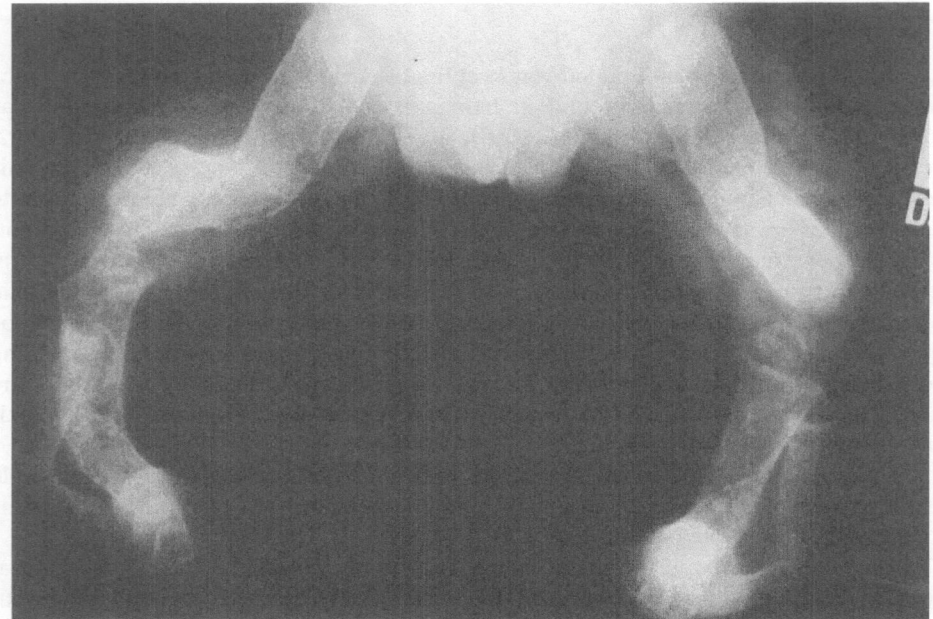

Figure 6.29. Osteogenesis imperfecta (OI) in a 3-year-old male with severe deformity and "ribbon-like" bones Radiographs like this one are usually associated with the "congenita" form of OI

The anterolateral tibial bowing or pseudarthrosis is usually manifest within the first 2 years of life and protection against fracture must be provided. Its cause is unknown. Bone grafting may be required (see Section 6.3.3.8). Leg-length discrepancies may require epiphysiodesis or other surgery.

6.3.5.4. Osteogenesis Imperfecta

Osteogenesis imperfecta is the result of a variety of defects in the production of type I collagen and is divided into four subtypes of which type I is most important. Type II is usually lethal in the perinatal period as a result of respiratory failure. Both types III and IV are rare. Type I patients are short with thin cortices, osteoporosis, and multiple long bone fractures, which occur most often between 2 and 3 years and during early adolescence. Skull radiographs reveal multiple small islands of bone, separated by sutures from each other, called *wormian bones* (the wiggly markings look like worms). Type I is an autosomally transmitted disease though it frequently represents a new gene mutation when, as often happens, the family history is negative.

Like other diseases with defects in collagen production, such as Ehlers–Danlos, patients with OI may exhibit hyperextensible joints, kyphoscoliosis, joint dislocation, bowed limbs, hernias, increased capillary fragility, thin skin, and scleras. The latter allows for choroidal pigment to show through, resulting in the characteristic blue scleras.

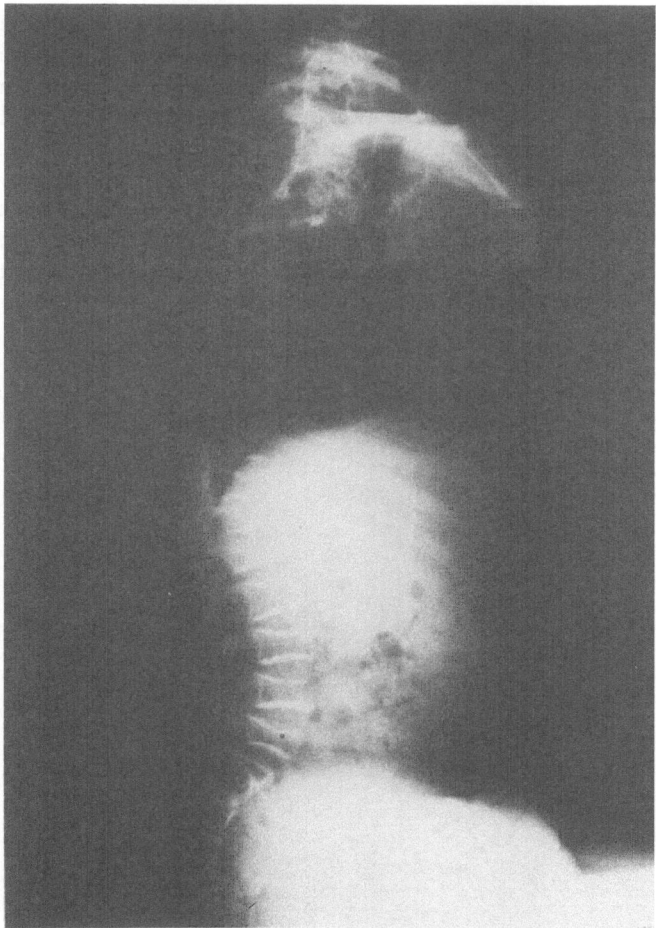

Figure 6.30. Lateral spine X-ray of a 3-year-old boy (not the same patient as Fig. 6.29) with osteogenesis imperfecta. Note biconcave compression of vertebral bodies. Scoliosis is common in OI as is short stature.

Deafness as a result of otosclerosis may make itself manifest in adult life. When dentinogenesis imperfecta is present, the patient is described as having type IB, when absent, IA.

Multiple fractures leading to deformity is the principal challenge and may require intramedullary rodding for support and to correct deformity.

6.3.5.5. Marfan Syndrome

Patients with Marfan syndrome are often tall with arachnodactyly and long, slim extremities (dolichostenomelia). The upper segment to lower segment ratio is decreased because the legs are long relative to the trunk (see Chapter 1). Identified now as caused by a defect in elastin (fibrillin), these patients exhibit scoliosis, joint hyperextensibility, striae, either pectus carinatum or excavatum, and hernias. Functionally important is the high frequency (80%) of upward dislocation of the lens. Survival is often limited by the serious cardiovascular problems, most prominently aortic dilatation and dissection, but also including mitral valve prolapse and other valvular insufficiencies. Though inherited as an autosomal dominant, there is considerable variability in clinical features and often a definite family history of disease is not present as an aid to diagnosis. When confronted with a tallish child (for their family background) who has scoliosis, thin extremities, and arachnodactyly, the question of Marfan syndrome should be raised. Echocardiography

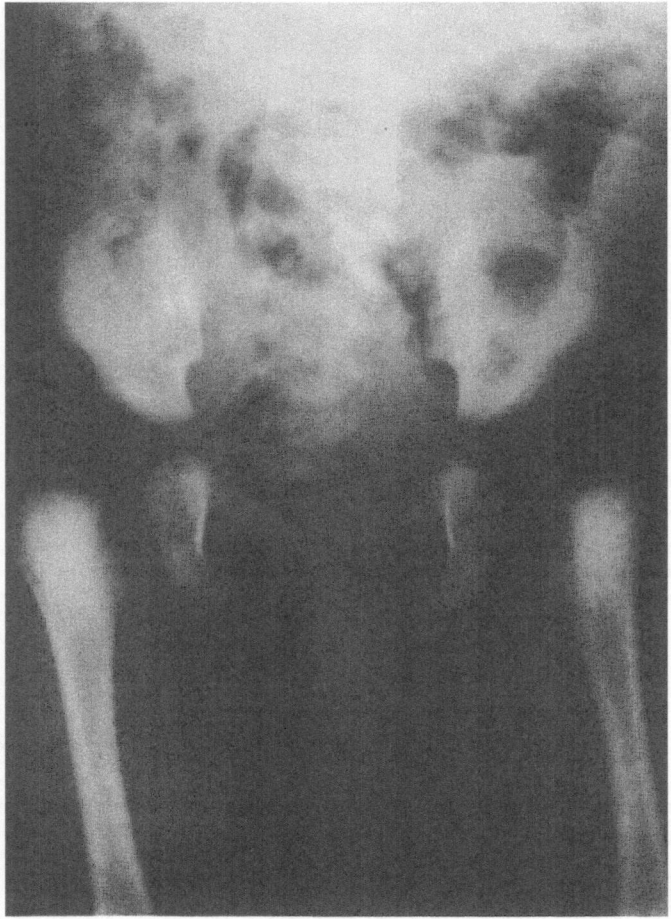

Figure 6.31. Bilateral dislocated hips in an infant with Larsen syndrome. This is the same child who later developed severe cervical kyphosis and progressive quadriparesis (see Fig. 5 5).

and a slit lamp exam should be considered, particularly if the midsystolic click and murmur of mitral valve prolapse is present. Additionally, both parents and siblings should be examined whenever possible.

6.3.5.6. Larsen Syndrome

Larsen and associates described six children with multiple dislocation of elbows, hips, knees, and wrists in 1950. Affected children additionally often exhibit clubfoot deformities, short metacarpals, tubular phalangeal bones, and other orthopedic abnormalities Cleft palate and congenital heart disease may be present as well. Cervical spine dislocations with cord compression may occur as the cervical vertebral bodies are small and misshapen. Both autosomal dominant and recessive modes of inheritance have been described. Treatment is primarily orthopedic.

6.3.5.7. Multiple Exostoses

Affected children demonstrate bony outgrowths, mostly at the metaphyses of long bones, resulting in deformity, asymmetrical long bone growth, disordered joint function, and reduced stature in some individuals. The exostoses are often noticed in early

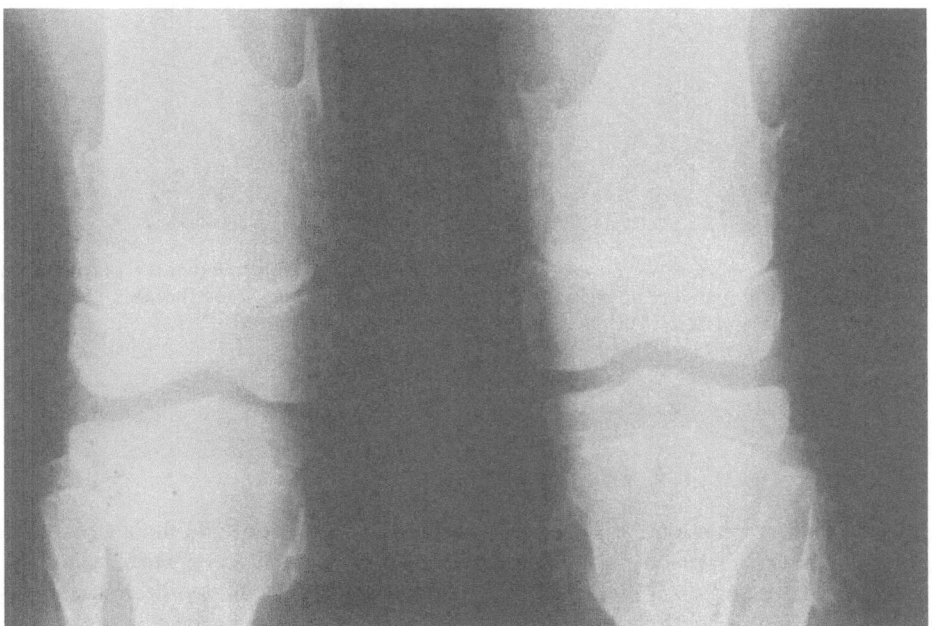

Figure 6.32. Multiple exostoses, also known as osteochondromas, in typical metaphyseal location near rapidly growing bones

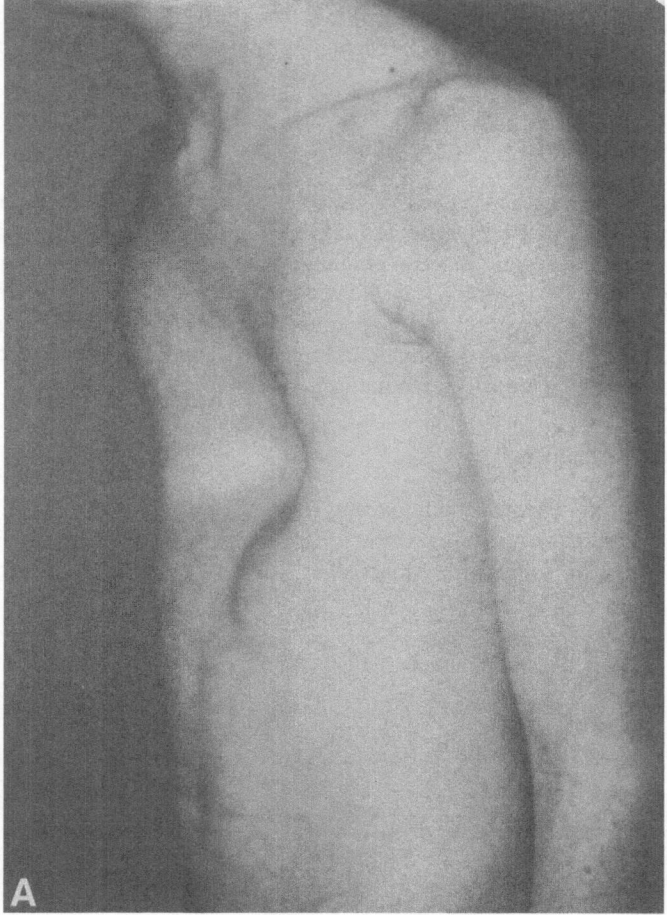

Figure 6.33. (A) Significant pectus excavatum is hard to define objectively. Like pornography, however, one usually knows it when one sees it. Most people would agree that this young man should probably be repaired. (B) Pectus carinatum.

childhood and will continue to increase in number and size until adulthood. Sarcomas developing from such lesions have been described with incidences between 2 and 10%.

Multiple exostoses is inherited as an autosomal dominant. One syndrome, Langer–Giedion, is associated with multiple exostoses though most patients have their exostoses as an isolated problem. Treatment is surgical and is directed toward removal of large lesions causing pain, limitation of movement, or deformity.

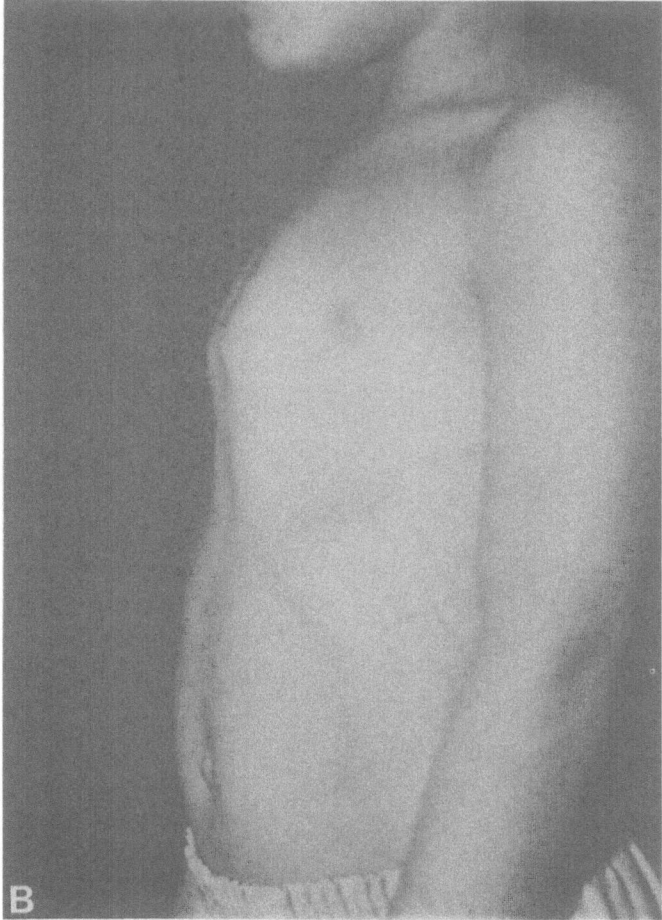

Figure 6.33. (*Continued*)

6.3.5.8. Pectus Excavatum and Carinatum

Pectus excavatum, when significant, represents a cosmetic and physiologic problem for the affected child. Cardiac function has been shown to be affected, with improvement after surgery (Beiser *et al.*, 1972). Defining what is significant, however, is the problem. In general, 2-cm depressions or greater are significant. Repair, when it is to be done, is best planned between 5 and 12 years. Occasionally, pectus excavatum is found associated with metaphyseal chondrodysplasia.

Pectus carinatum, on the other hand, is of purely cosmetic significance. Spondylo-epiphyseal dysplasia can cause this deformity though it is easy to spot considering the other manifestations of the disease.

7

Abnormalities of Skeletal Growth

7.1. INTRODUCTION

Perhaps including a chapter on growth in a book such as this one on pediatric orthopedics is a bit odd. Abnormal longitudinal growth, however, is a common complaint brought to the primary care provider and, at its most basic level, represents a major deficiency in skeletal function.

Ferreting out causes of overgrowth or undergrowth is important because such abnormalities of growth may be a major manifestation of systemic disease important in its own right. Marfan's syndrome and hypothyroidism are two such problems from opposite sides of the coin which come to mind. Additionally, the growth problem itself may represent a major problem for the child to deal with, regardless of cause.

7.2. MEASURING

Care must be taken in the measurement of children in the office if useful information is to be generated. This is true not only when the family presents worried about their child's growth, but should also be true when routine measurements are taken as part of regular preventive care. These should occur when the child is 2, 4, 6, 9, 12, 15, 18, and 24 months of age and yearly thereafter through adolescence.

Below 2 years of age, length measurements should be taken with the child supine, preferably on a measuring board made for the purpose. The child should be stretched comfortably to their full length with the soles of the feet perpendicular to the surface of the measuring table. An imaginary line from the lateral canthus through the external auditory meatus should also run perpendicular to the table with the length measured with the assistance of a right angle applied to the crown. Children older than 2 years should be measured upright with heels, buttocks, and occiput against a wall and height determined, as above, with one edge of a right-angled board applied to the crown and the other side held against the wall. Measurements should always be made with the patient shoeless and should be plotted on appropriate growth charts.

Significant growth problems can be reflected by a single point which is distinctly abnormal or a rate of growth which diverges significantly from the expectable rate. Growth abnormalities are most easy to evaluate if more than one measurement is available. This is often not possible, however. When only one point is available, for a growth problem to be considered, it should be significantly below the 5th or above the 95th percentile. As a rough rule of thumb, growth *deficiency* should be evaluated if a child's height age is more than 2 years below the child's chronological age. The height age is the age at which this child's height lies at the 50th percentile.

With two points on a curve available, growth velocity can be determined and compared with expectable norms on growth *velocity* charts. If such charts are not available, comparing actual growth rate with the expected rate using routine growth charts usually suffices. Regardless, children growing less than 3 cm per year between 3 and 13 years of age need to be investigated further.

Consideration in borderline cases should be given to the heights of the child's parents. Even a child at the 5th percentile and therefore theoretically "normal" may be exhibiting growth deficiency if both parents are at the 95th percentile for their heights. Statistically, the child's percentile extrapolated to his adult height should be between plus or minus 9 cm of the mean of the parents' percentiles. Another way of saying this is that a child at the 3rd percentile for height for his age has a normal height only if the mean parental height is less than 164 cm (about 5 feet 4 inches).

7.3. SHORT STATURE

Poor longitudinal growth may reflect psychosocial deprivation, serious systemic disease, endocrinologic deficiency, or primary dysplasia of bone. Many causes are remediable and more may be so in the future now that growth hormone is more available and the indications for its use are broadening. Regardless of cause, short stature is a burden that may be associated with significant psychological challenges for the individual and, as such, requires our attention to identification, diagnosis, and treatment.

7.3.1. Constitutionally Delayed Growth

Of course not everyone whose growth is below the third percentile has a problem. One pattern of normal growth which will often cause parental concern is that of constitutionally delayed growth, involving infants whose birth weight and early growth are solidly within the normal range but who then manifest slowing growth velocity. Bone age is delayed, though not severely so, and is consistent with height age. These children are never dramatically short, enter puberty late, and achieve, eventually, normal height. There is often a family history of normal height and delayed puberty.

7.3.2. Familial Short Stature

Because the distribution of height is a normal biological one in populations, the vast majority of children below the third percentile for height will be there because of their genes, not because they have a problem. These "physiologically small" children are never severely small. They are somewhat small at birth and will often have a family history of short stature. Their growth velocity will be normal throughout and their bone age will be equal to their chronologic age, not their height age.

Having said this, it's important to remember that there are some pathological causes for short stature which run in families though these are most often associated with more substantially deficient growth or other stigmata of genetic disease or both.

Some children seem to manifest both of the patterns described above, resulting in severe "physiological" growth deficiency unassociated with apparent endocrinopathy, systemic disease, or any other appropriate explanation. It is this group of children, at the border between physiology and pathology, who are currently the subjects of several trials regarding the efficacy of growth hormone for short children who are not, strictly speaking, growth hormone deficient.

7.3.3. Psychosocial Deprivation

Included here are all of the various situations which have an impact on the health, nutrition, safety, and well-being of the child. Both love and food are necessary for children to do well and a deficiency of either may result in poor growth. At its most severe and dramatic, psychosocial deprivation manifests itself in severe behavioral disturbances, including eating nonfood items or from garbage cans and drinking from

Table 7.1. Constitutionally Delayed Growth

Normal birth weight	Normal height expected
Growth problems not severe	Bone age delayed
Normal height in family	Bone age roughly equal to height age
Late puberty in patient	Slowed velocity of growth early on
Late puberty in family	

Table 7.2. Familial Short Stature

Growth problems not severe	Normal bone age
Small at birth	Puberty not delayed
Family members short	Short as adult
Normal growth velocity	

toilet bowls. More common and mundane, though no less serious, are such forms of family disorganization as results from parental drug addiction, alcoholism, mental illness, mental retardation, or other types of social dystrophy. Often children fail to thrive less from lack of emotional sustenance, love, and affection as from simple lack of appropriate calorie intake resulting from poverty or ignorance. Millions of children worldwide, and not only in the developing world by any means, are stunted not because their parents won't take care of them but simply because they can't.

7.3.4. Endocrine Causes for Growth Failure

There are three major endocrine causes for growth deficiency. Though less common than psychosocial deprivation or physiological causes for short stature, they are not uncommon and need to be specifically excluded when evaluating any child with short stature.

7.3.4.1. Hypothyroidism

Lack of thyroid hormone can be divided into congenital and acquired categories.

7.3.4.1a. Congenital Hypothyroidism. The most common type of congenital hypothyroidism results from either agenesis or hypoplasia of the gland. This occurs roughly once in every 4000 live births, is more common among girls, is not genetic, and results in low thyroxine levels and high levels of thyroid-stimulating hormone (TSH).

Occasionally (about 10% of the total), children will have a hypoplastic gland, with enough functional tissue present at birth to allow for normal thyroxine levels, though most often with high TSH levels.

Also in about 10% of children with congenital hypothyroidism, there exists a *biochemical* defect in the production of thyroxine. These defects are myriad and include such problems as decreased iodide trapping, defective organification or abnormalities in the metabolism of thyroglobulin, among others. As expected, there is often a goiter at birth and these defects are often inherited as autosomal recessive traits. As with an absent gland, TSH levels are elevated.

Congenital hypothyroidism may also be the result of maternal ingestion of goitrogens, including excessive amounts of iodide in the diet and medications like propylthiouracil, other drugs for maternal hyperthyroidism, radioactive iodine, or sulfonamides.

Rarely, congenital hypothyroidism results not from problems with the thyroid gland itself but with the pituitary, which produces TSH, or with the hypothalamus, which produces thyrotropin-releasing hormone, which stimulates the pituitary to produce TSH. These causes altogether represent a small minority of children with congenital hypothyroidism but are important because they result not only in low thyroxine levels but also in low TSH levels. Screening programs which rely solely on high levels of TSH to identify infants with hypothyroidism will therefore miss these children.

Typically, children with congenital hypothyroidism will variably exhibit the symptoms listed in Table 7.3. In the days before screening programs, many of these children suffered permanent central nervous system damage before the diagnosis was made because the signs and symptoms are easy to miss and the clinical picture is often incomplete. Things are better now though occasionally infants with hypothyroidism are missed on the newborn screen and subsequently incur significant permanent damage before someone tumbles to the diagnosis. It is wise never to assume that an infant with growth failure doesn't have congenital hypothyroidism only because they have a negative screen. Serum thyroxine and TSH levels will answer the question, but the question has to be raised.

7.3.4.1b. Acquired Hypothyroidism. Acquired thyroid deficiency is less likely to result in permanent CNS residua but no less likely to cause longitudinal growth failure and should certainly be included in the differential diagnosis of the older infant or child who is having trouble growing.

Specific causes include autoimmune (Hashimoto's or lymphocytic) thyroiditis, incomplete genetic metabolic defects as described above, dysgenetic or ectopic glands which function adequately initially but which the infant "outgrows" over time, pituitary or hypothalamic disease as a result of meningitis, trauma, or CNS tumors, exposure to goitrogens such as lithium or iodide-containing drugs, and dietary iodine deficiency which is rare in this country now that salt is supplemented with iodine. Acquired hypothyroidism is also more common than expected in such chromosomal aneuploidy syndromes as those of Turner, Down, and Klinefelter, in Noonan syndrome, and in cystinosis.

Acquired hypothyroidism should be considered in the child whose growth velocity diverges significantly from the norm or in the child whose height is significantly deficient, meaning height age more than 2 years below chronologic age. Symptoms of acquired hypothyroidism include muscle weakness, constipation, lethargy, and cold intolerance. Myxedema and muscle weakness may be apparent on examination as might

Table 7.3. Congenital Hypothyroidism

Prolonged jaundice	Hypotonia	Coarse facies
Hypothermia	Umbilical hernia	Growth failure
Enlarged fontanels	Constipation	Puffy face
Poor feeding	Bradycardia	Puffy extremities
Big tongue	Cool extremities	Big heart on X-ray
Hoarse cry	Lethargy	

paradoxical precocious puberty. Anemia is common and the delay in bone age is equal to or greater than the retardation in linear growth. The thyroxine level will be low and the TSH high, unless the pituitary–hypothalamic axis is disturbed.

7.3.4.2. Cushing Syndrome

Hypercorticalism has a profound effect on longitudinal growth in children and should be considered in the short child who manifests the other symptoms or signs of excessive adrenal steroid production, including hypertension, truncal obesity, hirsutism, moon facies, purple striae, hypogonadism, muscular weakness, excessive bruising, or such laboratory abnormalities as hyperglycemia, osteoporosis, or decreased bone age. It should be noted that distinguishing the short child with hypercorticalism from the exogenously obese child is usually easy because the latter children are almost always *tall* for their age rather than growth deficient.

These signs and symptoms result from several pathogenetic mechanisms which include benign or malignant adrenal tumors, excessive ACTH production related to abnormalities of the pituitary–hypothalamic axis (Cushing's disease), or iatrogenic exogenous corticosteroids or ACTH prescribed for arthritis, asthma, seizures, or a variety of other chronic illnesses.

Steroids affect growth by interfering with growth hormone production and/or insulinlike growth factor 1 (IGF-1; somatomedin C) action. The exact mechanism of poor growth may be different for endogenous Cushing's compared with iatrogenic hypercorticalism.

7.3.4.3. Growth Hormone Deficiency

Growth hormone affects longitudinal growth through its ability to generate IGF-1, produced by the liver and available systemically, but also produced locally at the growth plate. Growth hormone production is stimulated by hypothalamic growth hormone-releasing hormone (GHRH) and is inhibited by somatostatin. The cyclic nature of growth hormone secretion is a result of the complicated interaction of these controlling hormones. Growth hormone deficiency is most often the result of failure of the pituitary to produce adequate amounts of growth hormone. This in turn may be caused by developmental defects of the pituitary (sometimes associated with optic nerve hypoplasia, cleft palate, or other birth defects), tumors such as craniopharyngioma, or damage to the pituitary or hypothalamus from perinatal asphyxia or traumatic injury. Familial growth hormone deficiency of unknown cause has also been described.

Some children with severe deprivation and resulting dwarfism will manifest decreased growth hormone production after provocative testing and low IGF-1 levels, both of which return to normal after psychosocial rehabilitation.

Additionally, a variety of more rare defects in growth hormone function have also been described, including the production of biologically inactive growth hormone, deficiencies of growth hormone receptors, or other defects which interfere with the ability of growth hormone to generate IGF-1. Included here are Laron dwarfism, African pygmies, and endemic short stature in one group of indigenous residents of Ecuador.

IGF-1 levels will be low in these conditions in the face of normal or high growth hormone levels as opposed to both low growth hormone and IGF-1 levels in the usual forms of growth hormone deficiency

Children with growth hormone deficiency will often exhibit a decreased rate of growth from birth, and will be short and plump with round, immature faces Boys will exhibit small genitalia A history of breech delivery is often obtained Signs, symptoms, or laboratory evidence of panhypopituitarism may be apparent

Growth hormone deficiency should be considered when evaluating the short child with poor growth velocity. Growth greater than 5 cm per year virtually rules out growth hormone deficiency Diagnosing growth hormone deficiency is difficult and usually requires obtaining levels after pituitary stimulation It should be done by an endocrinologist experienced in the evaluation of children with growth deficiency

7.3.5. Chronic Illness and Malnutrition

Chronic disease is a common cause for growth failure in children Mechanisms may be different for each disease but involve some combination of poor growth resulting from decreased calorie intake and direct metabolic effects of the disease itself Examples of the latter include the hypoxemia of cyanotic congenital heart disease and the acidosis of renal tubular acidosis Initially wasted, these children will subsequently become both thin and short as compensatory mechanisms come into play to preserve what caloric energies are available for biologic processes even more important than growth As in children with chronic malnutrition from the developing world, children with growth failure secondary to chronic illness have been described as exhibiting lower than expectable levels of IGF-1 Exogenous growth hormone therapy has been described as improving longitudinal growth in several chronic illnesses, including renal disease and juvenile rheumatoid arthritis (juvenile chronic arthritis)

Common possibilities to be considered when evaluating a short child are included in Table 7 4 It has been well documented that growth failure as a result of chronic disease is relatively easy to diagnose with a thorough physical examination and a small number of routine laboratory examinations These include serum creatinine or BUN, electrolytes, complete blood count, ESR, urinalysis and culture, stool for ova and parasites, and tuberculin skin testing Exotic or intensive evaluations are not usually necessary nor are they particularly useful

Table 7.4. Chronic Illness and Growth Failure

Congenital or acquired heart disease	Juvenile rheumatoid arthritis
Cystic fibrosis or other chronic pulmonary disease	Other collagen vascular diseases
Renal failure, renal tubular acidosis	Inflammatory bowel disease
Chronic central nervous system disease	Malabsorptive syndromes
Chronic or recurrent urinary tract infections	Chronic liver disease
Tuberculosis	Depression or other psychiatric disease
Intestinal parasitosis	

7.3.6. Intrauterine Growth Retardation

The vast majority of infants who are born small are of not much greater risk than any baby of growing up to be short. This is certainly so for premature infants who are otherwise healthy. It is not so, however, for infants who are born after a period of intrauterine growth retardation (IUGR) and are thereby small for gestational age (SGA), defined for full-term babies as weighing less than 2500 g. Such infants are at particular risk for developing growth and neurodevelopmental problems as they get older. This is particularly so for infants whose intrauterine problem affected them for more than just the third trimester. Such infants are born quite short and their weight for height ratio may approach the norm. The potential for catch-up growth is limited to a greater degree than for those infants whose problems began relatively later in gestation. Such latter infants will paradoxically look worse at birth, thin and scrawny-looking with decreased subcutaneous tissue. Their height will be relatively better preserved, however, as will their head circumference and their potential for later normal growth and development.

Intrauterine growth may be affected by any one or more of a large number of pathological processes. They include any cause for placental insufficiency, including pregnancy-induced hypertension, toxemia, or diabetes mellitus predating pregnancy. Such mechanical types of placental insufficiency as thrombosis, placental infarction, or chronic abruption might be included here as well as any other process interfering with the efficient delivery of oxygen and nutrition to the developing fetus. These would include maternal malnutrition, high-altitude living, maternal cyanotic heart disease, and the placental steal syndrome which results when twin fetuses share one chorionic membrane with asymmetrical blood flow to one fetus at the expense of the other.

A toxic or infected intrauterine environment will also affect fetal growth. Maternal drug addiction including cigarette smoking, alcohol use, cocaine or amphetamine use, or narcotic addiction have all been implicated. Such prescribed drugs as phenytoin, warfarin, trimethadione, and folate antagonists have all been described as resulting in intrauterine growth problems as has radiation exposure during pregnancy. Intrauterine infections, including toxoplasmosis, rubella, cytomegalovirus, and syphilis, have also been well-associated with fetal growth deficiency. Intrauterine growth failure also occurs in pregnant women with untreated renal failure and in women who have phenylketonuria and who are not on a low-phenylalanine diet during pregnancy and before conception occurs.

Children with multiple congenital anomaly syndromes, including those caused by

Table 7.5. Intrauterine Growth Retardation

Placental insufficiency	Toxic environment
Toxemia	Cigarettes, alcohol, other drugs
Hypertension	Phenytoin, radiation
Diabetes mellitus	Congenital infection
Placental abruption	Maternal phenylketonuria
Maternal malnutrition	Maternal renal disease
Twins	Congenital anomaly syndromes
High altitude	

single gene defects or chromosomal abnormalities, are prone to low birth weight and will be discussed below.

7.3.7. Syndromic Causes for Growth Failure

Below is grouped a miscellany of other causes for poor longitudinal growth, together because they all manifest individual patterns of anomalies that affect not only skeletal growth but other organ systems as well. They include syndromes related to specific chromosomal abnormalities.

Children with Down syndrome are short but represent little difficulty in diagnosis. Their well-described stigmata will not be reviewed here and the reader is referred to standard texts for a description of the clinical presentation. Often, however, children with Down syndrome as well as other multiple congenital syndromes will have more than one reason for being short. Growth charts for children with Down syndrome are available and should be referred to. Unexpected deviation should in these children lead to attempts to discover if other pathology, such as hypothyroidism, is playing a role.

Turner syndrome is not only relatively common (about 1 in every 3000 girls) among all types of chromosomal aneuploidy but also causes significant growth difficulties and can be helped appreciably with treatment. The clinical manifestations present at birth, including peripheral edema, shieldlike chest with widely spaced nipples, prominent ears, high-arched palate, webbed neck with low hair line, short fourth metacarpal, increased carrying angle at the elbows, and hyperconvex nails, are often missed and continue to be overlooked until well into the teenage years when these children will present with primary amenorrhea or short stature made apparent by their classmates' pubertal growth spurts.

Earlier diagnosis will allow for more appropriate timing of estrogen replacement, growth hormone therapy, and improved growth potential. Because Turner's may be caused by a variety of chromosomal abnormalities other than XO, including ring chromosomes, isochromosomes, and deletions, buccal smears are inadequate to exclude the diagnosis and should be avoided in favor of formal karyotypes. As with Down syndrome, children with Turner syndrome are more likely than expected to be hypothyroid as well, most often as a result of autoimmune thyroid disease.

Other multiple congenital anomaly syndromes, either associated with chromosomal abnormalities or not, frequently manifest growth retardation as a cardinal sign. The list is long and includes the syndromes of Noonan, Aarskog, Bloom, Rubinstein–Taybi, Russell–Silver, and DeLange, among many others. Applying the precise label to these children is much less useful than knowing that a problem exists. A discussion of the details of each syndrome's anomalies is beyond the scope of this text. A careful physical examination performed on the child with short stature will identify those children with anomalies who need to be evaluated further by a geneticist. The combination of short stature with mental retardation, unusual facies, other birth defects, or a history of small size at birth should raise the possibility of a syndromic cause for the child's problems.

7.3.8. Bone Disease Causing Short Stature

Virtually all "primary" diseases of bone cause abnormal body proportions. Remember that under normal conditions the measured arm span is roughly equal to the child's height Since preschool children have slightly shorter limbs than adults, their arm spans will normally be 2 or 3 cm less than their heights The opposite is true for adolescents In virtually all of the causes for short stature described above, the normal relationship between height and arm span holds true, despite the shortness This does not hold true, however, when the short stature is a result of bone disease

In general, bone disease causes a disproportionate loss of extremity length relative to truncal height leading to arm spans significantly shorter than height, commonly termed short-limb or disproportionate dwarfism Good examples here include achondro-

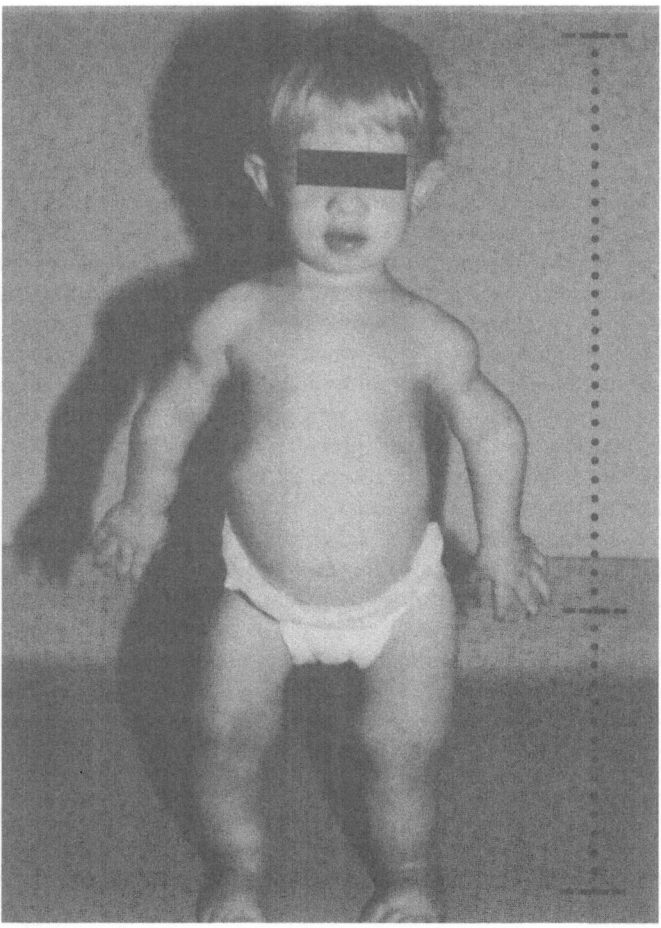

Figure 7.1. This little girl is short and was originally thought to have a metaphyseal chondrodysplasia Eventually she was found to have a very rare generalized enchondromatosis Regardless, she clearly has some kind of skeletal dysplasia, note increased upper segment–lower segment ratio, reflecting short-limb dwarfism

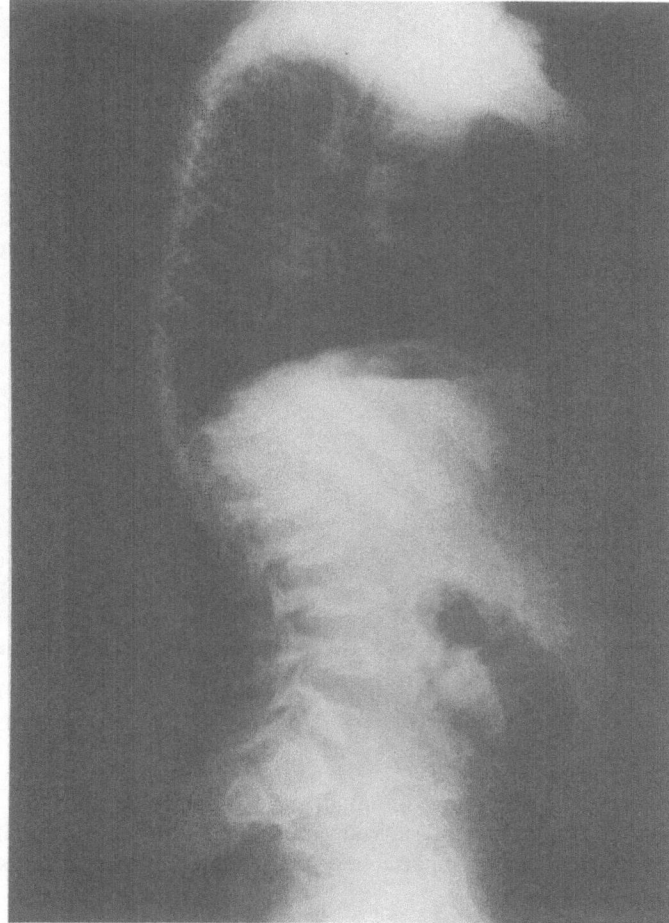

Figure 7.2. Children like this one with Morquio syndrome are short The platyspondyly (flattened vertebral bodies), however, causes a disproportionately short trunk and a decreased upper segment–lower segment ratio

plasia or metaphyseal chondrodysplasia. Occasionally, bone disease will affect spinal growth to a greater degree than extremity growth leading to an arm span greater than height, as occurs with spondyloepiphyseal dysplasia and several other skeletal dysplasias which affect the vertebral bodies.

The biochemical pathophysiology of many of these diseases is poorly understood and current classifications are based on clinical manifestations. Relevant to any discussion of growth failure related to constitutional bone disease are the osteochondrodysplasias. Included in this broad category are a widely varying group of diseases. Some have no spinal involvement (e.g., Ellis–van Creveld syndrome, metaphyseal chondro-

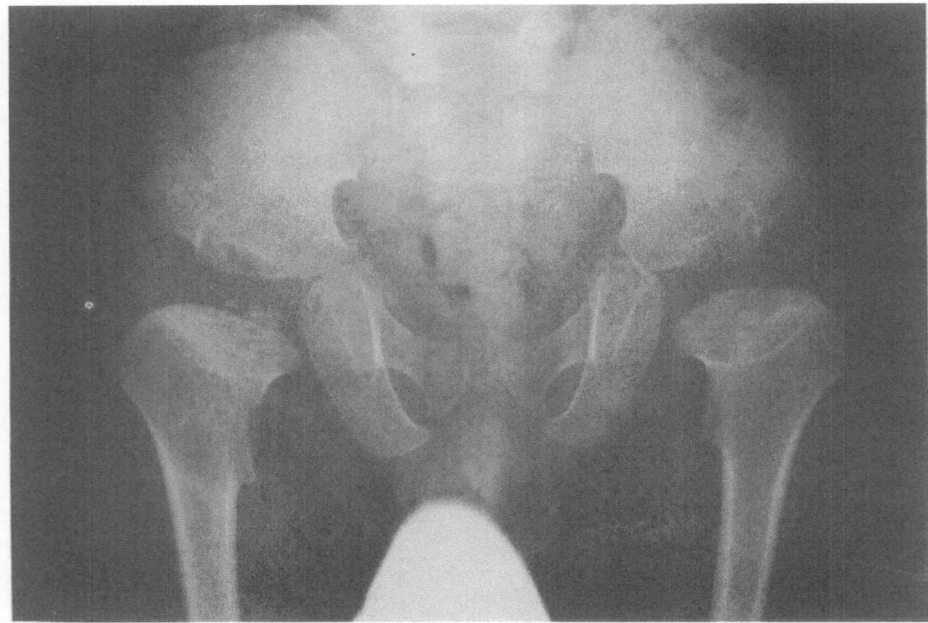

Figure 7.3. Spondyloepiphyseal dysplasıa ın a 4-year-old boy Note severely dysplastıc femoral heads, shallow and ırregular acetabula

dysplasia), some have considerable spinal disease (spondyloepiphyseal dysplasia, spondylometaphyseal dysplasia, Kniest syndrome), and some are potentially lethal ın the newborn period (osteogenesis imperfecta type II, Jeune's syndrome of asphyxiating thoracic dysplasia).

Most of the bone dysplasias have no known etiologic basis. Those with known causes include a varıety of defects of calcium and phosphate metabolism (like hypophosphatemic rickets), a variety of storage diseases (like Morquio syndrome, a mucopolysaccharidosis), and a variety of defects of collagen (as in osteogenesis imperfecta or some types of Ehlers–Danlos syndrome). Rickets is described in Chapter 4. Osteogenesis imperfecta is described in Chapter 6.

Storage diseases affecting bone include the mucopolysaccharidoses, the mucolipidoses, and the lipıdoses. They do not manifest themselves at birth but present at various times subsequently. Mucopolysaccharidoses are a family of diseases characterized by enzymatic deficiencies which lead to the storage of incompletely degraded glycosaminoglycans. Together with collagen, glycosaminoglycans are the stuff of which connective tissue is made. Short stature, progressive deformities, and skeletal dysplasia are major features. Additionally, all lead to impaired intellectual ability except for MPS IV (Morquio syndrome) and MPS VI (Moroteaux–Lamy). The mucolipidoses are similar though these patients are generally less severely affected. Gaucher disease is the only true lipid storage disease which manifests skeletal changes, which ıncludes

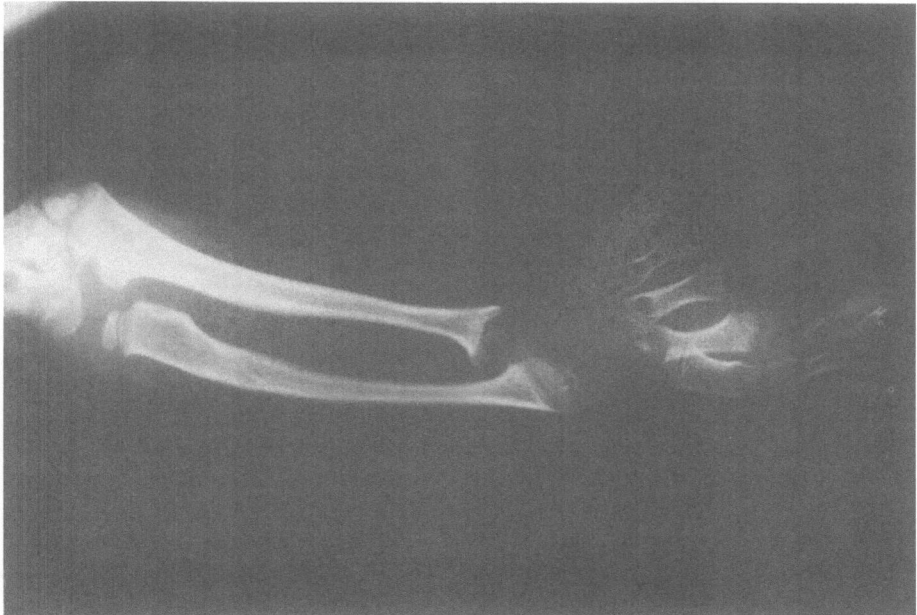

Figure 7.4. Morquio syndrome, one of the mucopolysaccharide storage diseases, causes shortening of the long bones, metaphyseal flaring, and fragmentation of the epiphyses.

pathological fractures, degenerative arthropathy, and osteitis. In general, only patients with the more mild form of adult Gaucher disease live long enough to manifest bone problems.

Diagnosis of any of the skeletal dysplasias depends on a low index of suspicion. Just as short stature and congenital anomalies beg the question of a multiple congenital anomaly syndrome (see above), the presence of short stature and impairment of body proportion, knee bowing, knock-knees, waddling gait, scoliosis, clubfeet, stooped posture, flat nasal bridge, or excessive lumbar lordosis should lead to a consideration of skeletal dysplasia.

X-rays would be a useful place to start, to include long bone films, hand, pelvis, and spine. Further evaluation, for storage disease or rickets, would then be based on abnormalities seen on radiography.

7.3.9. Diagnostic Approaches to the Short Child

An efficient evaluation of short children can be facilitated by asking and attempting to answer the following questions:

1. *Is the growth deficiency severe?* Severe growth deficiency may be functionally defined as a greater than 2-year spread between chronological age and height age and/or less than 3 cm of growth per year. Children with constitutional growth delay, genetic

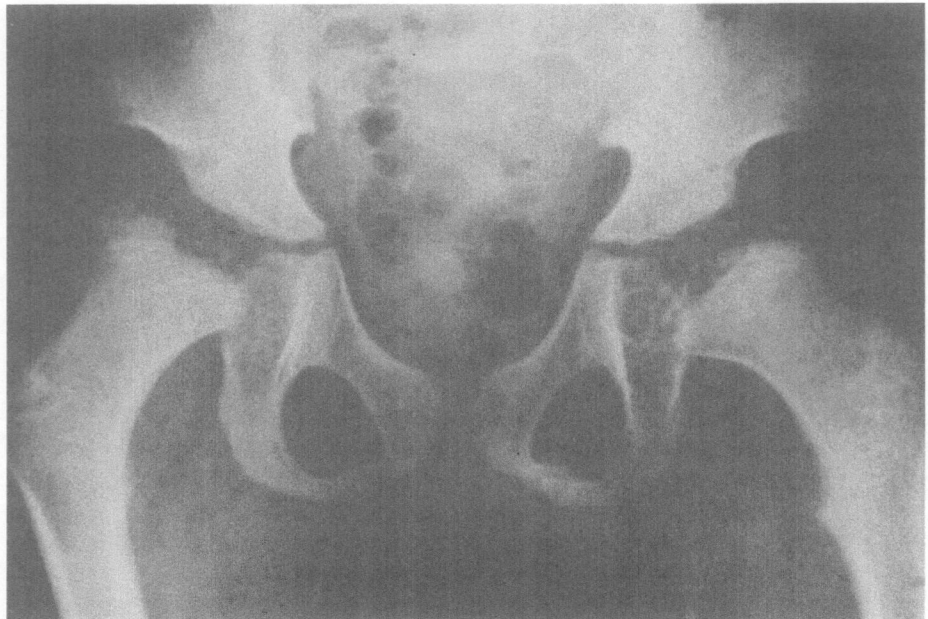

Figure 7.5. This AP view of the pelvis is of a young man with mucolipidosis type I Note irregularity, fragmentation, and failure of ossification of the femoral epiphyses The mucolipidoses clinically look like mucopolysaccharidoses but don't have excess mucopolysaccharide in their urine

short stature, mild forms of chronic illness, most forms of intrauterine growth retardation, many syndromes, and many skeletal dysplasias will exhibit less than severe growth deficiency.

2. *Is the history and physical exam normal?* Is there any evidence for neglect, chronic illness, malnutrition, multiple congenital anomalies, or dysplastic bone disease (genu varum or valgum, waddling gait, scoliosis, clubfeet, flat nasal bridge, excessive lumbar lordosis)?

3. *Are the screening labs normal?* If the evaluation is unrewarding to this point, perform the simple laboratory tests described above to rule out chronic illness or infection.

4. *Are thyroid studies normal?* If the growth deficiency is significant or signs or symptoms of hypothyroidism are present, thyroid studies should be performed. A much lower index of suspicion for hypothyroidism should guide the evaluation of growth problems in infants because of the disastrous effects of thyroid deficiency on the developing nervous system and the subtlety of the clinical manifestations.

5. *Is growth deficiency unexplained and significant or persistent?* If the height is not severely impaired and the initial evaluation is unrevealing, careful height measurements can be obtained periodically and the child can be followed for 6 months to obtain an accurate height velocity. Growth greater than 5 cm per year rules out an endocrine

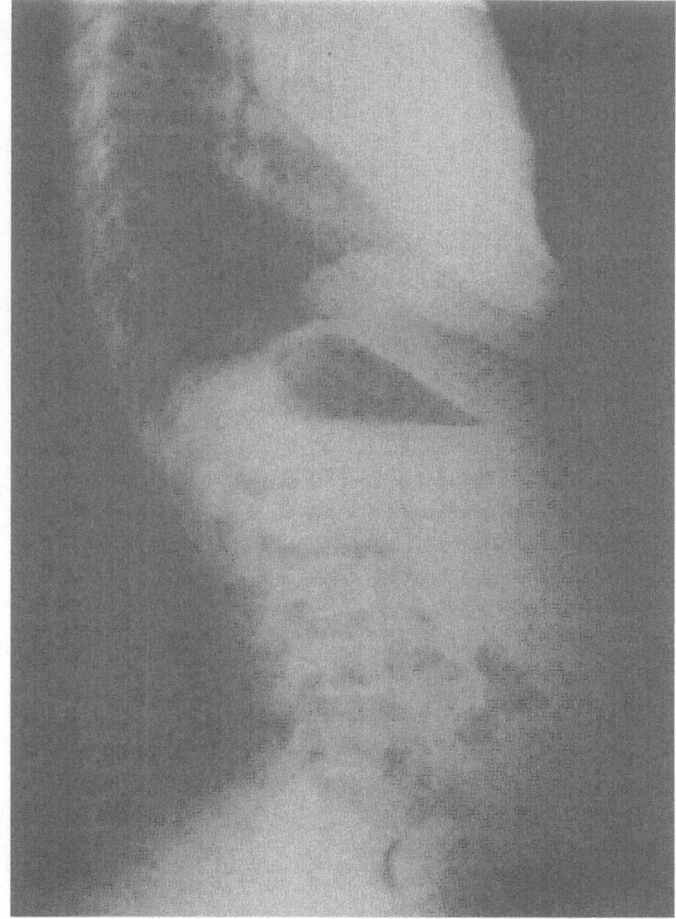

Figure 7.6. This 7-year-old female has achondroplasia Note excessive lumbar lordosis

disorder. Significant or persistent growth problems without an explanation require referral to someone experienced in the evaluation of childhood growth disorders, perhaps a pediatric endocrinologist.

7.4. THE TALL CHILD

Excessive growth only rarely is severe enough to cause concern and result in a visit to the physician. The concerns expressed are most often focused on self-image though occasionally the excessive stature will result from disease entities important in their own right.

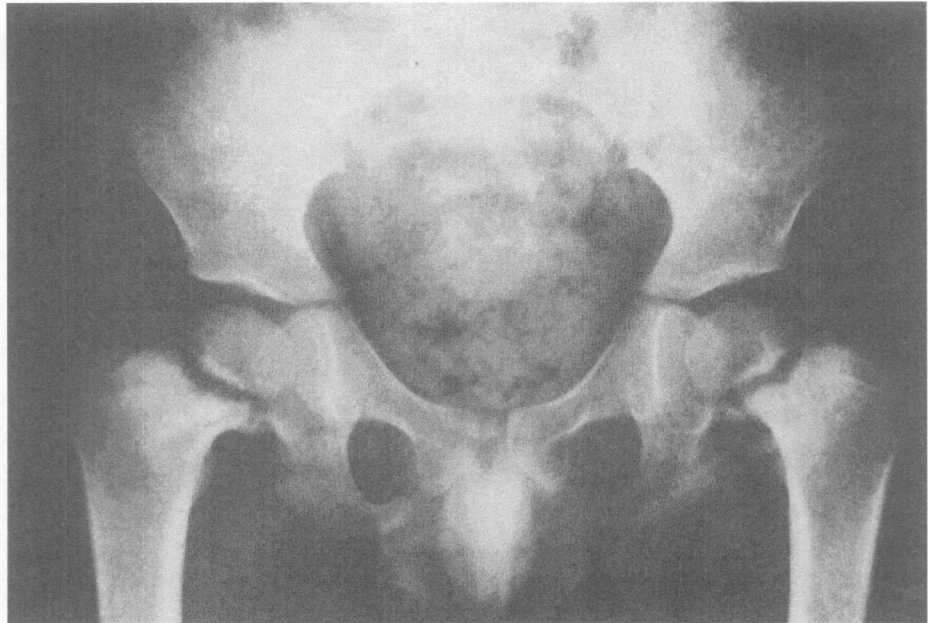

Figure 7.7. Metaphyseal chondrodysplasia in a 10-year-old boy. Note coxa vara and fragmentation of inferior and medial portion of metaphyses

The most common cause for large children is large parents. Other, much less common, causes include Marfan's syndrome, homocystinuria, Soto's syndrome or cerebral gigantism, hyperpituitarism, and a variety of sex chromosomal anomalies, including the XXX syndrome.

The clinical manifestations of Marfan's syndrome, inherited as an autosomal dominant disorder, include disproportionate long extremities, arachnodactyly, a high-arched palate, lenticular dislocation, joint hyperlaxity, pectus carinatum, excavatum, or other thoracic asymmetry, scoliosis, and a tendency to aortic dissection and aneurysm formation. About 15% of patients are thought to represent new mutations. The features of homocystinuria are similar, though it is inherited as an autosomal recessive and over half exhibit mental retardation.

Hyperpituitarism is rare in children and difficult to diagnose. Lateral skull films may show enlargement of the pituitary fossa and careful height observation over months demonstrates an ever-increasing rate of growth. Children with Soto's syndrome are big and clumsy and frequently have developmental problems. They are born big with large heads and facial features and they stay that way. Bone age is often advanced.

Children with an abnormal number of sex chromosomes are often tall, including girls with the XXX syndrome and boys with Klinefelter's syndrome (XXY). The girls exhibit some resemblance to children with Marfan's.

The boys often manifest excessive arm span relative to height. Because of their poor testicular function, they will continue to grow for a longer time than is typical and, though not excessively tall as children, will become very tall as adults.

Tall children with no family history of excessive stature or any of the physical findings described above should be evaluated for pathological causes for excessive stature. This may be best done through referral to a center experienced in the care of such children not only to confirm the diagnosis but to arrange for the most appropriate hormonal therapy thereafter.

8

Sports Injuries in Children

Brian Carney

8.1. INTRODUCTION

Organized sports for children and adolescents continues to increase in popularity. There are now an estimated 35 million nonschool sports participants in the United States between 6 and 18 years of age and an additional 5 million more students involved in high school sports. Large numbers of injuries may be inevitable considering the number of children involved. Our mission here is to provide a practical guide to the evaluation of the most common of these injuries.

A broader discussion of children's sports, including exercise physiology, psychological aspects of sports participation, as well as the role of the team physician, is beyond the scope of this chapter. Fortunately, there are a number of excellent sources for insight into these areas. The interested reader is referred to Dyment (1991), Micheli (1984), and Sullivan and Grana (1990).

8.2. EPIDEMIOLOGY

Sports injuries affecting children are common. One study found that 6% of all school children required at least first aid for a sports-related injury per year and that two-thirds were male. Regarding these injuries, 40% were the result of nonorganized sports, 38% occurred in physical education classes, and 22% occurred in organized sports programs at school or in the community (Zaricznyj et al., 1980). Most sports-related injuries involve the lower extremity (69%), at least in adolescents (DeHaven, 1978).

Although injuries increase with age and level of competition, the nature of the injury also varies with the sport. High school sports with the most injuries per participant are American football, wrestling, softball, gymnastics, track and field, basketball, soccer, and volleyball (Garrick and Requa, 1978). Ice hockey is frequently not included in school-based statistics but is apparently a dangerous sport. In youth hockey, Wilson found that 7% of children had sustained facial injuries during their careers. The same figure for high school athletes was 54%. Injuries included facial lacerations and nasal fractures.

Overuse injuries, like stress fractures, are more common in sports that require endurance training, like cross country.

8.3. GENERAL GUIDELINES FOR ACUTE CARE OF THE INJURED ATHLETE

Almost everyone today is involved in athletic activities. Pain or limp in pediatric athletes, however, is not necessarily related to their sport. Youthful soccer players get Legg–Perthes just like anyone else and hanging your diagnostic hat on an athletic injury may be premature unless your completed evaluation points you in that direction.

It's also worth remembering that prepubertal athletes have tendons, ligaments, and muscles that are stronger than their growth plates or muscular insertions. Significant trauma will more often, therefore, result in growth plate injury than ligamentous or tendinous injury; more often result in bony avulsion than a serious muscle injury. "Sprains" and "strains" are common explanations for extremity discomfort in young athletes. The hasty or inappropriate application of these labels may sometimes delay the identification of a more significant injury.

Initial care of acute athletic injuries should include *rest*, *ice*, *compression*, and *elevation* (RICE). Such treatment prevents further "secondary" injury to damaged tissues as a result of continued hemorrhage and edema.

Rest might include time off from participation and the use of a crutch or a splint with gradual weight-bearing. The typical inversion injury to the anterior talofibular ligament (ankle sprain), for example, usually requires prohibition of full weight-bearing for about 3 days.

Ice should be applied immediately and then four to six times daily for the next day or two. Application of ice for 15 to 20 minutes is most usually recommended. Wrapping the ice in a towel or a plastic bag makes it more easily tolerated and reduces the likelihood of superficial cold injury to the skin.

Compression is provided by the application of an elastic wrap or bandage or an air splint. The wrap should be wide enough and the concavities around bony prominences should be padded (gauze, tissues, a small towel) so that force may be exerted not only to prominences but also to surrounding soft tissue where edema is most likely to occur. Initial applications of ice can be made under a compression bandage also.

Elevation should be such that the lower extremity involved is higher than the athlete's heart.

Analgesics may be useful. Acetaminophen has minimal side effects and is often useful for mild pain. Aspirin and anti-inflammatory nonsteroidals may be useful for their antiprostaglandin effects. However, all of these drugs also inhibit platelet function and may worsen bleeding into an injured area. Dupont *et al.* (1987) found no difference between ibuprofen and placebo in outcome of ankle sprains. The use of nonsteroidals in children with acute athletic injuries is therefore a bit controversial at this time.

8.4. SPORTS INJURIES TO THE FOOT, ANKLE, OR LEG

8.4.1. Stress Fractures

Stress fractures occur when cumulative bone injury exceeds the bone's ability to repair, when too much training is done too soon. In general, overuse injuries such as stress fractures result from increases in training intensity or duration of greater than 10% per week. Any bone can be affected but the proximal tibia in runners and the pars interarticularis of the lumbar spine in gymnasts, football linemen, and weight lifters are affected most often.

Pain, localized tenderness, and swelling are typical. Radiographs are initially positive in only about 10% of cases. Technetium bone scanning may be necessary if immediate diagnosis is critical; for example, when a stress fracture of the femoral neck is suspected and failure to act may lead to displacement and disaster. Waiting 2 weeks for the radiograph to demonstrate a fracture works if time is not an important factor.

Treatment involves restriction of activity, and casting may be necessary for the uncooperative. Healing is usually complete in 2 weeks to 3 months, though tibial stress fractures can take longer, and full activities should not be reinstituted until pain is absent and radiographs reveal complete healing. Stress fractures, unless appropriately dealt with, can progress to frank fracture or even nonunion.

8.4.2. "Shin Splints"

"Shin splints" is a nonspecific term for pain in the tibia with exertion. It should be diagnosed only after more specific problems, like stress fractures and compartment syndromes, have been excluded (see below). Physical examination reveals localized tenderness affecting the medial border of the distal tibia. It is uncommon in younger children and is often bilateral.

Bone scanning may be necessary to rule out a stress fracture. A compartment syndrome must be considered as well. Anterior compartment syndromes are associated with more generalized pain and tenderness, a tense anterior compartment, decreased tibialis anterior strength, and decreased sensory perception over the dorsum of the foot and between the first and second toes.

Initial treatment of shin splints includes activity modification. Cross-training can include pool swimming, running, or the use of a stationary bike. Symptomatic care includes use of heat or ice and analgesics. Limb and foot alignment should be assessed. Shoe inserts may be beneficial.

8.4.3. Heel Pain

Heel pain can be related to a single, direct traumatic episode or to repetitive subacute trauma. Persistent pain resistant to conservative therapy (RICE, see above) indicates the need for radiographic evaluation. Bony calcaneal spurs are common nonspecific findings on X-ray and their presence should not be overinterpreted in children with heel pain. Similarly, increased radiodensity or fragmentation of the calcaneal apophysis is a **normal** finding on lateral radiographs of the foot (see below).

Chronic, repetitive traction on the calcaneal apophysis can lead to microfractures, apophyseal inflammation, and heel pain, known as calcaneal apophysitis or Sever disease. A **clinical** diagnosis, calcaneal apophysitis is similar in causality to another apophysitis, Osgood–Schlatter disease, but occurs in children a few years younger. Radiologic evidence of apophyseal sclerosis or fragmentation is a normal finding and not evidence for disease. Tenderness is apparent over the heel at the insertion of the Achilles tendon. Dorsiflexion at the ankle makes the pain worse. As with Osgood–Schlatter disease, calcaneal apophysitis is self-limited, with symptoms improving as the apophysis fuses with the main body of the calcaneus. While waiting for this to happen, a heel pad of foam rubber, stretching to reduce calf muscle tightness, ice, and reduction in activity are all helpful. Casting may be necessary in patients resistant to conservative therapy.

The plantar fascia extends from the calcaneus to the base of the phalanges and can become inflamed for many of the same reasons that shin splints occur. Heel pain, arch pain, localized tenderness, and pain on toe-walking result. Care includes rest, heat or ice, and the use of analgesics. A shoe insert may help with symptoms. Steroid injections have been utilized in adults but are not recommended in children.

Achilles tendonitis presents in a similar fashion though with tenderness localized to the posterior calcaneus at about the level of the ankle. It may be associated with thickening or nodularity of the heel cord. Training errors should be sought and corrected and activity modifications may be required. Symptomatic care includes heel cord stretching, heat, ice, and analgesics. Plaster immobilization can be employed for acute or resistant cases. A heel lift may be useful during the convalescent period.

Retrocalcaneal bursitis may occur with or without bony prominence (pump bumps). This irritation is usually related to shoe wear, and modification of the heel counter may be required. In those cases where bony prominence is associated with symptoms and resistant to nonoperative management, excision can be considered in the older child or adolescent.

8.4.4. Flat Feet

Flat feet are common, usually flexible (see Chapter 4), and should not predispose to injury or long-term symptoms. Flexible flat feet have free subtalar motion (inversion and eversion) and the arch reconstitutes when standing on the toes. Shoe inserts may be considered if there is foot or leg pain, skin calluses, or excessive shoe wear. Heel cord stretching should be performed if tightness is present.

8.4.5. Ankle Sprains

Ankle sprains are common athletic injuries usually caused by inversion. Tenderness and swelling are usually lateral. Tenderness medially may represent an associated deltoid ligament injury or if present laterally and proximally may represent an injury of the tibiofibular syndesmosis (high ankle sprain). Medial or proximal tenderness usually indicates a more severe injury with longer healing time and thus warrants more aggressive immobilization.

In children, the ligaments and their attachments to bone are stronger than the related growth plate (physis). For these reasons, injury may occur at the growth plate in cases initially thought to be sprains. Tenderness over the growth plate should lead to suspicion of a physeal fracture. Radiographs (AP, lateral, and mortise) should be taken. If there is a suspicion of a fracture, then immobilization and referral are appropriate because of possible growth arrest and deformity.

In older children, after growth plate closure, the pathology is similar to adults and involves injury to the joint capsule of the ankle, the anterior talofibular ligament, and the calcaneofibular ligament. Ankle sprains are graded from mild stretching with minimal swelling and limp (grade I) to partial disruption of ligaments and capsule with difficulty weight-bearing (grade II) to complete disruption with extensive bleeding and ankle instability (grade III).

Initial management of ankle sprains should include RICE. If radiographs show no fracture, then testing for instability can be done. This is accomplished with a drawer test.

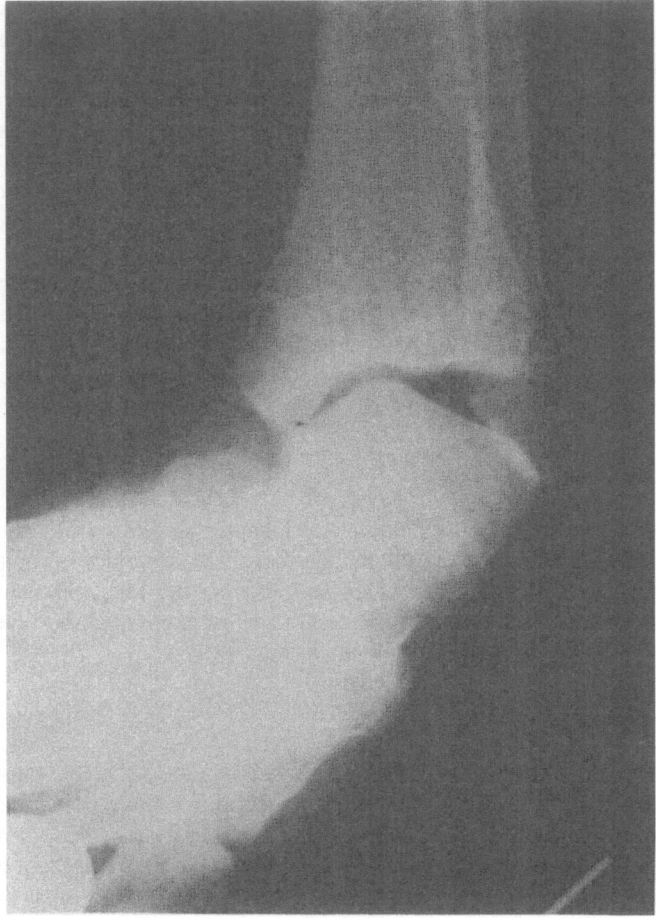

Figure 8.1. Grade III sprain of left ankle in 16-year-old boy, demonstrated by inversion stress view. Presence of symptoms chronically and failure of conservative measures would probably indicate need for surgical reconstruction

The heel is grasped firmly in the palm of one hand and the foot translated anteriorly on the tibia.

Repeat injuries are usually the result of too early a return to competition without adequate rehabilitation and strengthening. Grade I sprains require at least 1 week away from sports, perhaps with ankle taping on return. Grade II sprains require 2 weeks, with most of that on crutches together with an elastic sleeve for support. Grade III sprains may require casting or surgery and should be referred. Air splints are a convenient way to immobilize ankles with sprains. Even an uncomplicated ankle sprain requires 10 weeks to heal completely.

8.4.6. Osteochondritis Dissecans of the Talus

Osteochondritis dissecans most frequently affects the knee (see below). When the talus is affected, lesions may occur medially or laterally. Either may be seen with ankle trauma. In children younger than 12 years of age, immobilization and protected weight-bearing allow healing in the majority of cases. Clinical improvement may occur despite residual radiographic abnormality. Older children behave like adults and for them, spontaneous healing is less likely. Surgery may then be necessary to drill, pin, or remove the fragment.

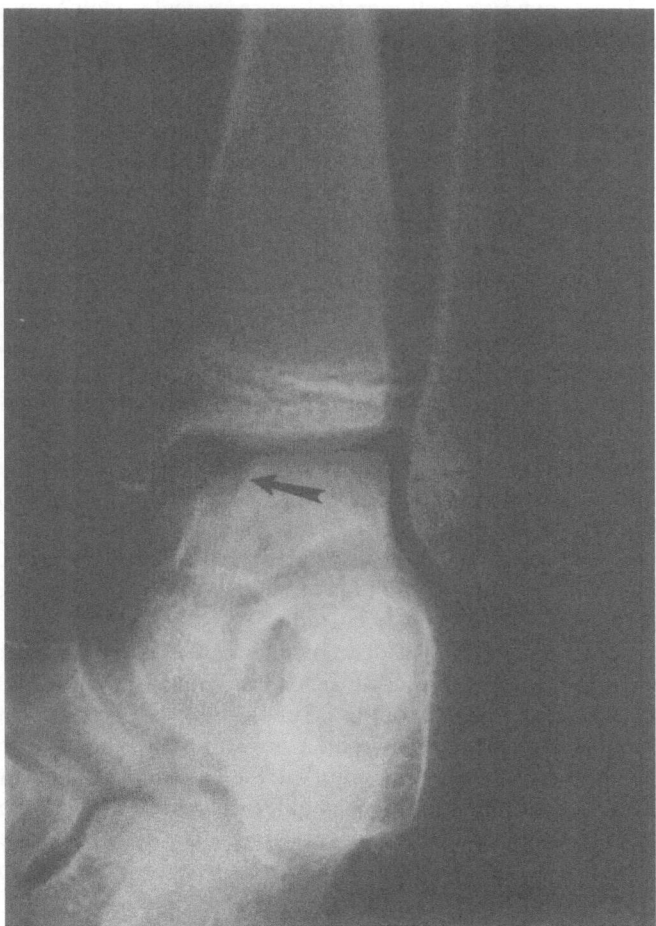

Figure 8.2. Osteochondritis dissecans of medial talar plateau (arrow); this is thought to be related to trauma by many authors though a history of a specific remembered traumatic episode is usually lacking. Like osteochondritis dissecans of the knee, osteochondritis dissecans of the ankle is more common in boys.

8.5. SPORTS INJURIES TO THE KNEE, THIGH, OR HIP

Hip pathology often presents as medial thigh or knee pain. Remember to examine and, as indicated, X-ray the hips of those young athletes presenting with knee pain. Slips of the capital femoral epiphysis (see Chapter 2), for example, can occur or worsen as a result of an athletic injury.

8.5.1. Ligamentous Injuries around the Knee

Acute trauma to the knee in younger children more often causes growth plate or other bony fractures than ligamentous injury for reasons described above. Adolescents, whose epiphyses have fused, however, will manifest more typical "adult" patterns of injury.

Medial joint line tenderness and swelling associated with a valgus stress to the knee are consistent with a medial collateral ligamentous injury. Check for medial–lateral instability with the knee flexed 20 to 30° (see Chapter 1). If there are no radiographic abnormalities (valgus and varus stress views may be useful) and the injury is localized to the ligament, the injury may be treated with immobilization and protection.

A good result is anticipated though return to full activity should not occur until there is full range of motion, normal strength, and no pain with gradually increasing activity. Follow-up will be required to ensure that physeal injury has not occurred. This is accomplished by a follow-up radiograph in 2 weeks' time and long-term follow-up for growth deformity or arrest.

Anterior cruciate ligament injury occurs from either deceleration with hyperextension or a blow sustained on a flexed knee while rotating. A "pop" is usually felt or heard. A hemarthrosis is often present, manifested by an acute effusion which occurs in minutes to a few hours. Tenderness is diffuse and there is markedly decreased range of motion. An anterior cruciate injury is confirmed on clinical exam by noting an increase in anterior movement of the tibia under the femur when the knee is flexed 20° (Lachman's test, see also Chapter 1).

X-rays (AP, lateral, sunrise, and tunnel views) should be obtained to rule out an associated fracture. Arthroscopy or MRI may be indicated to confirm the diagnosis and determine if a meniscal tear has also occurred.

The natural history of anterior cruciate ligament (ACL) injury is further instability and degenerative arthritis. For this reason, reconstruction is sometimes recommended, particularly with complete ACL disruption. Simple ligament repair has not improved stability in adults and results are no better in children. The concern with ACL reconstruction in children is the potential injury to the growth plate at the time of surgery with resulting limb length discrepancy or angular deformity. In children, this can be avoided by deferring surgical intervention until an older age or by altering surgical techniques. Procedures in children have been characterized by residual anteroposterior laxity but good functional results.

8.5.2. Injuries to the Meniscus

Persistent pain associated with a "click" or "pop" after a twisting injury is suspicious for a meniscal injury. Swelling, joint line tenderness, and locking are typical.

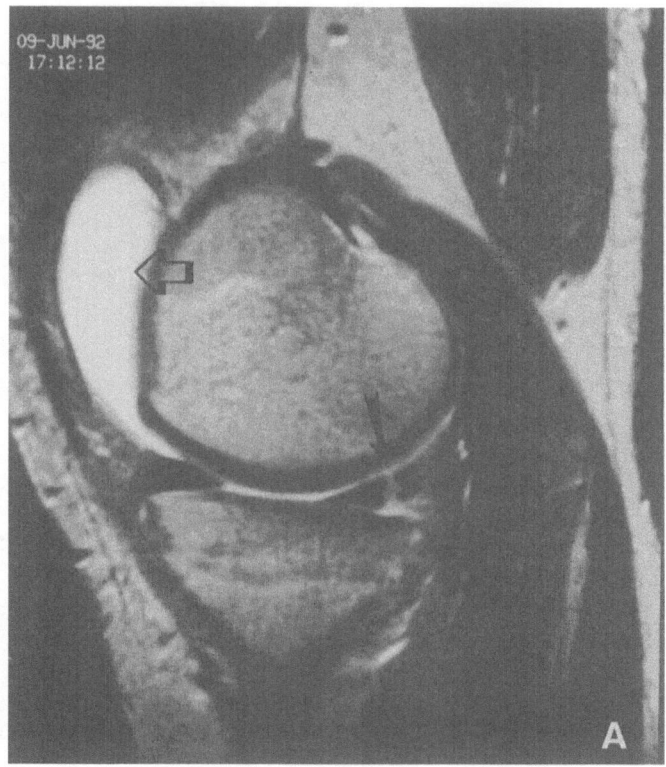

Figure 8.3. MRI of knee of 17-year-old male basketball player who incurred a twisting injury associated with a popping sensation, followed by instability. (A) Note large joint effusion in suprapatellar bursa (open arrow) and vertical tear of the posterior horn of medial meniscus (closed arrow) on sagittal image. (B) Medial collateral ligament injury is apparent on this coronal image as evidenced by hemorrhage and edema (arrow). (C) Sagittal section through intercondylar groove should show anterior cruciate ligament; its absence reflects complete tear. MRI courtesy of the Department of Radiology, University of Kentucky.

Meniscal lesions either can be acute tears or can be related to a congenital discoid meniscus. MRI scanning and arthroscopy are both diagnostically useful, the latter also providing the opportunity for treatment. Repair of meniscal tears is generally successful in children and removal of the entire meniscus should be avoided since it predisposes to later joint instability and arthritis.

8.5.3. Osteochondritis Dissecans of the Distal Femur

Osteochondritis dissecans is a lesion of articular cartilage and underlying bone. It affects the femoral condyles most commonly but also affects the ankle and elbow. Its etiology is obscure but may be related to repetitive trauma, abnormal ossification, or ischemia. Typical presentation is that of a young adolescent male with pain, history of a

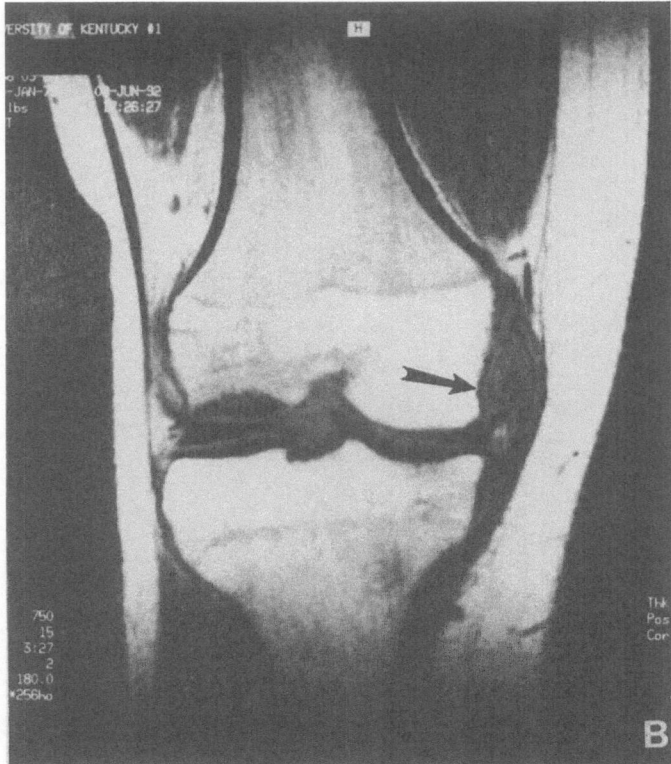

Figure 8.3. (*Continued*)

popping sensation, and mild joint swelling. X-rays are usually diagnostic, showing a lucent semicircle of bone surrounded by a slightly sclerotic margin.

If the anteroposterior film is normal, order a tunnel or notch view, which may show the more posterior aspects of the femoral condyles better. Sometimes normal variations in ossification, usually present posteriorly, can be confused with an osteochondritis dissecans lesion. This is particularly true in younger children. Technetium bone scanning or an MRI scan are useful if the diagnosis is in doubt.

The affected area, usually the lateral side of the medial femoral condyle, will most often heal in skeletally immature individuals with conservative management only, including reduced weight-bearing and immobilization. The prognosis in older individuals with closed growth plates is less good and fragment separation is more likely. Surgery, including drilling, fixation, or fragment removal, is often necessary.

8.5.4. The Patellar Pain Syndrome

The patellar pain syndrome (PPS), implying problems with patellofemoral tracking, is one of the most common causes of knee pain in adolescents. Chondromalacia

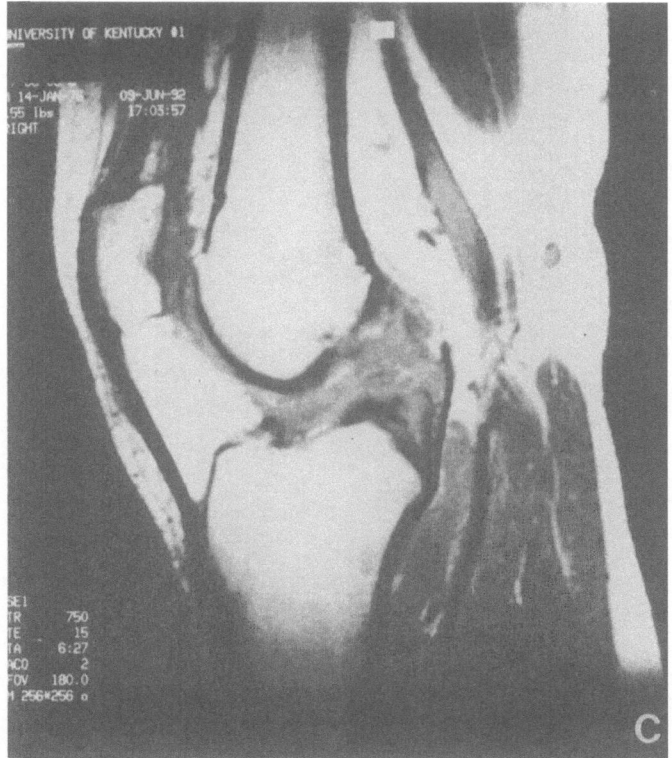

Figure 8.3. (*Continued*)

patellae is a severe subcategory of this disease reserved for those patients with histologically or arthroscopically defined damage to the patellar cartilage.

PPS usually manifests itself as diffuse anterior knee pain worse with activities that increase patellar compression against the femur, including prolonged sitting, stair climbing, or climbing uphill. There may be grinding, popping, or feelings of instability or giving way, though true locking is rare. Effusions may also be present. Patellar complaints are more common in loose-jointed or hyperlax individuals. Adolescent females appear to be most frequently affected.

As with other overuse syndromes, excessively rapid increases in endurance training may exacerbate preexisting minimal problems in athletes.

Evaluation should include assessment of overall limb alignment. Patellar problems are often seen in association with pes planus (flat feet), genu valgum (knock-knees), external tibial torsion, medial femoral torsion, and patella alta (high-riding patella). Excessive knee valgus can be quantitated with the "Q (quadriceps) angle," the angle subtended by the long axis of the quadriceps muscle and the patellar tendon. The Q angle is often increased in patients with patellofemoral pain. All of these accentuate the

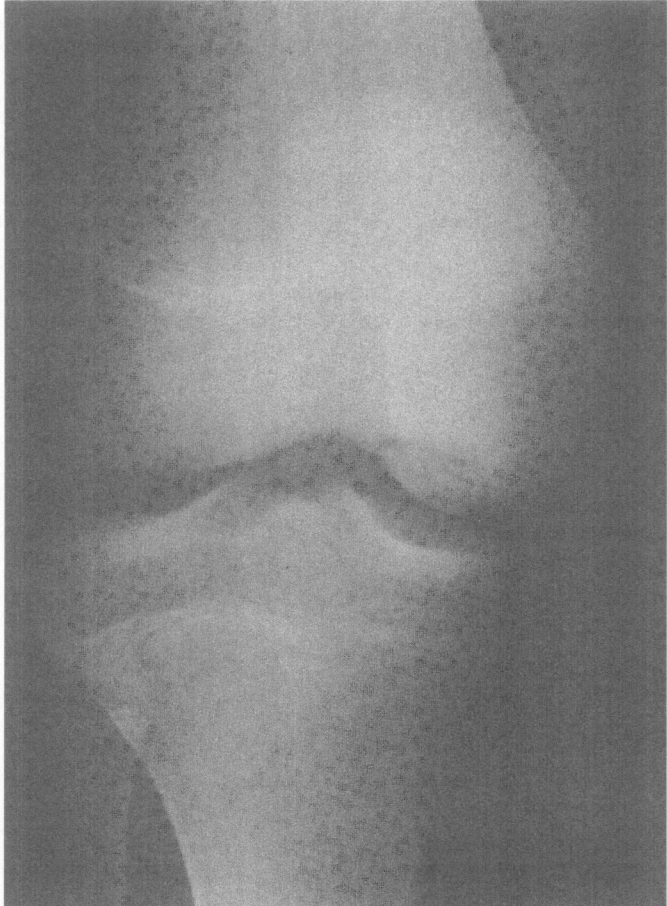

Figure 8.4. Osteochondritis dissecans of the distal femur in a 15-year-old boy. Note typical rounded subchondral lesion with obvious bone fragment and slight surrounding sclerosis. Lateral aspect of medial condyle is typical location.

tendency toward malalignment of the patella with excessively lateral tracking in the intercondylar groove.

Patellar mobility is assessed by medial and lateral movement of the patella with the knee in mild flexion. Often there is excessive lateral tightness of the patella such that the lateral border of the patella cannot be elevated. Patient anxiety during movement of the patella laterally represents a positive "apprehension" test and implies previous dislocation which the patient doesn't want to repeat, hence the apprehension. Crepitus, joint line tenderness, and iliotibial band tightness also may be observed. Retropatellar tenderness can be elicited by patellar compression during quadriceps contraction.

Thigh circumferences should be measured. Measure four finger widths up from the top of the patella on each thigh. Thigh circumferences should normally be within 1 or 2 cm of each other; atrophy is a good sign that "something" is wrong with the knee, be it patella or not. Medial quadriceps atrophy, in particular, is often apparent, reflecting chronicity and contributing to instability.

Abnormal patellar tracking may be noted by observing the patella as the patient slowly extends their knee from a fully flexed position while sitting at the end of the examining table. Look for lateral excursion of the patella or catching.

Radiographs should be obtained, including AP, lateral, and notch views of the knee and a sunrise (Merchant's) view of the patella to detect patellofemoral subluxation or other abnormalities.

Initial management should include quadriceps strengthening. This should be done initially in full knee extension (leg lifts 10 inches above the table for a 10 count) or from near terminal extension (less than 20° of flexion) against slowly increasing resistance. Extension from greater degrees of knee flexion should be avoided, to reduce compressive forces across the patella. A knee sleeve with patellar cutout may be useful. Persistent pain merits referral as does true patellar dislocation.

8.5.5. Pain Originating from the Patellar Tendon (Including Osgood–Schlatter Disease)

Anterior knee pain can also reflect pathology localized to the patellar tendon itself (patellar tendonitis or "jumper's knee"), the patellar tendon attachment to the tibia (Osgood–Schlatter disease), or the patellar tendon origin on the inferior pole of the patella (Sinding–Larson–Johansen syndrome).

All are overuse syndromes and all may be treated with reduced activity, heat or ice, and analgesics as necessary. Osgood–Schlatter disease results from patellar tendon traction on the immature cartilaginous apophysis of the tibial tuberosity. It typically occurs in early pubertal athletes with strong or tight quadriceps muscles and causes pain after exercise.

The child will localize the problem to the tibial tuberosity, which is usually prominent and tender. An X-ray is useful to exclude more substantial problems if doubt exists regarding the diagnosis. Symptomatic care is all that is generally required, including rest, reduced activity, and NSAIDs. Persistent symptoms may require cast immobilization but only rarely. A complete avulsion of the tibial tubercle has been reported but is rare. As bony maturation progresses, the process will heal itself with a residual prominence at the anterior tibial tubercle. No surgery should be undertaken until growth plate closure is complete. If, at that time, bony ossicles within the patellar tendon are symptomatic, they may be excised.

8.5.6. Intramuscular Hematoma and Myositis Ossificans after Trauma

A direct blow to the thigh can cause a hematoma within the quadriceps, resulting in swelling and muscle spasm. Treatment includes rest, ice, compression, and immobiliza-

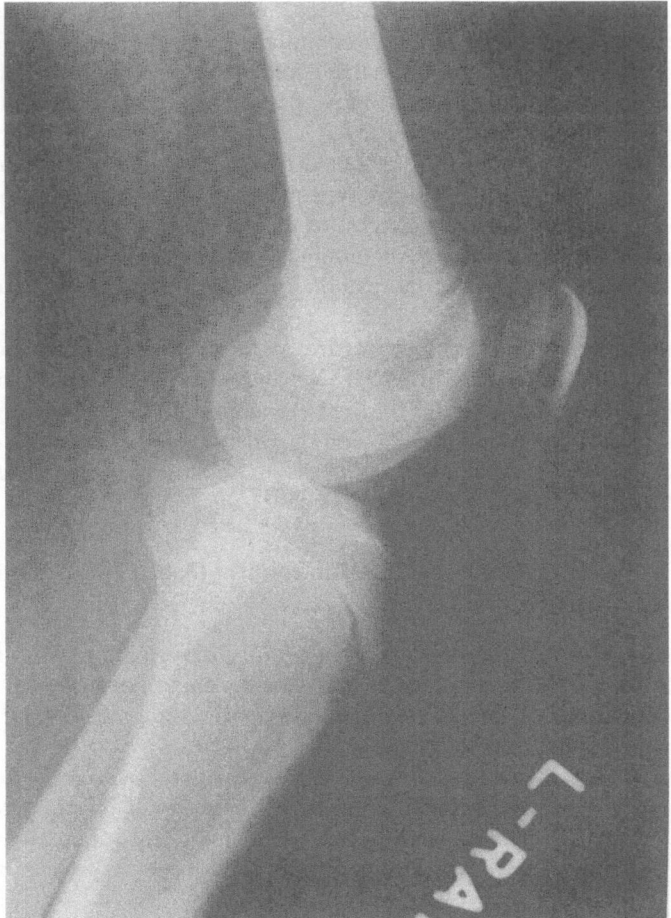

Figure 8.5. Radiography is not a good way to make the diagnosis of Osgood–Schlatter disease though it may be useful to rule out other causes of knee pain Normal, nontender tibial tuberosities will be prominent on X-ray but don't have irregular anterior surface

tion in knee flexion. Knee flexion keeps the quadriceps mechanism stretched and reduces the likelihood of fibrosis and shortening. Return to full activity should not be allowed until tenderness is absent and active knee flexion is at least 90°. Premature return can result in rebleeding and increase the possibility of heterotopic bone formation (myositis ossificans). Myositis ossificans as a result of trauma most often affects the quadriceps, the muscles around the hip, and the brachialis. Initially, the child will present with diffuse soft-tissue tenderness and swelling. Within several weeks of injury, a well-demarcated, rounded bony mass will appear on X-ray. Resolution without specific treatment is expectable but may take months. Appropriately padded thigh pads help prevent this problem.

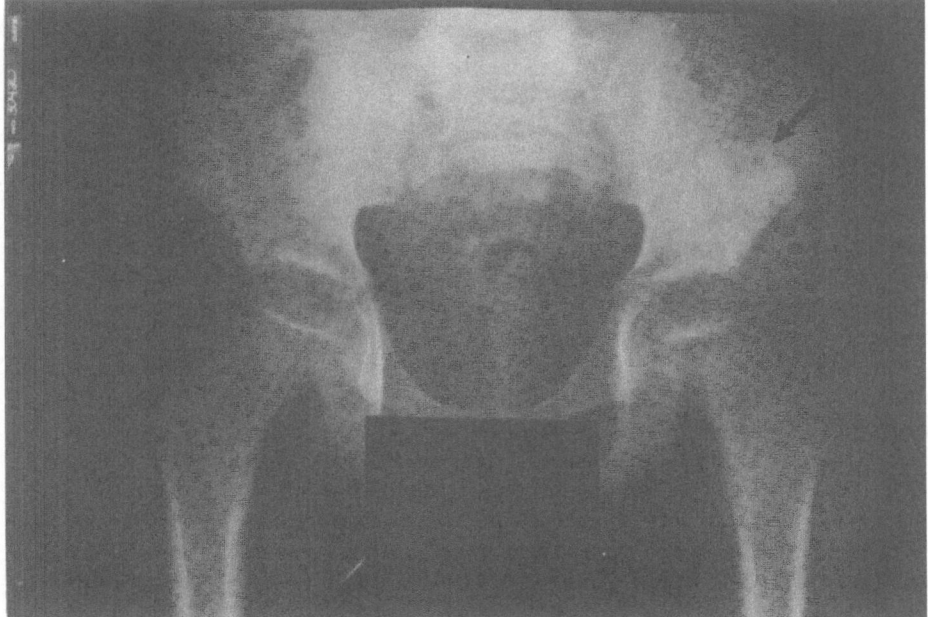

Figure 8.6. Myositis ossificans in the gluteal muscles of a 6-year-old boy is certainly unusual. Note well-defined, smoothly rounded ossific mass (arrow).

Various bone-producing malignant tumors, including osteosarcoma, are in the differential diagnosis of myositis ossificans. For this reason, appropriate consultation to an orthopedic surgeon is warranted if this diagnosis is being considered.

8.5.7. "Hip Pointers" and Other Pelvic Injuries

A direct blow to the ilium can cause an iliac crest contusion, a "hip pointer." These are tender to palpation and cause pain on lateral bending. Appropriately fitting football hip pads help to prevent this injury. Care is symptomatic.

Tendon attachments to the pelvis can be sites of avulsion fractures. Locations include the anterior superior iliac spine (sartorius), anterior inferior iliac spine (rectus femoris), ischium (hamstrings), lesser trochanter (iliopsoas), greater trochanter (abductors), and iliac crest (abdominal muscles).

Radiographs should be obtained to ensure that no underlying bone lesion is present. Differential diagnosis includes neoplastic disease and iliac crest contusion (hip pointer). These injuries should be treated symptomatically with heat or ice, and analgesics. Healing may not be complete for 2 months, and return to athletics is dependent on symptoms as activity is slowly advanced. Good results are expected even if bony union does not occur.

8.6. SPORTS INJURIES TO THE SPINE

Back pain in the young athlete may be the result of disease of the vertebral bodies, discs, or soft tissues.

8.6.1. Myofascial Back Pain

Myofascial back pain is a diagnosis of exclusion. As children grow, tightness of the lumbodorsal fascia plus weakness of the abdominal musculature may lead to a lordotic posture and "back strain." Most episodes of back pain on a myofascial basis can be treated with stretching of the posterior structures, including hamstrings together with strengthening of the abdominal musculature.

Bent-leg sit-ups are useful after the acute pain and spasm have resolved. Begin with isometric contraction of the rectus abdominis only, with minimal spinal flexion, before moving on to a few repetitions daily. Alternatively, have the child stand against the wall with heels, buttocks, and upper back in contact with the wall. Instruct the child to tighten the abdominal muscles to flatten the lower back against the wall and hold, at the beginning, for a five count. Behavioral modifications to reduce back strain are also useful. These include the use of a firm mattress, keeping one foot up on a stool when standing flatfooted, and emphasizing lumbar flexion, particularly by side-sleeping with the knees and hips in flexion.

8.6.2. Spondylolysis

Spondylolysis is the term given to a defect, stress fracture or lysis, of the pars interarticularis, the bony connection between the posterior elements of one vertebra and the superior facet joint of the next lower one. This occurs, usually without symptoms, in up to 5% of adolescents and is found with increased frequency in athletes, especially those specializing in diving, gymnastics, weight lifting, and football (linemen). Affected children are presumably predisposed to spondylolysis by some congenital weakness of the pars leading to a stress fracture after repeated trauma or, occasionally, after an acute traumatic episode. About 80% involve L-5, the remainder L-4. Most children with spondylolysis have bilateral disease and some of these will develop vertebral slippage with anteroposterior translation, a condition termed *spondylolisthesis*.

Symptomatic children with spondylolysis will present with postural abnormalities or with low back pain exacerbated by activity, particularly lumbar extension. Hamstring tightness may be severe enough to prevent normal hip flexion during the swing portion of the gait. Radicular pain should not present on straight leg raising, however, and such neurologic manifestations of nerve root compression as motor weakness, DTR changes, or problems with sphincter control should not occur with spondylolysis.

Lateral and oblique radiographs of the lumbar spine, technetium bone scanning, or computerized tomography can all be useful to confirm the diagnosis.

For the symptomatic athlete with spondylolysis, a temporary (6 weeks to 3 months depending on symptoms) reduction or cessation of those activities (like gymnastics) causing the trouble will usually reduce the child's discomfort. After acute muscle spasm

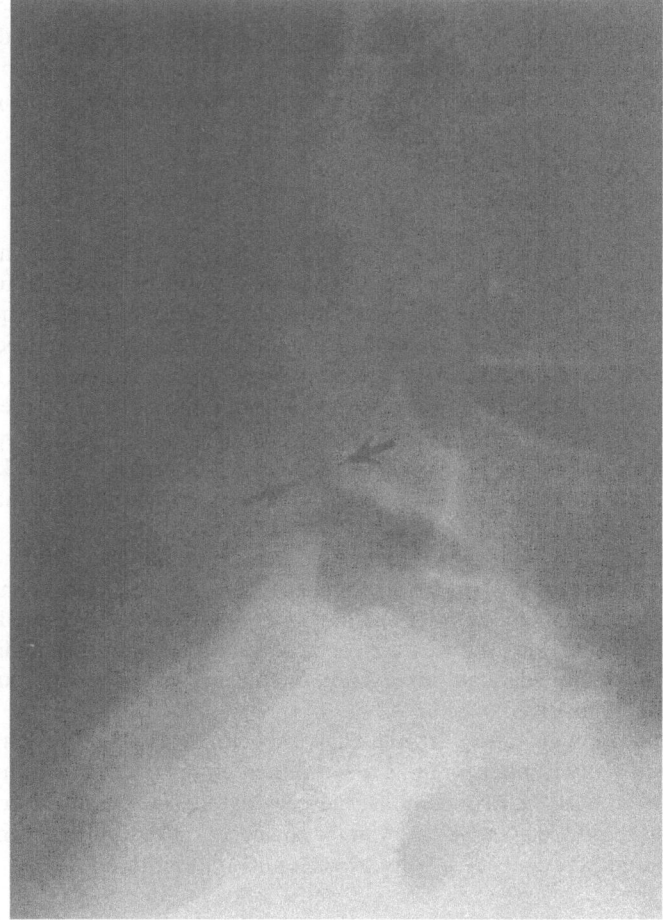

Figure 8.7. Spondylolysis of L-5 in a 15-year-old female, note defect in pars interarticularis (arrows). There is also a slight slip of L-5 on S-1 (spondylolisthesis).

is abated, hamstring stretching and rectus abdominis strengthening (see above) are useful. A back brace may reduce symptoms but is not associated with an increased likelihood of bony fusion.

8.6.3. Spondylolisthesis

Spondylolisthesis, slippage anteriorly of the superior vertebra on the inferior one, may lead to deformity and worsening pain. Symptoms and signs of nerve root compression (usually of L-5) may be present, including muscle weakness, sensory loss, and sphincter problems. Specifically, check for weakness of ankle dorsiflexion, since L-5 motor nerve roots provide innervation to the extensor hallucis longus muscle which is responsible for this function. Slippage of greater than 50% of the width of the vertebral body should lead to the restriction of contact sports. Worsening pain despite bracing, nerve root compression, or progression beyond this initial degree of slippage indicates the need for surgical stabilization.

8.6.4. Spinal Cord Injuries

Spinal cord injuries can be catastrophic and are most often cervical when incurred during athletic activity. Adequate medical coverage should be available for activities where there is significant risk of head or neck injuries and should include equipment for spine immobilization, cardiopulmonary resuscitation, and a plan for transportation to a medical facility with neurosurgical support. Any unconscious athlete must be assumed to have a spinal cord injury. Any conscious patient complaining of severe neck pain, weakness, sensory loss, or other neurologic symptom should have the spine immobilized. Helmets should not be removed nor chin straps loosened. The neck should not be moved until after radiologic clearance is obtained, remembering that vertebral instability with subluxation may be present even without a fracture.

In addition to sports with direct contact such as football, ice hockey, rugby, and wrestling, recreational diving (the No. 1 cause), gymnastics, and trampoline also represent significant risks. One-quarter of trampoline injuries requiring medical evaluation result in hospitalization. Injuries appear to occur when multiple individuals are on the trampoline without adequate supervision or spotting and are most common in the youngest individuals involved.

Transient quadriplegia often associated with paresthesias may occur after neck injury. Recovery usually is made within a few minutes though such symptoms should be taken seriously. Radiographs may demonstrate cervical stenosis or other bony narrowing. Neurological evaluation is mandatory and consideration should be given to removal from contact sports, especially if a bony abnormality is identified.

8.6.5. "Burners"

"Burners" occur with traction on the brachial plexus as might occur when a tackle forcibly laterally flexes the head and neck to one side. A sharp pain radiates down the arm, and a variable period of weakness and altered sensation follows. Repeated episodes can cause permanent weakness, especially in the C-5, C-6 distribution (elbow flexion, shoulder abduction, and shoulder external rotation). Affected athletes should not be allowed to return to competition until they have full painless range of motion of neck and shoulder and no altered sensation or weakness. The first episode and any subsequent episodes with a change in pattern of symptomatology should have radiographic evaluation. Repeated episodes should preclude participation.

8.6.6. Spine Instability in Children with Down Syndrome

Children with Down syndrome require cervical spine evaluations for participation in athletic competition, including Special Olympics. Instability is most prominent between the atlas and the axis. Lateral flexion and extension radiographs should be obtained prior to competition and about every 3 years in asymptomatic children. Atlanto-dens translation greater than 5 mm precludes sports that put the cervical spine at risk, such as tumbling and gymnastics. Neurological symptoms require further evaluation and consideration of surgical stabilization by bony fusion. Translation greater than 10 mm, even without symptoms, warrants surgical stabilization.

8.7. SPORTS INJURIES TO THE SHOULDER, ARM, OR ELBOW

8.7.1. Shoulder Dislocation

Anterior dislocation occurs as a result of trauma such as a missed arm tackle in football with a direct blow sustained on the abducted and externally rotated arm. As the humeral head is levered out of the glenoid there is immediate pain and guarding with a tender mass anteriorly. Hand sensation is altered in 10% of cases.

Immediately after dislocation, the patient may attempt self-reduction by holding both hands onto the flexed knee and providing longitudinal traction. If unsuccessful, manipulative reduction will be required once X-rays confirm the diagnosis. A sheet can be placed in the axilla and then across the patient's body. While an assistant holds counter traction, longitudinal traction is applied to the involved arm while in mild abduction. Rotation may be required. An alternative method using weights is accomplished by placing the patient prone. A weight or water-filled bucket is attached to the wrist and allowed to provide longitudinal traction.

Sedation should precede attempts at reduction. Following reduction, radiographs should be obtained and neurovascular status documented. Peripheral nerve function should actually be checked both before and after reduction, though the former is difficult because of the patient's discomfort. At the least, check sensation, wrist extension (radial nerve), wrist flexion (median nerve), and finger abduction (ulnar nerve).

Immobilization in internal rotation has been traditionally recommended for 6 weeks after reduction, though the length of immobilization has not been proven to reduce the high incidence of redislocation. Greater than 90% of individuals who sustain an initial dislocation when less than 18 years of age will sustain a second dislocation. With each episode less force is required. For this reason, surgical stabilization has been recommended for recurrent anterior dislocations. This entails either arthroscopic or open repair of the avulsed attachment of the capsule to the labrum (Bankart lesion), and possible capsular plication (tightening).

Anterior instability is determined by apprehension with the arm in an abducted and externally rotated position. Posterior instability is determined by increased posterior translation and apprehension when the arm is adducted and flexed across the body while supine. Inferior subluxation is noted where there is increased translation with direct longitudinal force inferiorly on clinical exam or radiographs. These instabilities alone or in combination often require arthroscopic evaluation to confirm the direction of instability.

Voluntary habitual subluxations may reflect underlying psychological problems. The subluxation is usually posterior but may be multidirectional and these patients seem to do poorly following surgical treatment.

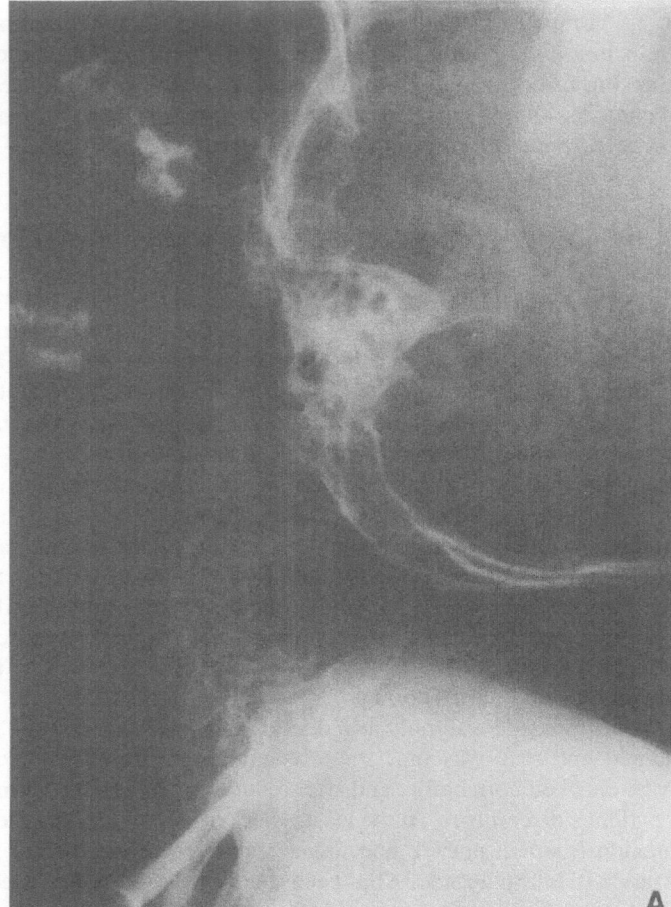

Figure 8.8. Flexion and extension views of cervical spine of 3-year-old boy with Down syndrome. (A) Note tight proximity of odontoid to posterior surface of anterior part of ring of atlas (C-1) in extension (arrow). (B) Note increased ring–odontoid distance (dotted lines) on full forward flexion, measuring 5 mm.

8.7.2. Shoulder Impingement

Shoulder impingement refers to the catching of certain structures, particularly the rotator cuff musculature, beneath the arch of the acromion and the coracoacromial ligament with resulting pain, tenderness, and shoulder weakness during abduction. It results from repeated overhead movement of the shoulder as might occur with competitive swimmers or baseball pitchers or with wheel chair athletes because of the high demands they make on their shoulders. It may be associated with shoulder instability and rotator cuff weakness. Pain is typically worse with full shoulder abduction above the

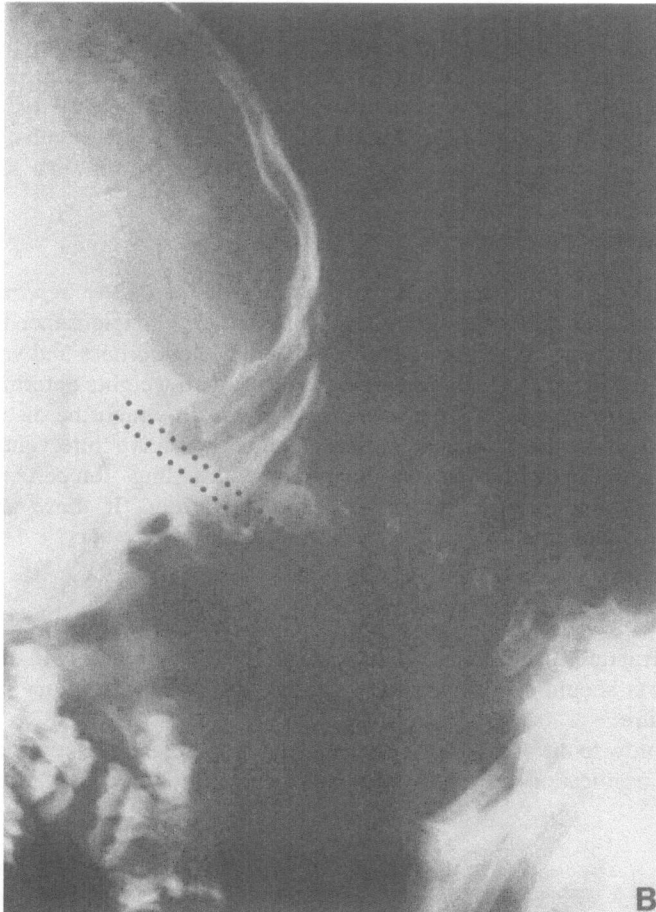

Figure 8.8. (*Continued*)

horizontal plane. Shoulder impingement should be treated with activity modification, heat or ice, and analgesics.

Therapy programs should include rotator cuff muscle exercises to improve strength; up to 6 months may be required for complete healing. Early intervention to curb excessive throwing in young athletes may be necessary to prevent progression to permanent changes.

8.7.3. "Little League Shoulder"

Pain associated with radiographic changes in the proximal humeral physis (epiphysiolysis) can occur with excessive throwing or other vigorous overhead activity "Little League shoulder"), typically in early teenage boys. Radiographic changes include widening and irregularity of the proximal humeral physis, presumably as a result of a stress fracture of the growth plate. Periosteal new bone formation may occur. Treatment is symptomatic and includes activity modification, such as moving to a position where less throwing is required. Completely restricting activity is probably not necessary but throwing should be limited for at least several months. Radiographic healing may not be complete for 4 to 6 months. There are no known sequelae.

8.7.4. Shoulder Separations

Injuries to the acromioclavicular joint are termed *shoulder separations* and are rare in preadolescents since children usually break their clavicle rather than injure the acromioclavicular joint. Separations are manifested by tenderness and varying degrees of elevation of the distal clavicle. Radiographs taken with weights determine the degree of displacement. Rare cases with severe displacement in which the distal clavicle has incarcerated itself in the trapezius muscle require operative intervention. The vast majority, however, can be treated symptomatically with a sling. Ten percent of cases will have residual symptoms after return to normal activities. If these are significant, resection of the distal clavicle with stabilization may be necessary.

8.7.5. Other Upper Arm Trauma

Clavicle fractures occur in child athletes usually as a result of a fall on the shoulder. Return to sports should be delayed for 4 months following the injury because of the risk of refracture.

A direct blow to the arm causing a hematoma of the brachialis muscle can progress to heterotopic ossification (myositis ossificans). Once injured, return to contact should

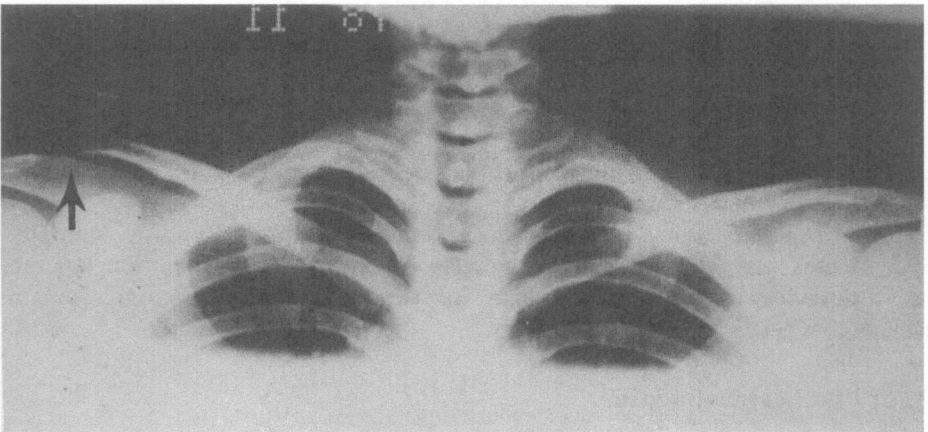

Figure 8.9. Acromioclavicular (shoulder) separation in a 16-year-old female (arrow) X-ray courtesy of the Department of Radiology, University of Kentucky

not be allowed until there is full pain-free range of motion at the elbow. Physical therapy should be avoided during the painful acute phase as rebleeding may occur. The differential diagnosis of myositis ossificans includes several malignant bone-producing tumors and for this reason orthopedic consultation is in order if the diagnosis is being entertained.

8.7.6. "Little League Elbow"

Both throwing things (balls) as well as yourself (gymnastics) lead to elbow valgus with compression of the lateral and distraction of the medial sides of the joint. Clinically this can result in medial epicondylitis or osteochondritis dissecans of the capitellum and/ or radial head laterally ("Little League elbow"). Children present usually with pain after throwing which progresses to pain all of the time and examination may demonstrate medial or lateral tenderness, grinding or locking with joint movement and a flexion contracture. Radiographs may reveal a variety of abnormalities including fragmentation and hypertrophy of the medial epicondyle, stress fractures of the epicondylar physis, calcifications of the ulnar collateral ligaments, and subchondral fragmentation of the capitellum or radial head. A similar lesion, though without subchondral fragmentation, can affect the capitellum in children who are slightly younger, without a history of repeated stress injury, and is known as Panner disease.

Treatment should include activity modification based on symptoms, usually for 2 months. Slow and graduated return to full activity should begin only after the elbow is pain-free and exhibits full range of motion. Throwing and gymnastic technique should be reviewed with an eye toward reducing valgus stress. If symptoms of pain or locking persist, evaluation for a subchondral fragment within the joint should be initiated and might include CT scan, arthrography, or arthroscopy. The best solution for this problem is prevention by restricting the number of pitches thrown by the young athlete. Many leagues wisely restrict pitching to two innings per game or six innings per week.

8.7.7. Elbow Dislocation

Elbow dislocations occur in athletics, usually as a result of a fall on an outstretched arm. Radiographs should be obtained to rule out fracture, including avulsion of the medial epicondyle of the humerus, which is commonly associated. Reduction is accomplished with longitudinal traction on the flexed elbow. Instability or redislocation is not a problem, although most will heal with some flexion contracture. For this reason, immobilization should be brief with active exercises initiated early.

8.8. SPORTS INJURIES TO THE FOREARM, WRIST, OR HAND

Children with forearm fractures should not be returned to contact sports for 4 months following injury because of the risk of refracture.

Epiphysiolysis of the distal radius can occur in young gymnasts, presumably related to stress fractures through the growth plate. Growth plate widening is seen on

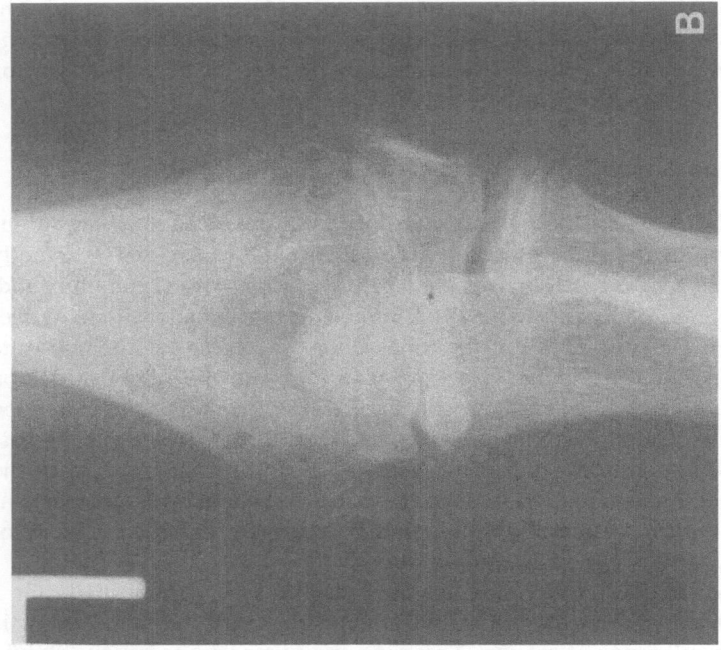

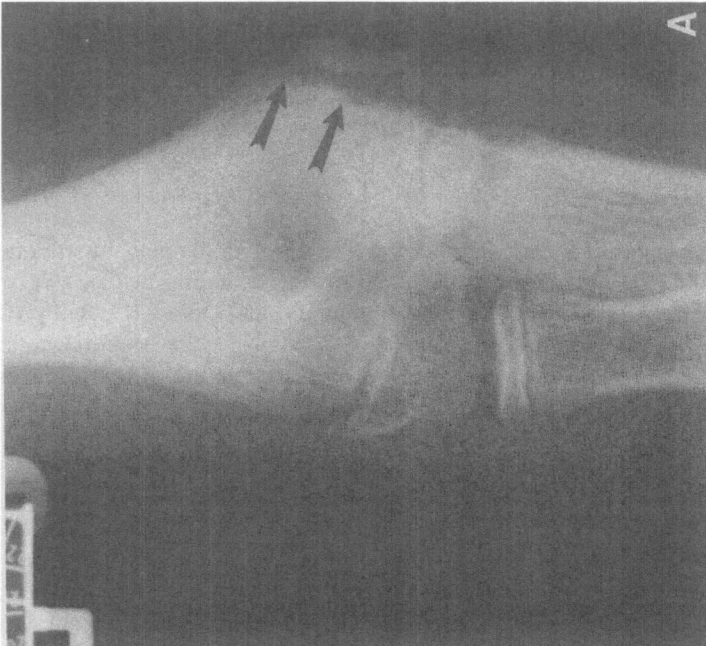

Figure 8.10. (A) Medial epicondylar fracture through physis of the right elbow of a 13-year-old male Little League baseball player (arrows) (B) Comparison view of normal (nonthrowing) left arm

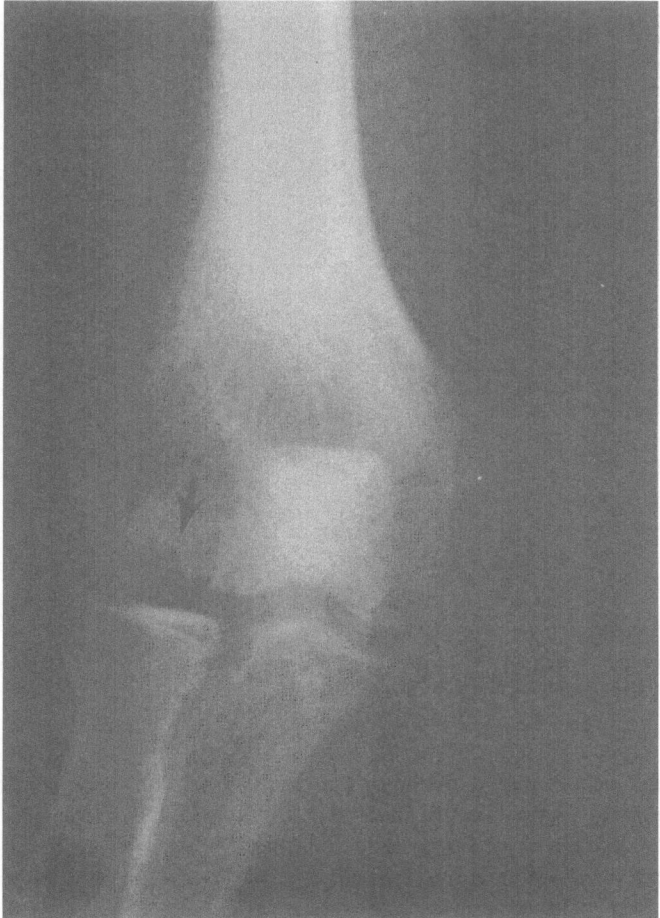

Figure 8.11. Osteochondritis dissecans of the right capitellum in a 16-year-old male (arrows). The radius is not involved. Panner disease is similar but occurs in younger patients and is not as associated with repetitive trauma. This and the preceding illustrate different manifestations of "Little League elbow."

X-ray, with clinical improvement and radiologic resolution occurring with reduction or cessation in gymnastic activities.

Scaphoid fractures after a fall on an outstretched hand often may not be evident on initial radiographs. Pain, tenderness, or swelling in the area of the anatomic snuff box should be treated conservatively with cast immobilization and repeat radiographs 2 to 3 weeks postinjury. Children seem to have better potential to heal this fracture and nonunion is much less common than in adults. Proximal or displaced fractures, however, are always difficult and may need a long-arm cast or operative intervention.

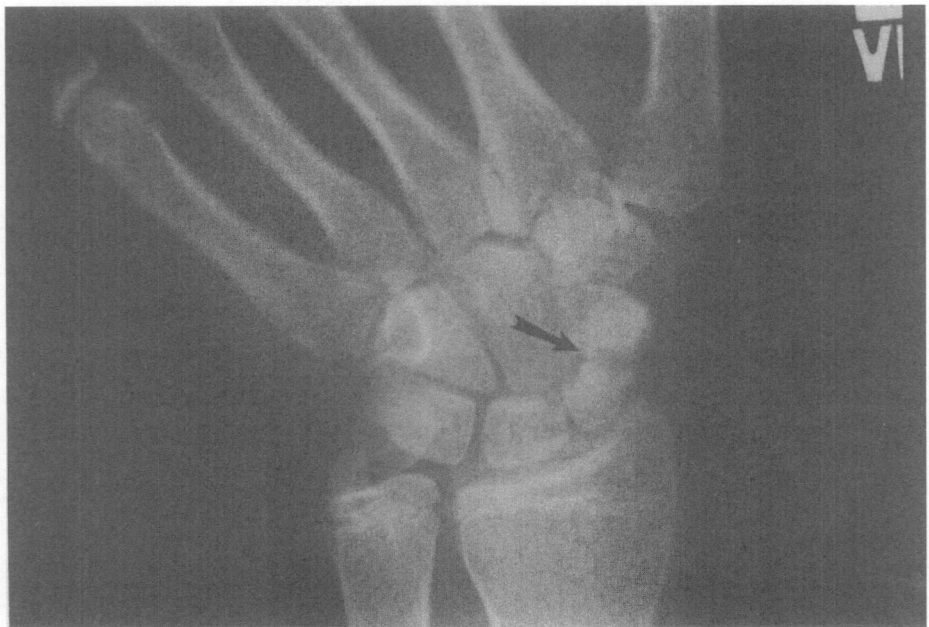

Figure 8.12. Scaphoid (navicular) malunion in a 16-year-old boy (arrow). The fracture was recognized early and treated appropriately, but failed to heal.

Mallet finger occurs with avulsion of the extensor tendon, with or without a bony fragment, from the distal phalanx. In skeletally immature individuals a physeal fracture of the distal phalanx may also be present. The injury results from longitudinal force applied to the extended finger as might occur catching a thrown ball. The ring finger is most often affected. The patient is unable to extend the distal interphalangeal joint. Immobilization of the distal interphalangeal joint in extension for 6 weeks usually yields good results. However, if a nail bed avulsion is present, the injury must be considered to be an open fracture. Additionally, even careful lateral radiographs (which should be done in all cases) may miss a physeal fracture since, in younger children, the epiphysis may not be ossified.

Interphalangeal dislocations are often reduced on the field. Radiographs should be obtained in all cases to ensure adequacy of reduction and ensure that no bony fracture has occurred. If the joint is stable, these can be treated with buddy taping. Middle finger should be taped to index and ring finger to fifth finger.

Injuries to the ulnar collateral ligament of the thumb usually occur as a result of forced abduction and extension, an injury known as "gamekeeper's thumb." Since children have stronger ligaments than growth plates, prepubertal athletes are more likely to experience a fracture through the growth plate of the proximal phalanx. Either fracture or ligamentous injury represents a serious injury, usually requiring surgery. Even partial tears require cast immobilization. Any injury of this kind merits referral.

9

Spinal Disease in Childhood

David B. Stevens

9.1. INTRODUCTION

Deformity, pain, or both are the predominant pediatric spinal complaints which prompt a visit to the primary care physician. This chapter will present a scheme to aid in the evaluation of these complaints, including the development of differential diagnosis, appropriate workup, and treatment options.

As vertebrates, we enjoy the highest differentiation of form and function in the animal kingdom. Our spine is unique in that we are the only true biped in the kingdom.

Because of this unique upright posture, our spine also has unique characteristics, particularly so as we develop. We are all familiar with the infant spinal posture, a gently rounded "C" shape as they cuddle. After achieving an upright posture, the toddler initially manifests an exaggeration of the normal spinal curve, with greater lordosis than in the adult The increasing kyphosis evidenced by many adolescents is accentuated in some, contributing to such characteristic teenage back problems as postural roundback, Scheuermann kyphosis, and spondylolysis

Patients seen for apparent abnormalities of form or appearance comprise the largest group This is particularly so with the advent of mandatory school screening for scoliosis in many states It is estimated that a spinal deformity is suspected in about 10% of children screened Of these, only a few will have a true spinal deformity Primary care physicians are well-positioned to provide the next stage of evaluation after school-based screening

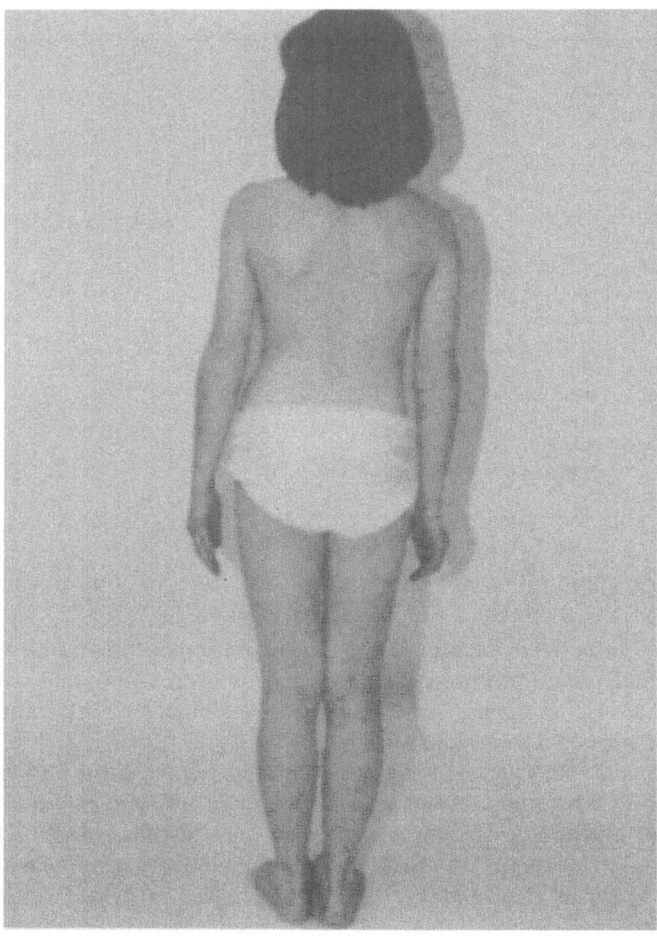

Figure 9.1 Note slight asymmetry in the way the arms hang at the sides of the torso, slightly lower right shoulder and right scapula, slight pelvic obliquity To pick up mild asymmetries, the child's knees and ankles must be together and they must be looking straight ahead

9.2. PHYSICAL EXAMINATION

The patient needs to be examined standing, from the front, the back, and the side. This is best done with the patient draped appropriately without clothing or with whatever clothing modesty absolutely requires. The patient is inspected noting apparent curvatures, deformity, or truncal shortening.

Shortening or webbing of the neck and a low hair line may reflect cervical vertebral abnormalities (Klippel–Feil). In school-aged children, the distance from the top of the head to the pubis (upper segment) should be roughly the same as the distance from the pubis to the floor (lower segment). A decreased upper segment–lower segment ratio may reflect congenital defects of the spine or spondyloepiphyseal dysplasia.

Are the cervical and lumbar curves appropriately lordotic; the thoracic curve appropriately kyphotic? Look for asymmetry of shoulder height or scapular height, pelvic obliquity or differences in the shapes of the narrow triangles made by the medial border of the arm and the lateral border of the thorax and abdomen. The skin should be carefully inspected for hemangiomas, café-au-lait spots, neurofibromata, hairy patch, lipomatous mass, or sinus tract, particularly noteworthy if in the midline. Check for excessive skin elasticity suggestive of Ehlers–Danlos.

Are the shoulders centered over the pelvis? If not certain, check with a plumb bob. If the patient is decompensated, the bob will not fall through the sacral crease. Palpate for tenderness or masses. Focal tenderness is particularly noteworthy. Is there punch tenderness over the sacroiliac joints, the surface markers for which are the dimples of Venus?

Examine the patient in the forward bending position. Ask them to clasp their hands and bend forward so that the hands are midway along the shin bones. This usually results in the C-7 vertebra and the sacrum being level and the trunk parallel to the ground. Any rib humps or paravertebral humps suggestive of scoliosis can be easily visualized in this posture. The spine should be inspected from the side noting any exaggeration of thoracic kyphosis. If present, differentiation must be made between a short, sharp angular curve and a long, gradual curve.

Ask the patient to walk in order to observe the gait. Look for subtle signs of hemiplegia, pain during stance phase, a leg length discrepancy, short steps suggestive of hamstring tightness, a foot drop, or a truncal sway. With the patient on the table, check the straight leg raising test, deep tendon reflexes, sensation, muscle strength, Babinski reflexes, and leg lengths. Cavus deformities of the feet or clawing of the toes or fingers may also suggest a neuromuscular problem, either generalized or related to an intrinsic lesion of the cord. Limb lengths and joint range of motion should also be noted.

9.3. SPINAL DEFORMITIES

9.3.1. Scoliosis

Scoliosis, lateral spinal curvature, may be congenital or acquired. It may be idiopathic, like most adolescent curves, or related to a particular pathologic process such as a malformation of one or more vertebral bodies or a neuromuscular disease, like

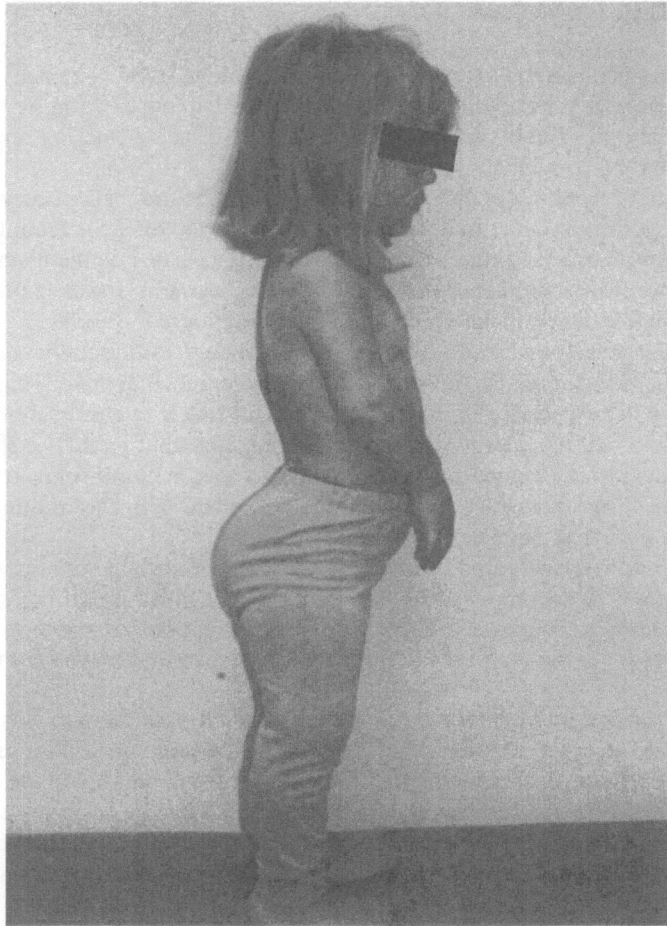

Figure 9.2. Little girl with hypochondroplasia; this is a distinct bone dysplasia characterized by short-limb dwarfism. It is milder than achondroplasia, but similar in some respects Note excessive lumbar lordosis and increased upper segment–lower segment ratio

cerebral palsy or muscular dystrophy. A listing of different categories of scoliosis is included in Table 9.1.

The Scoliosis Research Society has adopted definitions for measurement of the curve and the general curve patterns as they appear on standing anteroposterior X-rays of the thoracolumbar spine. The angles made by lines perpendicular to the endplates of the vertebrae at either end of the curve provide a measure of the severity of the curve. The end vertebrae are the last ones at the top or bottom of the curve which tip toward the concavity of the curve. The disc spaces at these end vertebral bodies are parallel.

Mild curvatures are 20° or less, moderate ones are between 20 and 40°, and severe

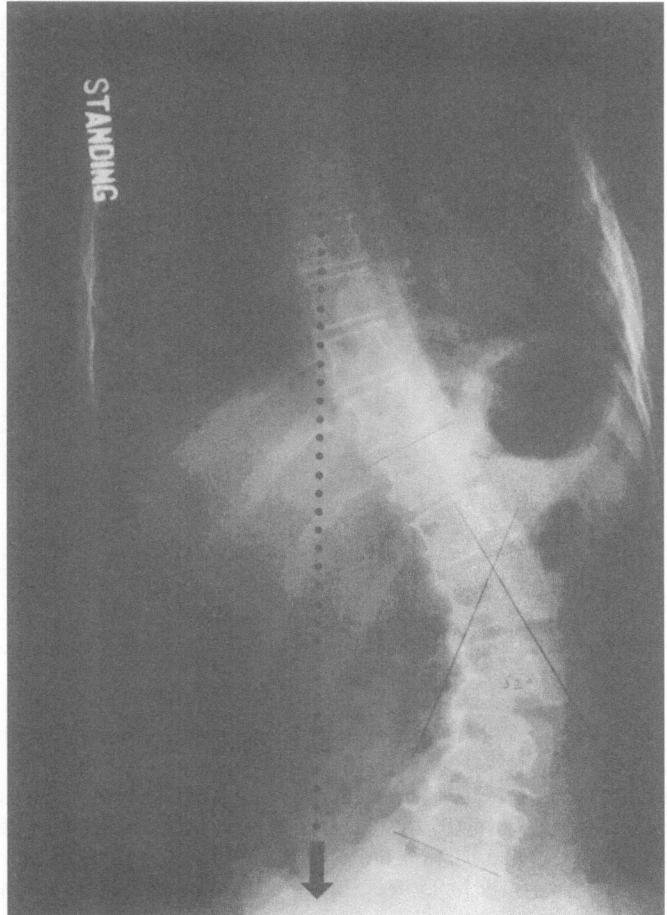

Figure 9.3. This teenage girl has spinal muscular atrophy and a typical "C"-shaped neuromuscular curve Note that her curve is decompensated and that her shoulders are not over her pelvis

ones measure greater than 40°. Most curves greater than 10° can be detected easily by careful physical examination.

9.3.1.1. Idiopathic Scoliosis

Most idiopathic scoliosis is painless and exhibits thoracic convexity to the right, the so-called "right thoracic curve." Though of unknown causation, the theory now most popular is that idiopathic scoliosis is related to some disorder of postural regulation. Though idiopathic scoliosis can be subcategorized by age as infantile, juvenile, or

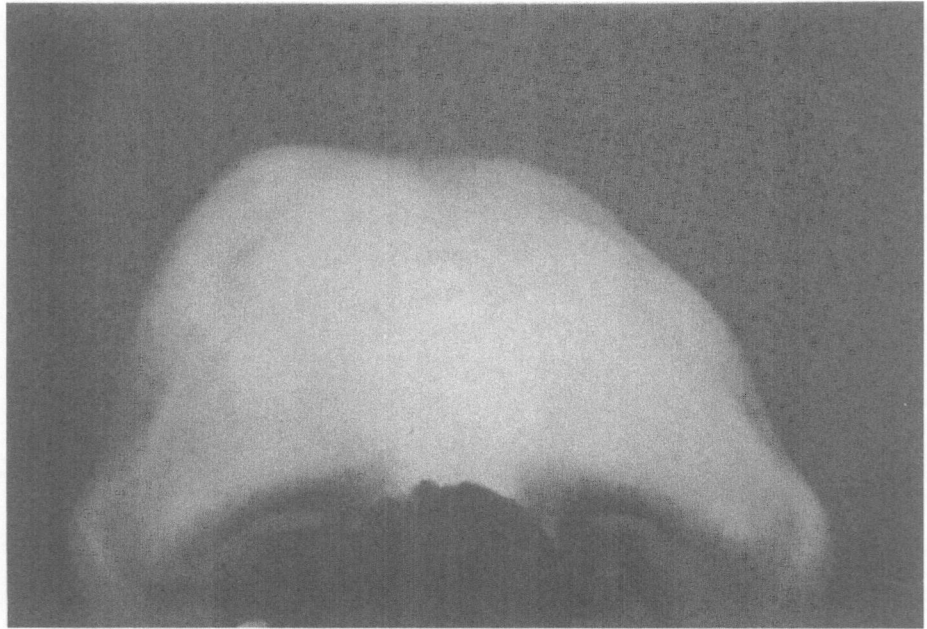

Figure 9.4. Forward bend test here reveals mild right-sided paraspinal prominence

adolescent, most is adolescent. Most patients who progress are female, with a sex ratio of about 8 to 1.

By definition, idiopathic curves are ones in which all specific causes have been ruled out. The increasing use of MRI has allowed for the identification of children with inapparent abnormalities of their spinal cords. In the absence of bony abnormalities, these children in the past would have been labeled "idiopathic" (see below).

Table 9.1. A Simple Classification of Scoliosis

Type	Clinical example
Postural	Leg length discrepancy
Structural	
Idiopathic	Most common, usually right-sided adolescent curve
Congenital	Hemivertebrae, bar
Neuromuscular	Cerebral palsy, Duchenne muscular dystrophy
Other	Spina bifida
	Marfan syndrome
	Neurofibromatosis
	Osteogenesis imperfecta
	Cord tumor
	Spondyloepiphyseal dysplasia
	Osteoid osteoma (painful)
	Ehlers–Danlos syndrome

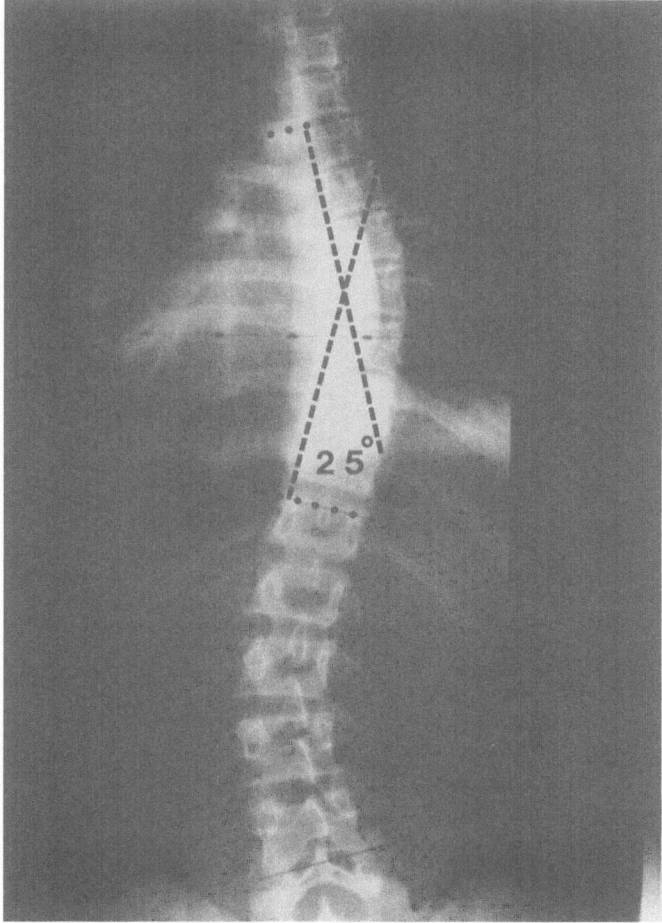

Figure 9.5. The Cobb angle is formed by the intersection of the two perpendiculars from the end vertebral bodies of this thoracic curve. In the typical "S"-shaped idiopathic curve both the thoracic and lumbar curves are measured separately. Monitoring for progression in this 14-year-old female would be by radiologic examination every 4 to 6 months.

9.3.1.2. Congenital Scoliosis

Since congenital scoliosis is frequently more severe and because the patient will be at risk for progression throughout growth, its early detection is important. All children should have their spines checked carefully as part of every "well-child" physical examination. In many states, screening programs have been developed to do school-based screening in the first and sixth grades. The early screening is designed to detect congenital scoliosis and the sixth grade screening to detect acquired idiopathic curves.

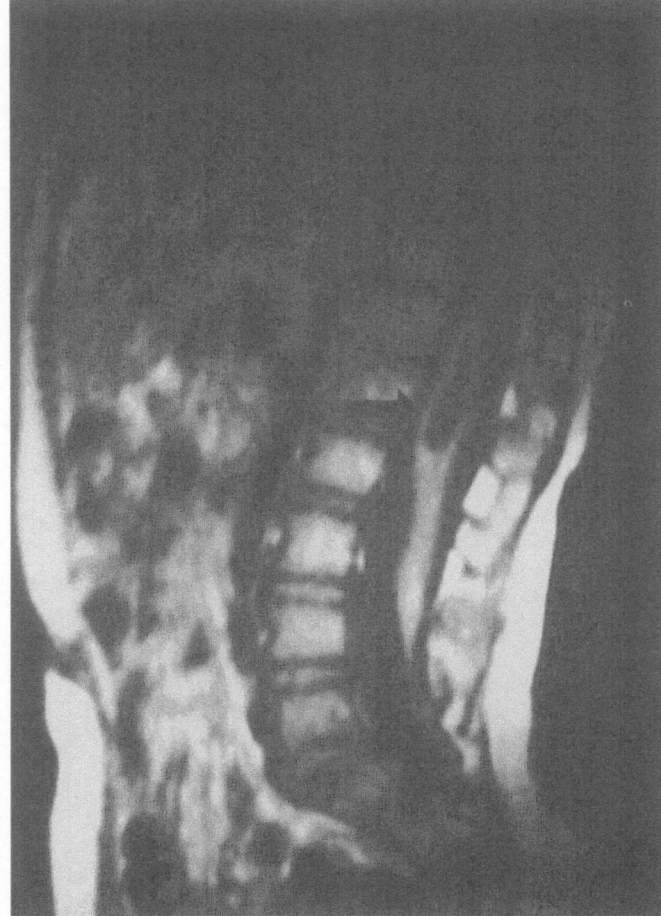

Figure 9.6. Syrinx (arrow) in the spinal cord of a 4-year-old girl.

Congenital scoliosis requires careful radiography to define the pathological anatomy. Hemivertebrae, a congenital anomaly in which half of the vertebral body is absent, are often associated with congenital curves.

Other congenital anomalies associated with scoliosis include unilateral unsegmented bars which "tether" one side of the vertebral column while allowing the other side to grow, butterfly vertebral bodies, and such dysraphic processes as spina bifida and diastematomyelia, in which a fibrous or bony septum in the spinal canal separates the cord into two halves.

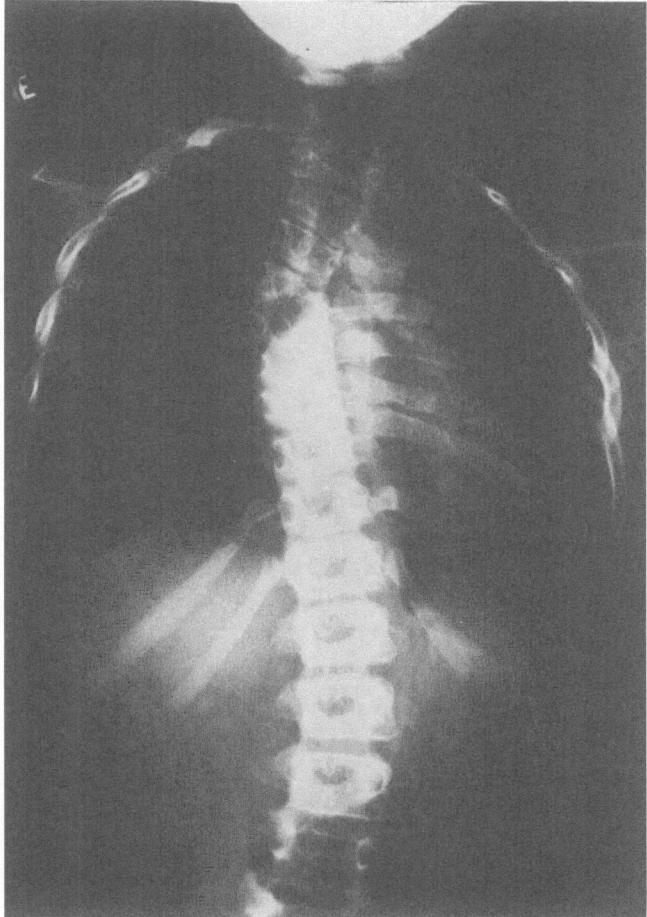

Figure 9.7. Congenital scoliosis in a 9-year-old female; note hemivertebra in midthoracic area and abnormal ribs. This patient also has cervical spine abnormalities (Klippel–Feil syndrome). The presence of vertebral abnormalities is associated with renal anomalies and the kidneys should always be checked by ultrasound or an IVP.

9.3.1.3. Treatment of Scoliosis

The standard treatment now for scoliosis is one of the three "O's": **observation**, **orthosis** (bracing), or **operation**. Observation is indicated for the mild, idiopathic curve measuring less than 20°. Serial clinical and X-ray examinations every 6 months to establish if the curve is static or progressive are mandatory. Such observation needs to be continued until the patient is skeletally mature.

The risk factors for progression of idiopathic curves in adolescence or young

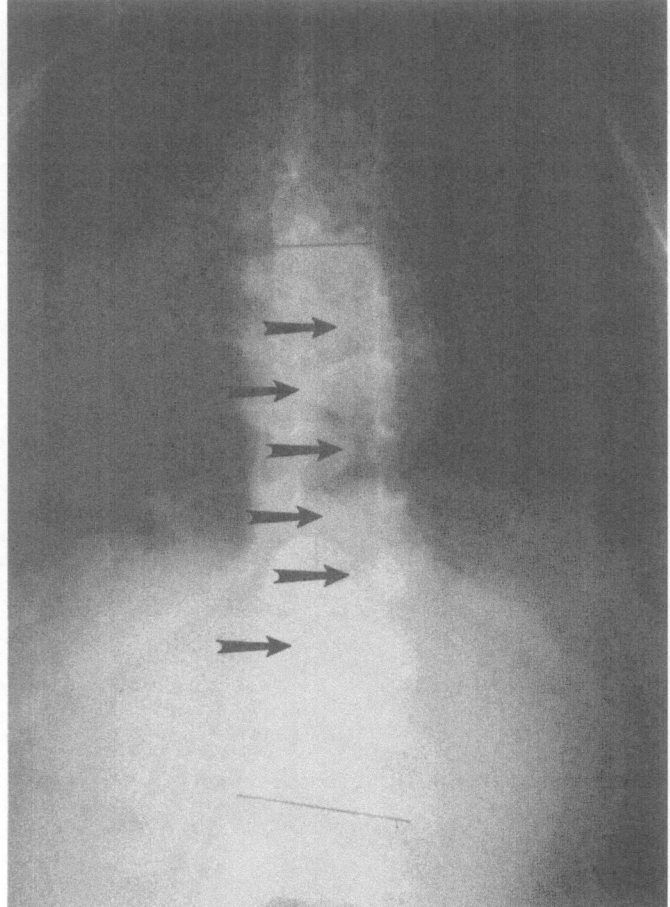

Figure 9.8. Congenital scoliosis in a 2-year-old male. The butterfly vertebrae (arrows) in this boy represent the presence of sagittal clefts within each vertebra, leaving two hemivertebrae at each segment. Happily the presence of two hemivertebrae at each level more or less balance each other out and the scoliosis here is mild, at least for now.

adulthood have been pretty well established. If a patient has not reached bony maturity, is premenstrual, and has a curve of 20° or more, the probability of progression is over 60%. On the other hand, if a patient is skeletally mature, is past menarche, and has a curve of 20° or less, the probability of progression is about 2% (Lonstein and Carlson, 1981).

Orthoses are indicated for children in whom the curve is considered acceptable at diagnosis but in which progression of the curve is either proved or probable. If successful, the brace will prevent worsening of the curve but will not permanently reduce the size of a curve. Braces come in many varieties, are difficult to construct, and are even harder to wear. However, studies have shown that a well-constructed brace properly fitted and built and used most of the day and night will prevent progression in a significant portion of patients.

In those patients who have curves over 40° or who have significant cosmetic deformities, operation usually is indicated. Prior to the use of metal spinal instrumentation, prolonged bed rest in a body cast was required and failure of fusion rates of 50% were common. Spinal fusion, originally done in 1910 by Russell Hibbs, is the goal of the operation, that is, to convert the curvature from a flexible, progressing deformity to a solid, fused mass of bone through a posterior approach along the laminae. The advent of Harrington rods, followed by Luque fixation. Cotrel-Dubousset, Texas Scottish-Rite, Isola, and now Modulock instrumentation, among others, have made spinal surgery for scoliosis a complicated and expensive process. These various systems each have their advantages and disadvantages. With proper application the success rate is high, though no long-term follow-ups are available for the newer systems and even the Harrington rod has been in wide use only since the late 1960s (see Fig. 9.13).

9.3.1.4. Associated Anomalies

In the past, before MRI, most patients thought to have idiopathic scoliosis, did not have studies of the central nervous system prior to operation. The recent introduction of MRI has documented a much higher rate of structural neurological abnormalities of the cord in these patients than previously expected. These have included hydromyelia, syringomyelia (see Fig. 9.6), and the Arnold–Chiari malformation, among others. An MRI should be seriously considered for any scoliosis patient:

1. With neurological findings; look in particular for loss of abdominal cutaneous reflexes
2. With a left thoracic curve pattern (convexity to the left) since most idiopathic scoliosis is right thoracic
3. Younger than 10 years of age
4. With a rapidly progressive curve, or
5. With vertebral abnormalities

Renal anomalies occur with increased frequency in children who have congenital scoliosis or any other vertebral abnormality. A good renal ultrasound or IVP or both is therefore indicated. Similarly, congenital heart disease is associated and deserves at the least a careful listen. Any murmur present should be considered serious until excluded by an appropriate evaluation.

Dwarfing skeletal dysplasias frequently cause scoliosis. These include spondylo-epiphyseal dysplasia, the mucopolysaccharidoses, and diastrophic dwarfism. Children with achondroplasia, in addition to scoliosis, have pathologically increased dorsal kyphosis and lumbar lordosis sometimes with spinal canal stenosis and an increased risk of paraplegia.

Patients with neurofibromatosis also should be carefully evaluated since they have a higher incidence of scoliosis (see Fig. 1.10). When present, it is thought to carry with it a

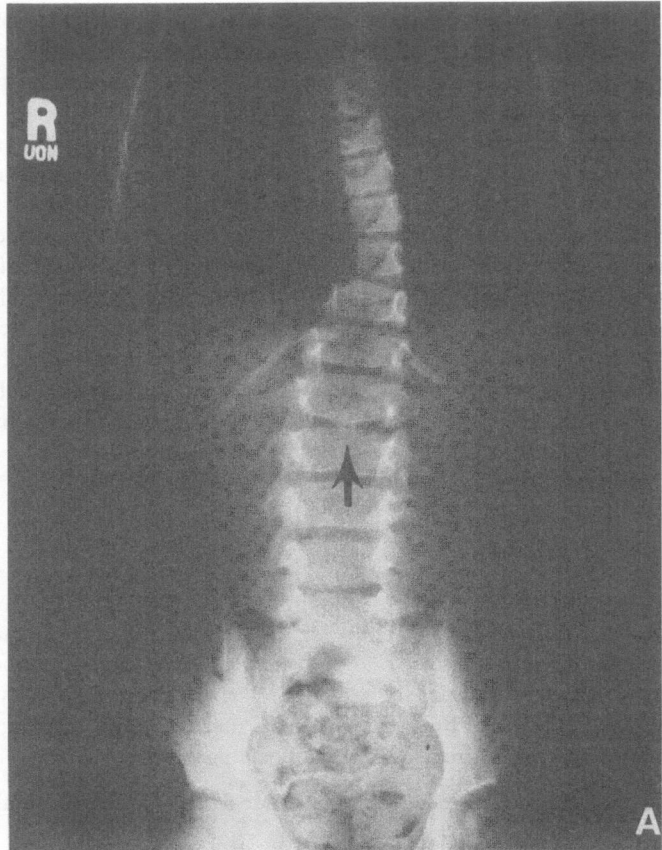

Figure 9.9. (A) Scoliosis in a 5-year-old female with a diastematomyelia (arrow). (B) Tomogram demonstrates midline spiculation of bone well. Diastematomyelia refers to the split in the cord rather than midline spiculation itself, which is not always present, and the upper lumbar cord is a typical location. Patients with diastematomyelia may present with a scoliosis, worsening neurologic function as tethering occurs with growth or with a midline hemangioma, hairy patch, or sinus tract.

greater risk of progression than an idiopathic curve of the same magnitude. Other associations with scoliosis include Marfan syndrome (see Fig. 9.14), Ehlers–Danlos syndrome, homocystinuria, osteogenesis imperfecta, and such causes of weakness as muscular dystrophy and spinal muscular atrophy (see Fig. 9.3), among many others.

9.3.2. Thoracic Kyphosis

There are two primary deformities of the thoracic spine in the sagittal plane. One is postural roundback which makes its appearance in early adolescence. With this condition the patient has increased thoracic kyphosis together with excessive lumbar lordosis.

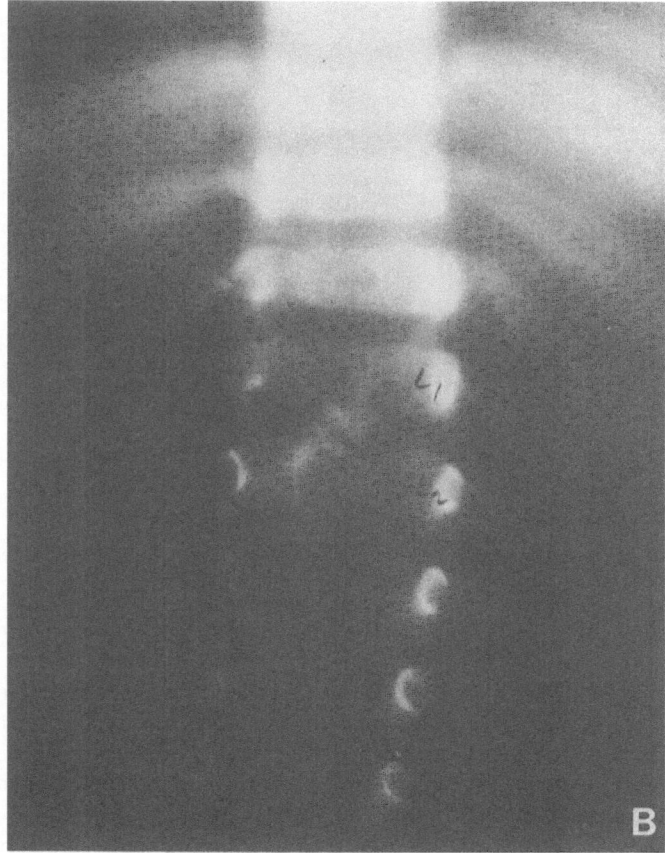

Figure 9.9. (*Continued*)

Such a deformity is flexible and decreases in severity with recumbency or with forward bending.

Fixed roundback deformity, or Scheuermann disease, is a rigid kyphosis of the dorsal spine (see Fig. 1.4) associated with endplate fragmentation and anterior wedging of at least three adjacent vertebrae. Presumably because of associated excessive lumbar lordosis, spondylolysis (see below) among patients with Scheuermann kyphosis occurs with increased frequency.

Patients with either type of kyphosis typically present with deformity, pain, and back fatigue in early adolescence. Physical examination should note the flexibility of the curve, with self-correction, examiner correction, and forward bending. Check for scoliosis which is common but usually mild and for hamstring tightness which seems to be worse the more rigid the curve.

The benefits of intervention for postural roundback have never been demonstrated.

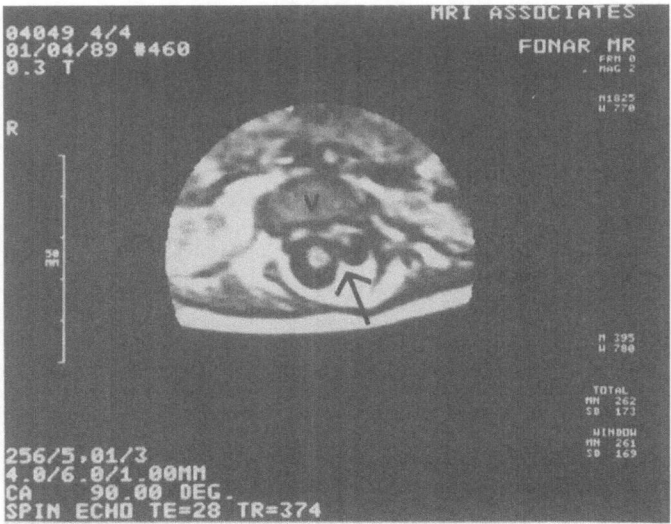

Figure 9.10. MRI showing diastematomyelia with splitting of spinal cord (arrow), each portion of which is covered by its own meninges. v, vertebral body.

If the young person is interested in improving their posture, then reinforcing this awareness, stretching their hamstrings, and improving trunk hyperextension by lying on the floor prone, will certainly not hurt. Sometimes, however, such focusing merely provides one more opportunity for parental nagging. Under such circumstances the exercises may do more harm than good.

The skeletally immature patient with true Scheuermann kyphosis can be treated in a three-point orthotic system which reduces lumbar lordosis with a well-molded pelvic mold, applying a posterior force just below the apex of the curve and an anterior force over the upper sternum. Assuming compliance, some correction can be obtained as the child grows. This condition is sometimes painful though long-term follow-up studies in adults are equivocal and many patients have little, if any, pain over the long run after skeletal maturity has occurred. Spinal instrumentation, a significant undertaking usually requiring anterior disc excision as well as posterior fusion, might be considered for severe cases.

9.4. PAINFUL LESIONS

Pain in the back is the second way in which pediatric spine disease may present. A good history should define the nature of the pain, its location, radiation, and relationship to activity; whether it is constant, intermittent, or nocturnal. The presence of painful scoliosis in particular is a red flag since most adolescents with idiopathic scoliosis are pain free. A careful physical examination is equally essential.

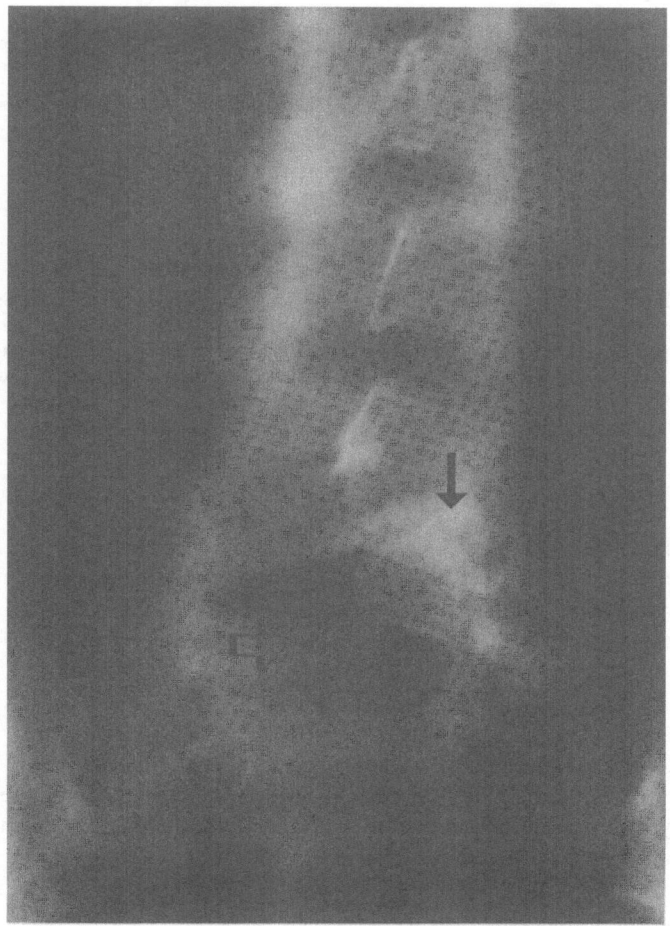

Figure 9.11. This 4-year-old girl presented with mild weakness of her right lower extremity and some measurable calf and thigh atrophy. X-ray reveals a lateral bar affecting L-4 and L-5 (arrow) and spina bifida occulta of L-5 (open arrow). Her spine is straight for now though such segmentation problems may reduce growth on the side with the bar leading to scoliosis as the patient grows.

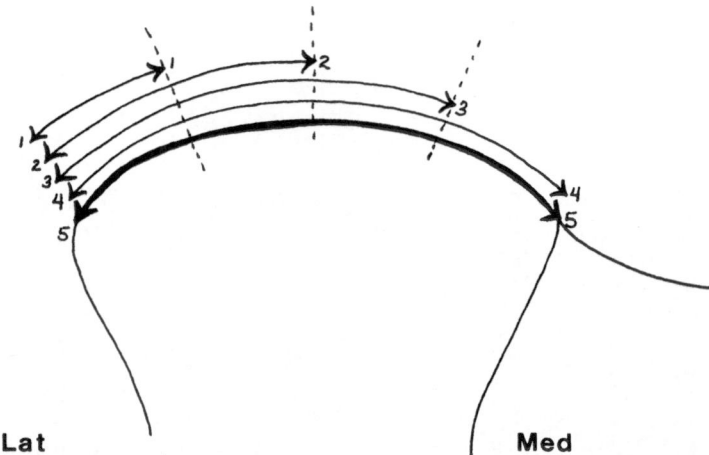

Lat   **Med**

Figure 9.12. Skeletal maturity is a major factor in predicting progression of scoliosis. The Risser method is convenient since it uses the iliac apophyses which are usually seen on the spinal films. Iliac ossification progresses laterally (stage 1) to medially (stages 2 to 4) before it fuses (stage 5). By the time Risser stage 1 is evident, menarche has just occurred or is just about to occur and the patient is growing at her maximum rate. By the time Risser stage 4 has occurred, longitudinal growth is virtually complete.

In an analysis of 100 children with back pain, Robert Hensinger of Ann Arbor, Michigan, determined that one-third had some lesion related to trauma, one-third had some deformity such as Scheuermann disease or postural roundback, 18% had an infection or tumor, and 15% could not be diagnosed (Hensinger, 1985).

9.4.1. Staged Evaluation

Careful X-ray examinations of the spine are indicated, including AP, lateral, and oblique projections. If these are negative, a technetium bone scan should be considered as well as an erythrocyte sedimentation rate. If these do not show any abnormalities, then MRI or CT should be considered.

9.4.2. Discitis (see also Chapter 2)

Discitis, an inflammatory process of the intervertebral disc, may be associated with localized pain, refusal to walk, abdominal pain, anorexia, and irritability in infants and young children. Examination will reveal a stiff back with spasm and localized tenderness, most often over L-4–L-5. The ESR is usually increased though the leukocyte count is most often normal. Radiography is not helpful early on but will eventually demonstrate narrowing of the intervertebral disc space, with erosion, irregularity, and sclerosis of the adjacent vertebral endplates after about 3 weeks (see Fig. 2.22). Technetium bone

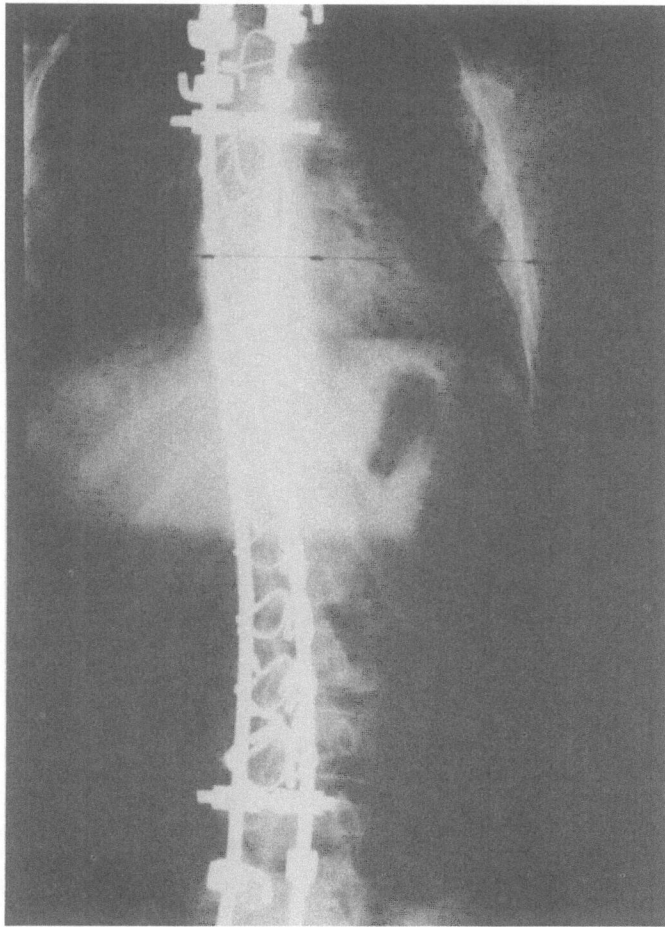

Figure 9.13. Same patient as in Fig. 9.3, now postop after spinal instrumentation. Internal fixation allows for earlier mobilization after surgery and obviates need for prolonged casting.

scanning will often reveal an area of focal uptake and MRI scanning may be useful if the bone scan is not.

Discitis is presumed to be a bacterial infection though blood cultures are almost always negative and direct aspiration of the disc space reveals a pathogen, usually *Staphylococcus aureus*, in only a minority of cases.

True vertebral osteomyelitis is a different, more dramatic disease with more toxicity and a sicker patient. Vertebral bodies themselves, rather than the interspace, are involved. In either case, tuberculous disease of the spine needs to be ruled out with a tuberculin skin test.

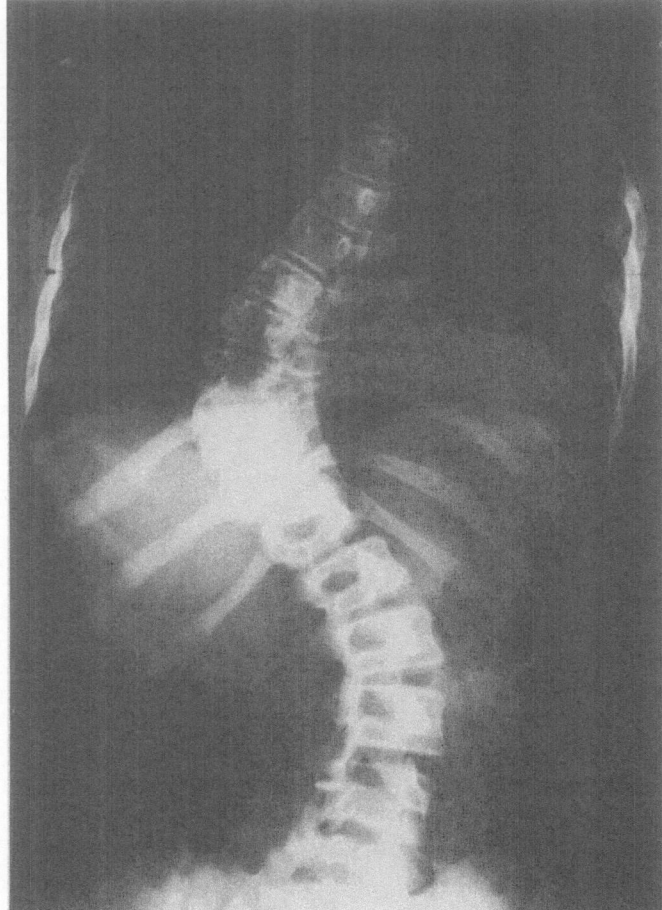

Figure 9.14. Moderately severe scoliosis in this 11-year-old girl with Marfan syndrome.

The use of antistaphylococcal antibiotics in children with discitis is a source of constant discussion and some controversy. Certainly it would be reasonable to see how the child did without them, at least initially. Immobilization is usually self-imposed. If the child is very uncomfortable, a corset, plaster body cast, or molded plastic orthosis may be useful. Nonsteroidal anti-inflammatory medications (see Chapter 11) may be necessary.

Resolution of symptoms may take weeks to months but is complete in children with typical discitis. Later symptoms of back pain are uncommon. Though the disc space may be completely lost, with follow-up films showing fusion of the contiguous vertebral bodies, the disc space will most often reconstitute itself completely.

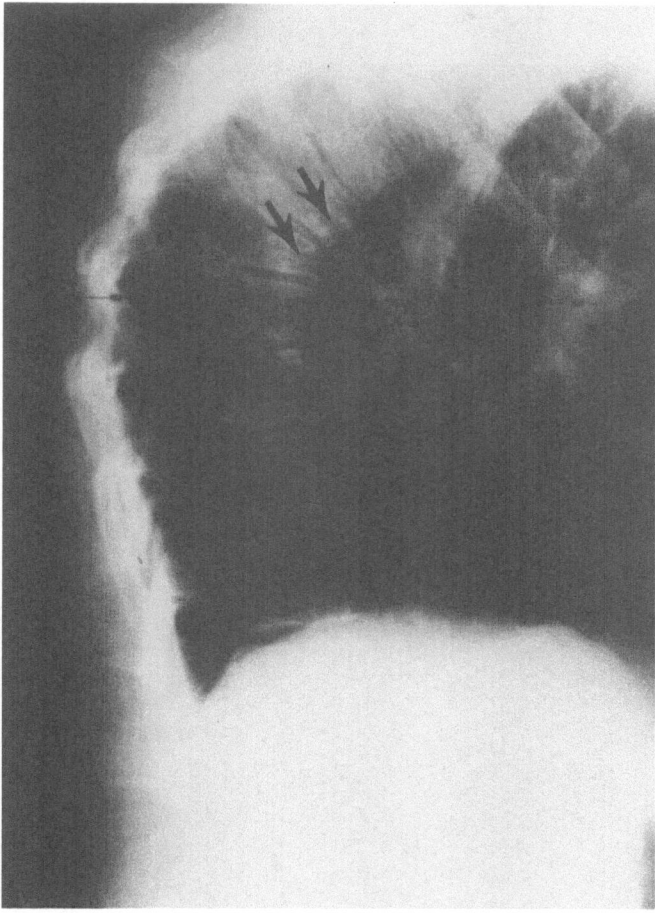

Figure 9.15. Severe kyphosis with anterior wedging of multiple vertebral bodies (arrows) is typical of Scheuermann disease as in this 19-year-old male.

9.4.3. Spondylolisthesis and Spondylolysis

Spondylolisthesis means slipped spine. One of the lower lumbar vertebrae, usually L-5, literally slides anteriorly across the next lower vertebral body. This slippage is a result of bilateral bony defects or stress fractures of the pars interarticularis, which is part of the posterior elements of the spinal arch. The presence of such defects is termed *spondylolysis*. It is hypothesized that the affected child is born with a propensity to develop such a defect which is then actualized with repeated stressful activity (see also Chapter 8). The frequency of spondylolysis in the general population is as high as 6% (Fredrickson *et al.*, 1984) and it is sometimes difficult to know if the child's back

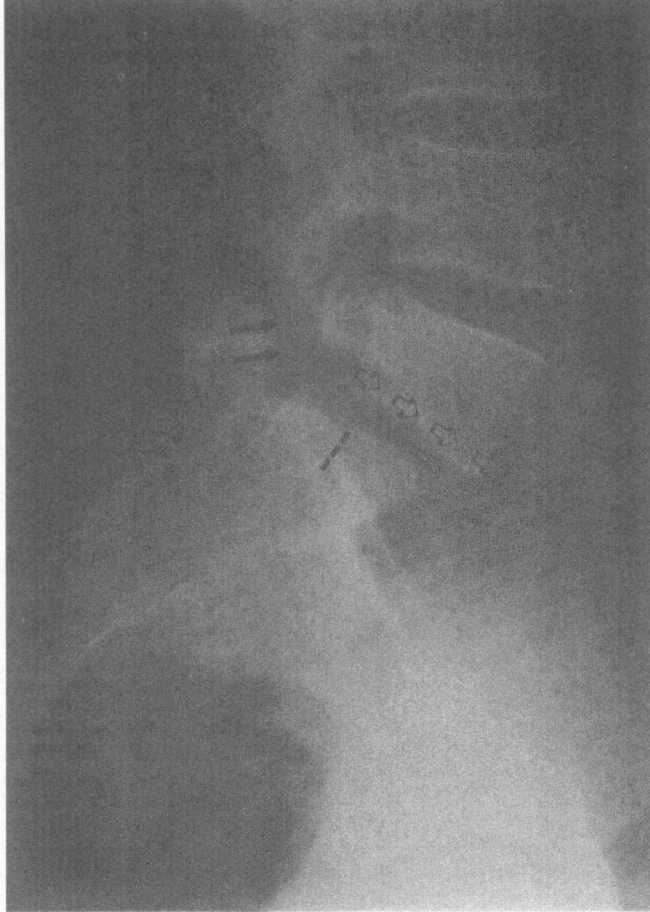

Figure 9.16. Spondylolysis (arrows) and spondylolisthesis (open arrows) in a 16-year-old male The slip is more than ¼ of the surface of the sacrum, but less than ½, and therefore is a grade 2 slip

complaints are related to the presence of the pars defect or whether the latter is only coincidentally present Similarly it is not known why some children with spondylolysis will slip while many others won't

Frequently the pain is related to nerve root compression with radiation to the lower extremities Spondylolisthesis of sufficient magnitude to cause significant pain is usually obvious on physical examination with the child demonstrating loss of the normal lumbar lordosis, "shortening" of the waist resulting from prominence of the iliac wings posteriorly and tight hamstrings with a shortened stride length and a tendency to crouch at the knees. Scoliosis, if present, is not usually structural but more often related to asymmetrical muscle spasm.

Spondylolysis is sometimes difficult to see radiographically, even when oblique films of the lumbar spine are obtained. Technetium bone scanning may be useful if symptoms have been present for less than a year. CT may also be useful if the need for an immediate diagnosis is compelling. When spondylolisthesis is present, lateral X-rays of the lumbosacral spine usually show the deformity without difficulty. Severity is graded based on the approximate fraction of the lower vertebral body traversed by the slip: grade 1 = ¼, grade 2 = ½, and so on.

Treatment should be based on symptomatology. Spondylolysis usually requires some modification, usually temporary, of activity, nonsteroidal anti-inflammatory medications, and hamstring stretching. Spondylolisthesis which is mild to moderate (slips less than 50% of vertebral width) and associated with minimal symptoms requires only observation with repeat standing lumbosacral films every 6 months. Restriction of those activities likely to exacerbate the slip (like gymnastics, weight lifting, or football) would be reasonable. In cases with more substantial slips and significant symptomatology, surgical fusion between the fourth and fifth vertebrae and the sacrum results in relief of symptoms and restoration of adequate function. Some spine surgeons now recommend true reduction of the spondylolisthesis, though it probably is not necessary in the majority of patients.

9.4.4. Intervertebral Disc Disease

Disc herniation does occur in adolescence, frequently manifested by significant paravertebral muscle spasm, tight hamstrings, and diffuse, poorly localized pain, sometimes radiating into the distal lower extremity. Most occur either between L-5 and S-1 or between L-4 and L-5. Affected children may have neurologic deficits, including weakness and decreased DTRs, which may overshadow the pain. This is in contradistinction to adult disc herniation in which pain is the primary and major symptom.

The patient will exhibit positive straight leg raising tests bilaterally, will stand with forward flexion of the trunk, and may have unilateral paravertebral muscle spasm with a list to one side or the other. Frequently, the onset of symptoms is gradual and there is usually no discrete traumatic or lifting event remembered.

Plain films are usually unrevealing. In a patient with persistent back pain, particularly if radicular and associated with spasm, MRI should be considered if ESR, bone scan, and plain radiographs are unrevealing (see Fig. 9.17). Most often, patients with disc herniation will respond to adequate rest in a body cast.

9.4.5. Intrathecal Lesions

Primary intrathecal lesions are not as common as brain tumors in children but do occur and manifest themselves by neurological findings and back pain without discrete radiographic findings. Listen for a history of increasing bowel or bladder difficulties; look for DTR changes, weakness, sensory loss, or abnormalities of tone. In these patients, the MRI and myelogram can be of great help.

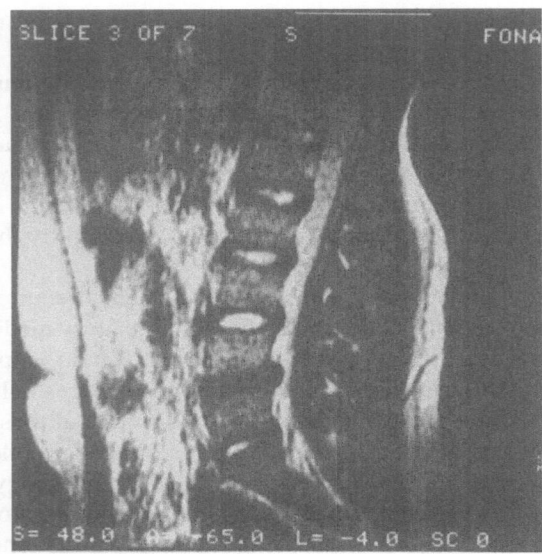

Figure 9.17. L-4–L-5 disc prolapse in a 20-year-old male is easily seen on this MRI scan.

9.4.6. Chronic Arthritis

Juvenile rheumatoid arthritis (JRA) and juvenile ankylosing spondylitis both cause spinal disease in children. In the polyarticular form of JRA, the majority of children have stiffening and even ankylosis of the cervical spine as a result of facet joint synovitis. Atlantoaxial instability may also be present as a result of C-1–C-2 synovitis and may be of concern neurologically if hyperextension of the neck is necessary during anesthetic intubation.

Ankylosing spondylitis occurs predominantly in adolescent or young adult males and is manifested by pain, lumbar flattening and stiffness, limitation of chest expansion, and reduced lateral flexion of the spine. It is associated with sacroilitis and HLA B-27 positivity. X-rays may lag clinical disease by years (see also Chapter 11).

9.4.7. Pathologic Fractures

Pathologic fractures, often compression fractures, occur in the spine of children and adolescents, causing pain, spasm, and deformity. Included here are such disorders as eosinophilic granuloma (now grouped under Langerhans cell histiocytosis), sarcoidosis, and neuroblastoma. Careful workup, including referral as needed, should result in an appropriate diagnosis in these patients.

9.4.8. Tumors of the Spine

Two specific tumors of the spine are associated with both deformity and pain. Aneurysmal bone cysts occur about the pelvis and throughout the spine and are

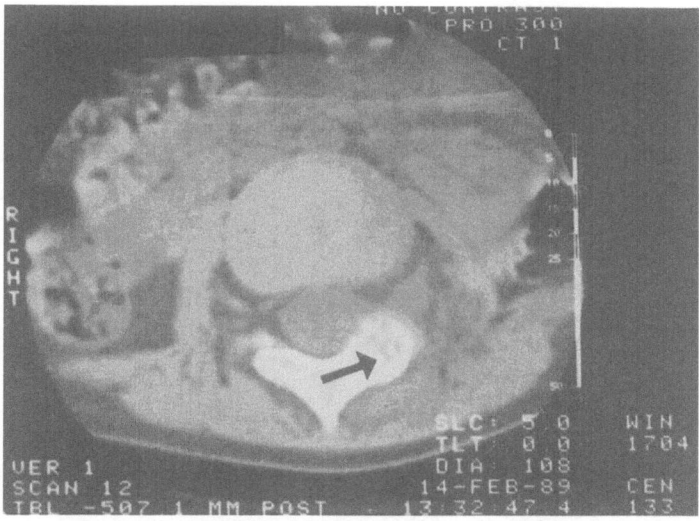

Figure 9.18. Osteoid osteoma in a vertebral pedicle (arrow), a typical location. Nidus is frequently calcified on CT scans when not detectable on plain films

associated with pain and an expanding lytic lesion on X-ray. Curettage and bone grafting is the preferred treatment. In some surgically inaccessible areas, X-ray treatment may be useful.

Osteoid osteoma and its big cousin, osteoblastoma, are benign skeletal tumors, characterized by a nidus of osteoid tissue surrounded by densely reactive sclerotic bone. They occur not infrequently in the posterior element of a vertebral body, and cause localized pain with muscle spasm and secondary scoliosis, usually with the curve concavity on the side of the lesion. Pain is worse at night and has traditionally been relieved by the use of aspirin (not as good a sign as it used to be since few children receive aspirin any more). It is difficult to diagnose because it frequently is not visible on plain radiographs. Technetium bone scanning reveals an intense area of focal uptake, however (see Fig. 2.18). Surgical excision results in relief of pain and resolution of the scoliosis.

9.5. OTHER SPINAL CONDITIONS

9.5.1. Os Odontoideum

The embryologic development of the first and second cervical vertebrae is complicated. The dens or odontoid process, which is the finger of bone projecting from the top of the body of C-2, articulates with the front of the ring vertebral body (C-1) and provides stability to the upper cervical spine. It originates from three separate ossification centers which fuse to produce a solid piece of bone from the top of the dens down through the body of C-2. *Os odontoideum* is the term used to describe failure of the

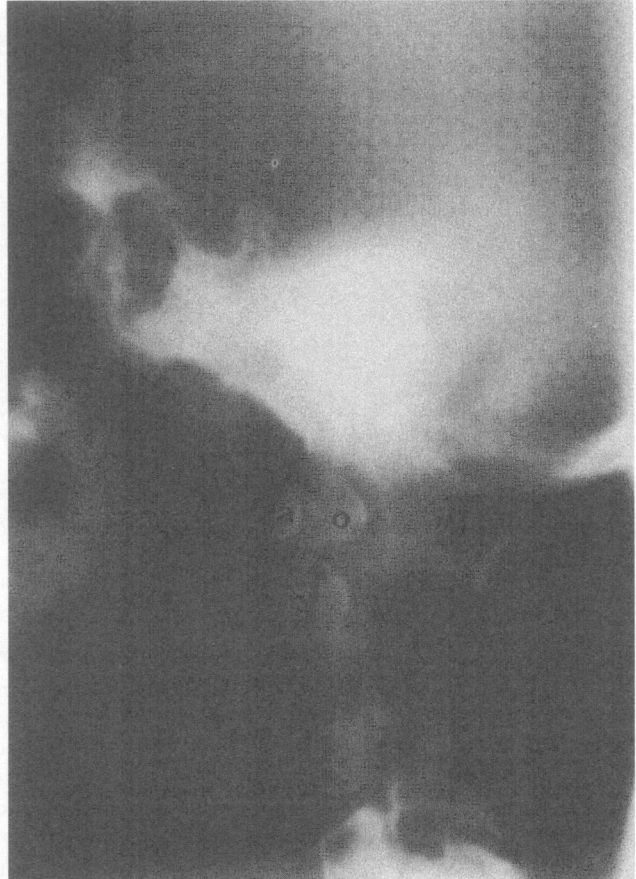

Figure 9.19. Os odontoideum affecting a 14-year-old male is readily apparent on this tomogram (arrow). Note separate odontoid fragment (o) which moves with atlas (a).

fusion process, with a structurally weakened odontoid allowing for increased mobility between the first and second vertebrae, analogous to, and difficult to tell the difference from, the nonunion of an odontoid fracture.

Children with os odontoideum or other congenital or acquired abnormalities of C-1–C-2 may present with local neck symptoms such as torticollis, progressive quadriplegia, transient neurologic symptoms, or incidentally, when a lateral neck radiograph is obtained after an episode of trauma.

Surgical fusion is indicated for children with neurologic signs or symptoms, progressive or excessive instability, or persistent pain or limitation of neck motion. Excessive instability is defined variably by different experts but is usually considered to be present when there is greater than 5 to 7 mm of distance between the posterior surface of the anterior ring of C-1 and the anterior surface of the odontoid. Perhaps as important as any absolute distance is the presence of a substantial increase in the atlanto-dens distances from extension to flexion.

9.5.2. Down Syndrome and Cervical Spinal Instability

Presumably secondary to ligamentous laxity, instability between C-1 and C-2 and also between C-1 and the occiput is more frequent in children with Down syndrome (see Fig. 8.8). Additionally, some children with Down syndrome have actual loss of the transverse atlantal ligament which is designed to keep the odontoid snuggled up against

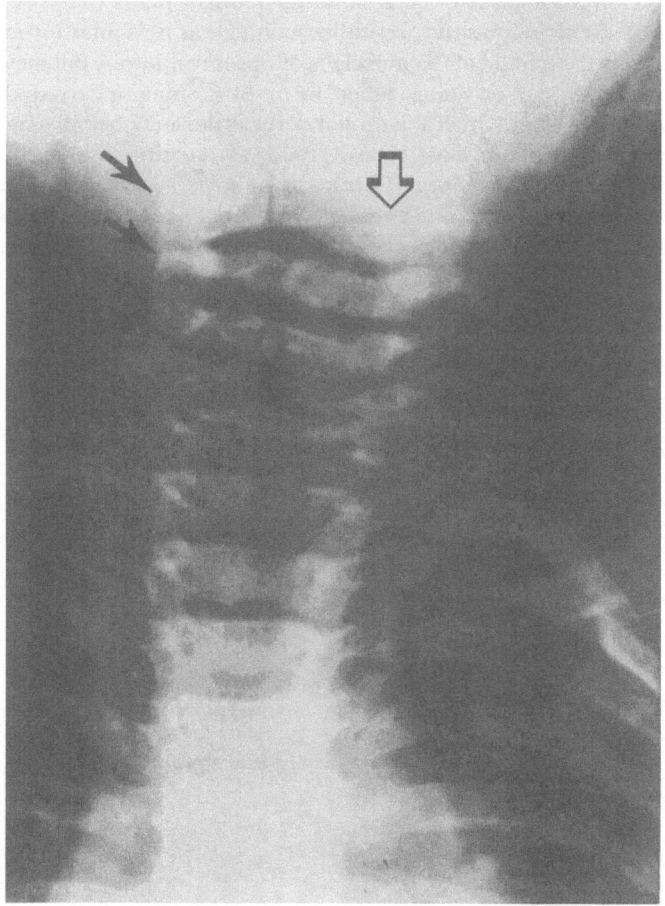

Figure 9.20. Klippel–Feil syndrome, note lateral bar (arrows) of C-2, C-4, and C-5 on right and hemivertebra of C-3 on left (open arrow)

the anterior ring of C-1. Neurologic signs or symptoms, happily, are much less common than radiographic abnormalities.

Lateral cervical spine flexion and extension films should be periodically obtained on children with Down syndrome, perhaps every 3 years in school-age children. This is particularly so if they are engaging in athletic activities which involve contact or neck flexion or are to undergo general anesthesia requiring neck hyperextension for intubation. Many organizations require a medical certificate that cervical instability does not exist before participation in athletics is permitted.

9.5.3. Torticollis

Torticollis (literally, twisted neck) is complicated in its etiology but refers to abnormal posture of the head in relation to the shoulders, usually with lateral flexion and rotation of the head. In most cases of congenital torticollis, this is caused by a fibrous contracture of the sternocleidomastoid, so-called congenital muscular torticollis. This fibrous tumor (olive) in the middle of the muscle is of obscure etiology but may be related to a compartment syndrome or some other form of trauma incurred during late intrauterine life or during labor. Other positional deformities may be present, including hip dysplasia (see Chapter 6). In most cases, gradual stretching and tincture of time result in a satisfactory outcome. Surgical release of a persistent contracture of the sternocleidomastoid, however, may be necessary and should be done before the patient develops facial asymmetry and ocular accommodation to the abnormal posture.

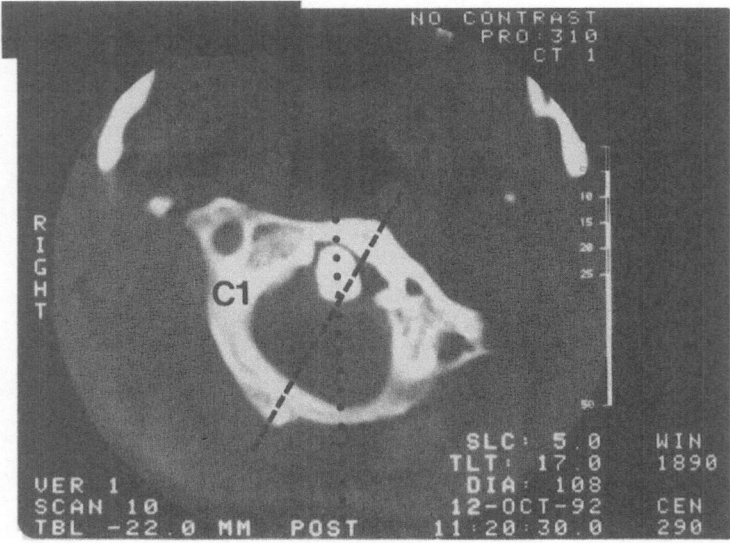

Figure 9.21. Rotatory atlantoaxial subluxation in this teenage female as demonstrated by CT. C-1 is rotated clockwise about 30° relative to C-2, as judged using long axis of odontoid.

Primary congenital anomalies of the cervical spine, including Klippel–Feil syndrome, odontoid hypoplasia, or os odontoideum, may also present with torticollis (see above). Failure to make the correct diagnosis may result in neurologic catastrophe if physical therapy is attempted injudiciously.

Acquired torticollis can result from serious cervical trauma but is more frequently related to such benign causes as minor soft-tissue trauma or viral myositis. Rotatory atlantoaxial subluxation is not rare in children and may be related to an upper respiratory tract infection or to chronic inflammation of the C-1–C-2 joint as occurs with JRA.

Other, less common causes of torticollis include gastroesophageal reflux, cervical disc disease, ocular strabismus, cervical syringomyelia and tumors of the posterior fossa, brain stem, spinal cord, or vertebral column.

Plain radiographs (AP and lateral) of the cervical spine should be obtained on all infants with torticollis before therapy is attempted. CT (for bony lesions) or MRI (for cord lesions) scanning should be considered when radiographic abnormalities, neck webbing, low hair line, or neurologic abnormalities are in evidence or when no sternocleidomastoid abnormality is apparent.

Therapy can be performed at home by gentle but persistent lateral flexion of the head to stretch the contralaterally tightened sternocleidomastoid muscle. Rotation of the head toward the side with the tightness can be done simultaneously. Ten to twenty repetitions, holding momentarily at maximal range, will usually suffice if done three or four times daily. Physical therapy is a good idea in order to monitor progress and compliance.

10

Musculoskeletal Trauma

10.1. INTRODUCTION

It is our purpose here to review common musculoskeletal injuries seen in children and to offer suggestions for treatment or referral.

Traumatic injuries discussed below will generally be those of relatively modest degree rather than the high-velocity trauma likely to result in multiple-system trauma presenting in the emergency room. It is axiomatic, but well worth mentioning again, that all physicians have a responsibility not only to appropriately treat traumatic injuries but to try to prevent them as well through anticipatory advice given at routine visits and by supporting such legislative efforts as mandatory seat belt and bike helmet laws.

10.2. COMMON PEDIATRIC MUSCULOSKELETAL INJURIES

The immature skeleton responds to trauma in ways that are significantly different from the mature one:

1. Traumatic dislocations are uncommon in prepubertal children because their joints are more strongly put together than the adjoining growth plates. Force applied to an extremity is more likely to result in a fracture through the growth plate than a dislocation.
2. Severe sprains (ligamentous injuries) and strains (muscular injuries) are similarly uncommon in prepubertal children for the same reason.
3. Damage to the entire growth plate may result in complete arrest of growth and severe shortening. Damage to a portion of the growth plate may result in uneven arrest of growth and an angular deformity.
4. Angular deformities may also result from a diaphyseal or metaphyseal fracture itself, though a growing child's bone will correct angular deformity to a surprising degree. The younger the child, the greater is the ability to correct angulation.
5. Fractures that result in rotational deformities are more of a problem and do not correct nearly as well.
6. Fractures may result in overgrowth as well. For reasons incompletely understood, fractures will stimulate growth at the physis of the fractured bone.

Evaluation of pediatric trauma requires attention to the details of the injury. If the injury occurred several days ago, has the pain and tenderness improved?

Is there discoloration or localized tenderness? Is there evidence for neurologic damage with loss of sensation and paralysis or arterial injury with pallor, pain, and a cold extremity? Mild strains or sprains with diffuse tenderness and discoloration may need only rest, elevation, ice packs, and analgesia.

Weakness, joint instability, or a joint effusion or hemarthrosis may imply a more significant soft-tissue injury requiring referral.

Fractures may be **buckle**, with both cortices intact, **greenstick**, with one intact, or **complete**, with both disrupted. They may be **comminuted**, with three or more fragments, or **compound**, with the skin punctured. They may be **transverse**, **oblique**, **longitudinal**, or **spiral**. They may affect the diaphysis, the metaphysis, the physis, the epiphysis, the articular surface, or more than one of the above.

Knowing the Salter–Harris classification of different types of epiphyseal growth plate fractures is important but less important than knowing that such a growth plate fracture has occurred. This is not always easy since such fractures are difficult to see radiologically. Growth plate injuries should be suspected when soft-tissue swelling is significant, particularly in the presence of a hemarthrosis, even with negative X-rays. Technetium bone scanning may be more sensitive and referral is always indicated when a growth plate injury is suspected.

Finally, don't forget to ask yourself "why" this injury happened, a slightly different question than "how" it happened. Is this a child who is pathologically hyperactive or impulsive? Is there evidence for enough social disorganization of the family to prompt a concern regarding child abuse, intentional or related to malignant neglect (see Chapter 3)? Is there evidence for intrinsic bone disease like osteogenesis imperfecta, Ehler–Danlos, osteoporosis, cysts, or steroids?

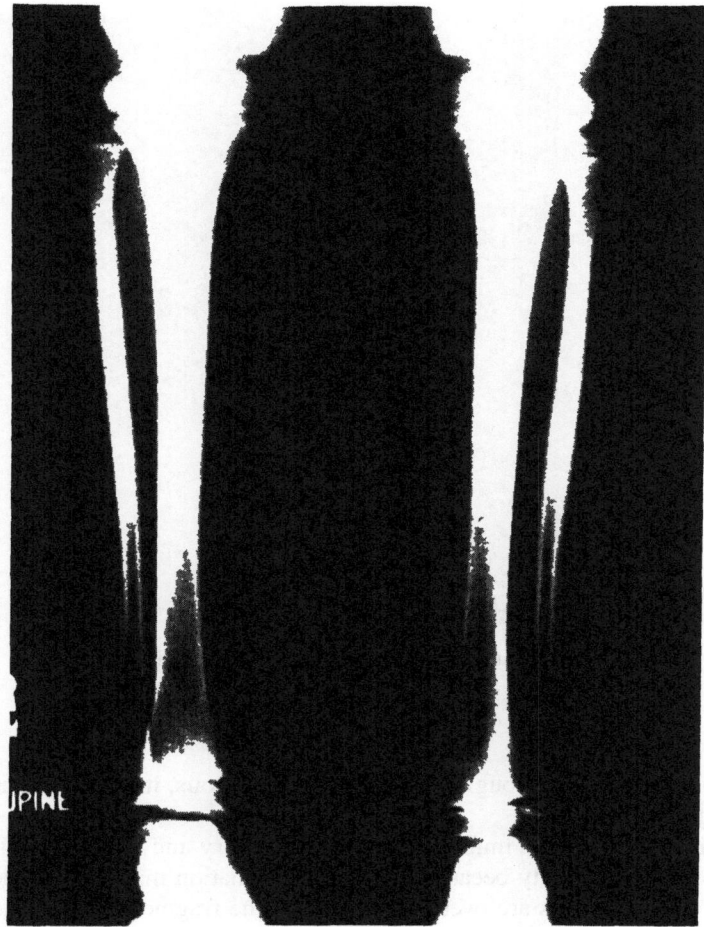

UPINE

Figure 10.1. Note well-healed torus fracture to medial aspect of distal left tibia Fracture has caused medial overgrowth with a leg-length discrepancy and obliquity of the ankle joint

10.2.1. Fracture of the Clavicle

One of the most commonly broken bones in the body is the clavicle. Its function is to serve as a strut to connect the pectoral girdle to the axial skeleton. A compressive force applied to the side of the shoulder or transferred through an outstretched upper extremity is the most common cause of this fracture. The clavicle is most commonly broken in the midshaft but fractures occur anywhere along its length. A fracture may be combined with a dislocation of either the sternoclavicular joint medially or the acromio-

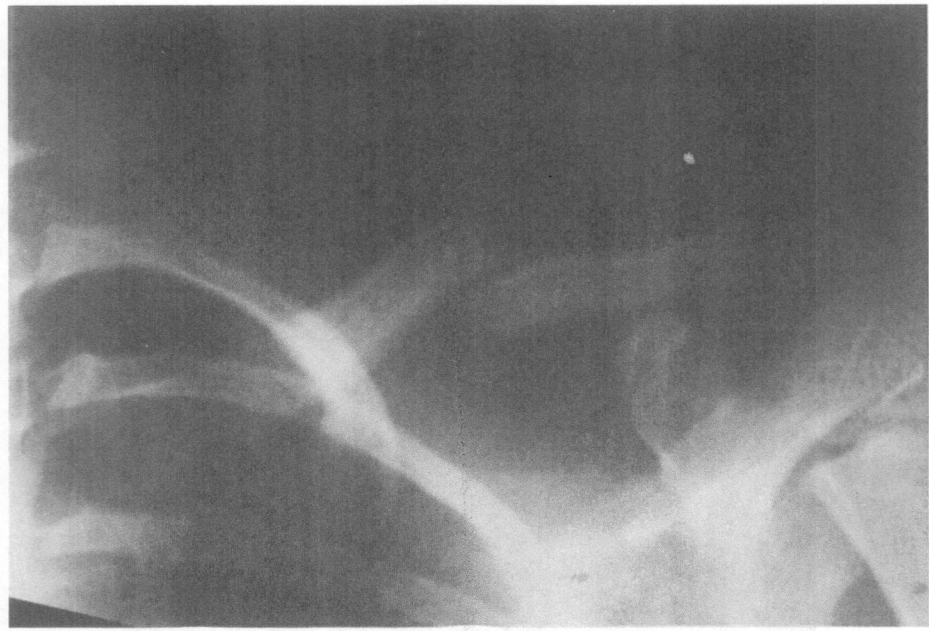

Figure 10.2. Fractured clavicle beginning to show callus formation.

clavicular joint laterally. Although the bone is subcutaneous, it is rather unusual for the fracture to puncture the skin.

The child will complain immediately after the injury and will be unable to abduct (elevate) the upper extremity because of pain. Examination may reveal a bony prominence if the two fragments are overriding. Even if the fragments are aligned, there is usually swelling resulting from a hematoma. There is always tenderness to palpation at the fracture and even passive manipulation causes pain. It is very unusual for nerve or vessels to be damaged but examination of peripheral pulses and a neurologic exam should always be done.

The child will complain of pain with passive or active movement of the shoulder. Sleeping is troublesome because rolling on the involved shoulder causes pain. Fortunately, sufficient union of the clavicle occurs in 7 to 10 days for pain to lessen and function to return. Radiographically, early union is seen at 3 weeks. Any residual deformity or bony prominence usually spontaneously corrects in children under 10 years of age.

There are many treatments recommended for a fracture of the clavicle and none are very effective. In an effort to reduce overriding, various figure-of-eight straps, casts, and bandages have been suggested to force the shoulders back. Unfortunately, the constant pressure required and the constriction of the axillae caused by these appliances are often intolerable and sometimes inflict more discomfort than the injury. Usually a simple sling for 10 days to 2 weeks with appropriate oral pain medication is sufficient treatment. The child will even discard this when the pain diminishes. There are few significant residuals of a fractured clavicle in a child. Repeat or follow-up X-rays for alignment or healing are not necessary.

10.2.2. Fracture of the Humerus

In general, these fractures should be referred for orthopedic consultation because the treatment may be complex. It is important to emphasize that one of the more serious fractures occurring in children is a supracondylar fracture of the humerus. This fracture occurs immediately proximal to the condyles of the humerus through the relatively weak epicondylar ridges. Any displacement or rotation may result in an angular deformity referred to as a cubitus varus or "gunstock" deformity. Although this deformity does not result in any loss of function, it is unsightly.

The most common age for this fracture to occur is between 2 and 12 years. The child presents after falling off a swing, out of a tree, off a bike, and the like. There is immediate swelling and loss of function. The severity of the fracture varies. In some, there is only a crack through the humerus just above the condyles of the humerus and no displacement. Indeed, at times it is difficult to see the fracture on X-ray. However, swelling, pain, and point tenderness just above the elbow should lead the physician to suspect an undisplaced supracondylar fracture of the humerus. Should this be the case, a simple posterior splint can be applied initially with the elbow at 90° of flexion and the child referred.

Should the initial X-ray examination reveal any angulation or displacement of the distal fragment, the child should be referred to an orthopedist immediately. A displaced supracondylar fracture of the humerus is a serious injury. The immediate concern is a compartment syndrome of the forearm (Volkmann's ischemic necrosis) which can lead to serious loss of function. Improper reduction can also lead to deformity.

10.2.3. Nursemaid's Elbow

This injury is not a fracture but rather a subluxation of the radial head from the confining annular ligament associated with a transverse tear of the ligament. The history is usually given that the child was being pulled or lifted by the hand. A click is sometimes felt or heard as the child screams with pain and refuses to use the involved extremity. It is rare after 5 years of age.

The examiner will see an unhappy whimpering child who holds the arm immobilized, usually with the elbow in flexion and the forearm pronated. There is no swelling but the child is very apprehensive that the examiner will try to palpate or manipulate the elbow. The only physical findings are tenderness over the head of the radius and resistance to supination of the forearm.

X-ray examination is not necessary with a typical history and will show no pathology. If radiographs are taken to rule out an associated fracture, the child will not

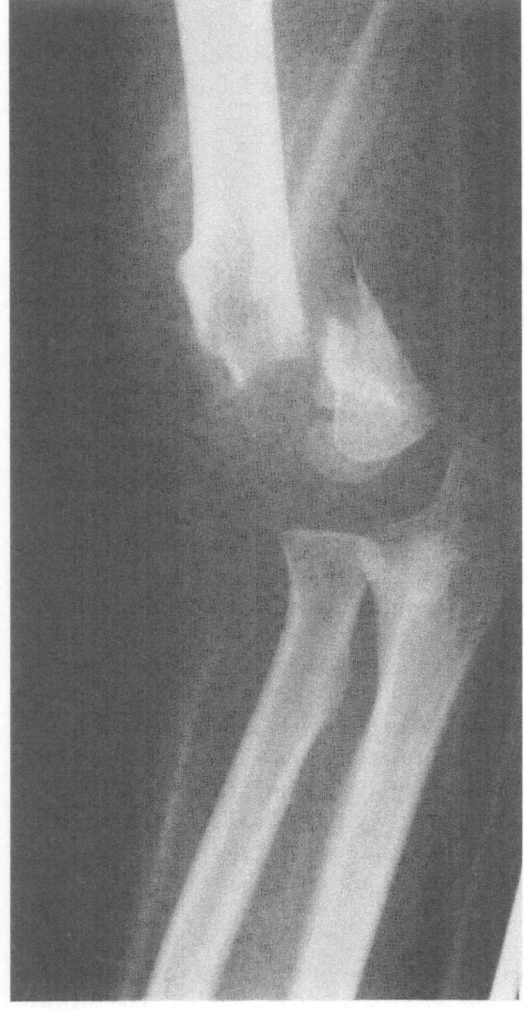

Figure 10.3. Supracondylar fracture of the humerus; such an injury represents a neurovascular risk of major proportions and should be splinted and referred immediately

infrequently return with normal function of the elbow. This is because the X-ray technologist has supinated the forearm in order to obtain an anteroposterior view of the elbow. This maneuver frequently reduces the radial head and relieves the symptoms.

Regardless, reduction is usually not difficult. No anesthesia is necessary. After gaining some confidence, grasp the child's arm with one hand just above the elbow with the elbow flexed 90°. With the other hand, grasp the thumb and radial side of the hand. While applying gentle traction, rotate the forearm firmly into full supination. A click may or may not be felt as the head reduces, but the child is usually relieved and starts using the extremity normally within a few minutes. Repeated attempts at reductions are only very occasionally necessary and sometimes full return of function doesn't occur for 2 to 3 days. If no improvement becomes evident after watching the child for a reasonable length of time, alternative explanations for the child's difficulties should be sought. Some children have recurrent dislocation until they reach the age of 4 or 5 years.

10.2.4. Monteggia Fracture of the Forearm

This specific fracture is mentioned because failure to diagnose this injury can lead to permanent loss of function. A Monteggia fracture is defined as a fracture of the ulna, usually midshaft, with a dislocation of the head of the radius, usually anteriorly. In children under the age of 7 years the ulna can undergo a volar plastic deformation without obvious fracture accompanied by an anterior dislocation of the head of the radius. The symptoms are not dramatic and the swelling can be quite subtle.

Pathomechanically, a fall on an outstretched arm sufficient to fracture the ulna (even if a greenstick) must do something to its bony forearm roommate. If the radius is not also fractured, it is essential to look for a dislocation of the radial head. The child presents with discomfort, holding the forearm flexed and pronated at the elbow. Examination will reveal some loss of passive supination of the forearm.

X-ray examination will reveal some anterior bowing of the ulna and close inspection will show anterior dislocation of the head of the radius. Radiographs should be done at both the elbow and wrist in order to avoid missing radial dislocation. Remember that the long axis of the radius proximally should always pass through the capitellum.

If a Monteggia fracture dislocation is present, the patient should be referred. Similarly, an isolated fracture of the ulna, even without apparent radial dislocation, should be seen by an orthopedist. On occasion, the child with this diagnosis will be missed and the mother will then bring the child in about 6 to 8 weeks after the injury noting a firm lump laterally at the elbow. This is the dislocated head of the radius. Even at this time some corrective surgery can and should be done to restore normal function.

The opposite scenario also occurs. Isolated fractures of the radius should be checked thoroughly for disruption of the distal radioulnar joint. On physical examination the distal ulna may appear protuberant or hypermobile. With radial fractures, radiographs of the distal radioulnar joint should always be obtained.

10.2.5. Buckle (Torus) Fracture of the Radius

These are common and occur as a result of a fall on an outstretched arm. There is initial pain but no deformity. It is not uncommon for parents to ignore the injury, considering it to be one of the many bumps and bruises of a growing child. There is little discomfort as long as the extremity is not used but symptoms persist and parents then seek medical attention.

On examination there is minimal swelling over the distal radius, no deformity, and normal passive but not active motion of the hand. The child will resist passive flexion and extension of the wrist and pronation and supination of the forearm elicits pain. The most important clinical finding is point tenderness to palpation of the radius about 1½ inches proximal to the wrist. The physical findings and the history of reluctance to use the extremity should lead to an X-ray examination.

Such an examination will reveal a buckle fracture of the dorsal cortex of the radius just proximal to the end of the bone. There is no significant angulation and no displacement. This fracture would heal with no treatment at all but the physician should apply some sort of forearm splint to increase comfort, and to remind the child of the fracture and hopefully avoid a complete fracture should another injury occur soon. The child's symptoms disappear within a week and the fracture is healed sufficiently in 3 weeks to allow removal of any immobilization.

10.2.6. Spiral Fracture of the Tibia

This injury to the midshaft of the tibia without fibular injury is seen in children 12 to 30 months of age. It is caused by a rotation stress applied to the tibia occurring during a fall. The fall does not have to be impressive and may occur during play. The rotational stress causes an undisplaced, usually long, spiral fracture of the tibia that does not cause deformity and the child is usually rather quickly pacified but simply refuses to walk.

On examination there is surprisingly little found. The child may or may not show discomfort with deep palpation of the tibia. There is no significant swelling. Some-

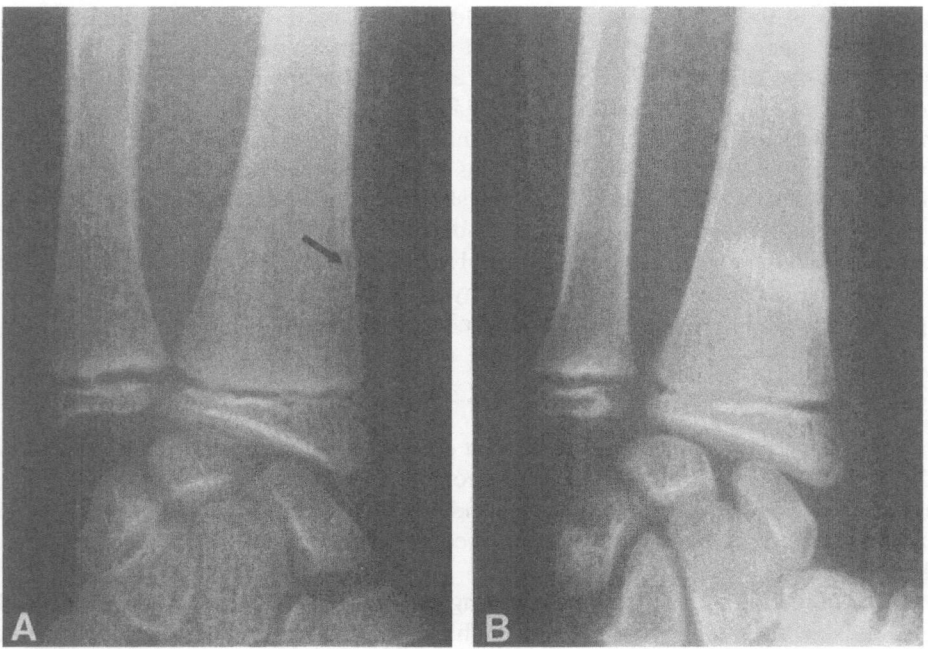

Figure 10.4. (A) Torus fracture of distal radius represented by a barely perceptible buckle of cortex (B) Follow-up injury demonstrates true nature of transverse bony injury

times a twist applied to the foot causes the child to wince but this does not localize the pain. The diagnosis is that of exclusion. A child in this age range who refuses to walk, is afebrile, and has a normal joint examination must be considered to have an undisplaced spiral fracture of the tibia.

X-ray examination is often useful though the standard anteroposterior and lateral radiographs may not always show a fracture. Under such circumstances, a 45° oblique film may. If still in doubt, a technetium bone scan is more sensitive than plain radiographs early on.

External immobilization in a weight-bearing plaster cast for 3 to 4 weeks is all the treatment required.

Child abuse is in the differential diagnosis, particularly so in the young infant who is not walking or even standing.

10.3. BIRTH TRAUMA

Birth may be a traumatic event for the neonate as well as the mother. Injury may occur to the brain, skull, face, spinal column, abdominal viscera, brachial plexus, muscles of the neck, or the long bones. This section will deal with damage to the brachial plexus and injuries to the long bones.

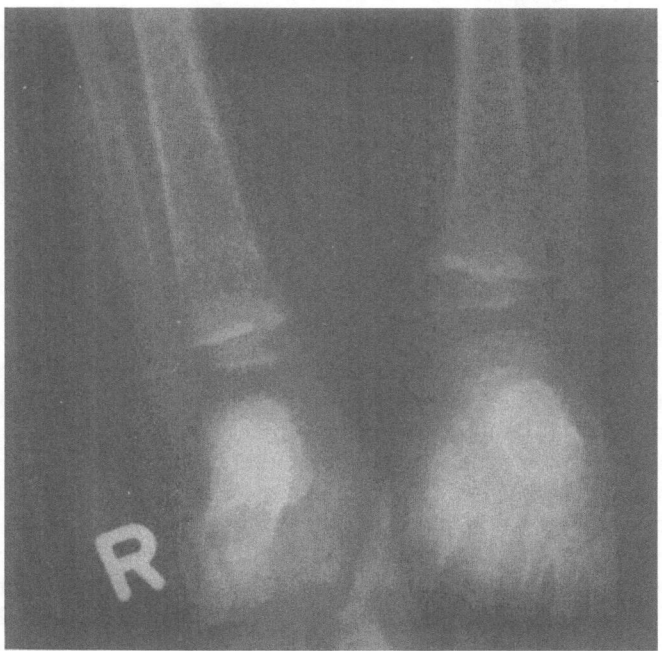

Figure 10.5. Spiral fracture of right tibia. When difficult to see on conventional AP and lateral films, spiral fractures may sometimes be seen on oblique view.

10.3.1. Brachial Plexus Injury

Injury to the brachial plexus is caused by traction on the head during delivery complicated by shoulder dystocia secondary to macrosomia. The incidence of this injury is 0.37 to 0.87 per 1000 live births (Donn and Faix, 1983). Upper brachial plexus palsy involves the C-5 and C-6 nerve roots and is called Erb or Erb–Duchenne palsy. Sixty to seventy percent of all brachial plexus injuries are of this type. About 25% of the injuries involve the lower roots C-8 to T-1 (termed Klumpke paralysis) and in 10%, the entire brachial plexus is involved. Bilateral involvement occurs in about 10%. There is an accompanying clavicular fracture in 10% (Jackson *et al.*, 1988).

The injury is often noted by the parent, or by the physician during a Moro reflex, if one upper extremity does not move normally. Closer examination will reveal that the abductors and external rotators of the shoulder are paralyzed, and the infant cannot flex the elbow or extend the wrist (the waiter's tip posture). Sometimes there is an accompanying paralysis of the ipsilateral hemidiaphragm. The grasp reflex is normal with Erb paralysis.

A lower brachial plexus injury results in absence of grasp. Frequently accompanying this injury are manifestations of Horner syndrome (ptosis, miosis, enophthalmos, and anhidrosis) caused by cervical sympathetic nerve paralysis.

Differential diagnosis includes injuries to the arm serious enough to cause a pseudoparalysis as a result of pain, such as fracture of the humerus or clavicle, shoulder dislocation, or epiphyseal separation (see below).

Although either of these injuries is alarming to the family at the outset, the bright side of the picture is that between 70 and 90% completely recover. Recovery usually occurs by 1 year. If no recovery has occurred by 2 years, the prognosis for any further improvement is not good.

The only initial treatment indicated is passive stretching exercises to prevent the development of contractures. This is usually done by the parents after instruction by a physical therapist.

10.3.2. Birth Injury to the Spine

Injury to the spinal column during delivery fortunately is rare but when it occurs, it is all too often devastating. The cervical spine is the most commonly damaged but fracture dislocations of the thoracic spine have also been reported (Gresham, 1975). Seventy-five percent of birth injuries to the spine occur with breech deliveries. In the cervical spine, C-5 to C-7 are the most frequent levels involved.

When examining any baby who is "floppy," quadriplegia must be differentiated from other causes of hypotonia, including cerebral causes and disease of the motor unit. The child's generalized flaccid appearance is common to all. With a cord injury, however, the astute observer will note a sensory level with decreased sensation and sweating below the injury. With a C-5 lesion, checking the ulnar side of the hand with a pin elicits no response. Testing the thumb side of the hand produces a painful response. Respiratory depression, paradoxical respirations, and urinary retention may also occur.

X-ray examination of the cervical spine may or may not show pathology. Frequently, the damage is caused by dislocation and hemorrhage after which the dislocation spontaneously reduces. The prognosis for any significant recovery is poor.

10.3.3. Fracture of the Clavicle at Birth

Nadas and Reinberg (1992) suggest that obstetrical maneuvers during delivery, cesarean section, prolonged labor, and prematurity are the principal risk factors for skeletal fractures incurred during delivery. Others continue to report, however, at least for clavicular fractures, that macrosomia and shoulder dystocia are major causes (Gonik *et al.*, 1991).

Clavicular fractures are by far the most common fracture caused by birth trauma, occurring in about 3% of live births (Solonen and Uusitalo, 1990). Ten percent of these will have accompanying brachial plexus injuries (Oppenheim *et al.*, 1990). Clavicular fractures are usually recognized by a large fusiform swelling over the clavicle in the first few days of life and by failure of the child to move the involved extremity normally. The prognosis for union and normal function is excellent. A little sling can be fabricated by pinning the sleeve of the involved arm to the body garment in order to make the baby a little more comfortable. Symptoms subside within a week. The callus formation is rather profuse but the contour of the bone returns to normal in several months.

Congenital pseudarthrosis of the clavicle is a rare condition which may be confused with fracture of the clavicle (see Chapter 6). The right clavicle is affected 90% of the time. It is thought that clavicular growth is interfered with embryologically by anomalous formation of the great vessels in the right hemithorax. Left-sided pseudarthrosis is a marker for dextrocardia (Gobson and Carroll, 1970). A nontender mass is easily palpated in the midshaft of the clavicle. There is usually no accompanying loss of function. Radiographs show a nonunion of the midshaft of the clavicle with the distal fragment displaced inferiorly and a hooklike deformity at the nonunion site. Callus is not present.

10.3.4. Fractures of Long Bones at Birth

Fractures of the humerus, femur, or tibia occur in about 0.03% of births (Solonen and Uusitalo, 1990). The presence of a fracture of any of these bones is recognized by swelling of the extremity, warmth, deformity, tenderness, and decreased movement. X-ray examination will usually show some angulation, an observation which should not cause alarm. The fracture is treated for a week or two by the simplest splint possible—a folded towel or very small pillow. The child's extremity returns to normal function quickly and angular deformities of up to 45° correct spontaneously in a few months. Complete return to normal is expectable.

10.3.5. Epiphyseal Separation of Long Bones from Birth Trauma

Sometimes the force required to deliver a baby is sufficient to separate the cartilaginous end of a long bone, the epiphysis, from the shaft. It is almost impossible to forcibly dislocate a major joint in a newborn. The stabilizing ligaments of the joint are stronger than the junction between the epiphysis and the diaphysis of the bone.

Clinically, the infant will demonstrate swelling of the end of the long bone and will have limited function because of pain. The epiphyseal separation may occur at the proximal or distal end of the humerus or femur. Involvement of the proximal is the most difficult to discern clinically because of the thicker soft tissues in the region but here too swelling does occur. Any passive or active movement of the extremity causes pain.

Early on, the X-ray picture is usually confusing because it often gives the appearance of a dislocation of the adjacent joint. After a week or 10 days, X-rays will show a large amount of periosteal new bone and callus. Most of these injuries are handled appropriately by simple splinting for comfort. The only challenging injury is at the elbow where the epiphyseal separation is equivalent to a supracondylar fracture (see above) and may require reduction and splinting in flexion.

11

Evaluating the Child with Arthritis and Other Joint Problems

11.1. INTRODUCTION

This chapter concerns itself with the evaluation of the child with arthritis and related conditions. Because of its complexity, arthritis has been given a separate chapter. For the evaluation of extremity pain in general, refer to Chapter 2. Our emphasis here will be on the process of diagnosis. Treatment will be only briefly discussed. Suggestions for further reading dealing with the details of treatment of each condition are listed in the Bibliography.

Synovial joint lining reacts to inflammatory processes in a limited number of ways: swelling, pain, warmth, and limitation of motion. The latter, limitation of motion, represents objective evidence for arthritis even in the absence of other signs and should be searched for carefully. Limitation of motion may be particularly important when dealing with arthritis of the hip since the hip is difficult to observe directly and swelling and warmth are not often apparent.

Though redness, the other cardinal manifestation of inflammation, does occur with joint inflammation, it does so only with acute processes as bacterial infection in the joint. Chronic joint inflammation, as in juvenile rheumatoid arthritis (JRA), usually does not cause red joints.

Since many processes can cause swelling around, rather than in, the joint, consideration must also be given to this possibility when evaluating presumed arthritis. For example, cellulitis in the soft tissue around a joint can look remarkably like an intra-articular process as can the swelling of the fingers which occurs with sickle-cell dactylitis.

11.2. PRESENTATION

Children with arthritis of any kind may present with pain, swelling, or limited motion in the joint affected. They may also be brought to the primary care physician with a joint contracture, refusal to walk, low back pain, a limp, swelling of an individual finger, fever, weight loss, rash, chronic eye irritation, or a leg length discrepancy.

11.2.1. Presentation of JRA

JRA will not uncommonly cause swelling and stiffness of a single joint. Many parents and physicians not aware of this fact will ascribe the swelling to trauma instead or to a "congenital" contracture. This may unfortunately lead to unnecessary and detrimental immobilization. Additionally, many children with chronic arthritis will not complain of much pain. This may be confusing to physicians who commonly hear their adult patients, friends, or colleagues complain with arthritis. Dactylitis, or swelling of a finger caused by chronic inflammatory arthritis, may be the initial manifestation of JRA and may be mistakenly thought to be related to bony infection, particularly if phalangeal periostitis is present. Unnecessary biopsy may result.

On the other side of the coin, hip pain may be prematurely labeled as resulting from JRA without a complete workup if the physician doesn't realize that monarticular hip disease is a most uncommon way for JRA to develop in a young child. Potentially serious delays in diagnosis or inappropriate therapy may result.

11.2.2. Inflammatory versus Biomechanical

In general, any chronic inflammatory process involving a joint will cause morning stiffness or stiffness after inactivity. The opposite is true for biomechanical or traumatic

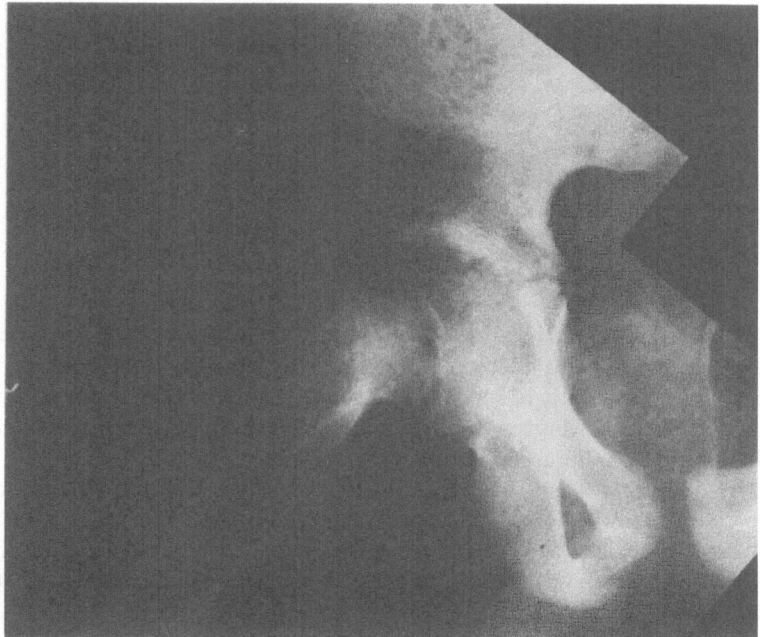

Figure 11.1. Slipped capital femoral epiphysis in a young adolescent male. Relevant to hip disease in this age group are several important caveats: (1) don't blame hip pain or stiffness on JRA—it rarely presents as isolated hip disease; (2) don't forget that hip disease will not infrequently present with thigh, knee, or even buttock pain; (3) strains and sprains as causes for chronic symptoms are unlikely in children before bony maturation has been achieved—get an AP of the pelvis and frog-leg laterals if there is any question.

processes which will cause increased pain after activity and for which rest will provide relief.

11.3. DIFFERENTIAL DIAGNOSIS

By paying attention to several historical and examination features (see Table 11.1), an organized approach to diagnosis can proceed stepwise from more common to less common, without being either too aggressive (and expensive) diagnostically or, on the other hand, too cursory.

11.3.1. Timing Is Everything

It is useful to categorize disease by acuity (see Tables 11.3 and 11.4). However, all things have to begin sometime and sometimes a chronic problem is noticed acutely. The story told is that the swelling has been present for only a few days, when in actuality it's been present much longer. When confronted with confusion regarding the onset of

**Table 11.1. Diagnosis Is
Facilitated by Attention to:**

Timing (chronic versus acute)
Age at onset
Pattern of joint involvement
Preexisting disease
Associated symptoms and signs
Screening laboratory tests

symptoms, look for associated features of chronicity. Children with chronic joint disease usually have had a chance to develop muscle atrophy, synovial thickening, soft-tissue contractures, bony deformity, or localized or generalized growth problems. Radiologic changes of osteoporosis, overgrowth, early bony maturation, or loss of articular surface, among others, may also be useful in assaying for chronicity.

JRA, by definition, has to be present for 6 weeks, in children 16 years of age or younger, only after all other causes have been ruled out. Most types of acute or postinfectious viral arthritis are gone by 6 weeks as is the arthritis of acute rheumatic fever, Kawasaki disease, serum sickness, and the acute, transient hip inflammation which occurs with toxic synovitis.

Table 11.2. Age of Onset for Selected Joint Diseases[a]

Joint disease throughout childhood and adolescence
    Polyarticular and systemic onset JRA
    Osteomyelitis or septic arthritis
    Viral arthritis
    Lyme disease
    Arthritis caused by leukemia or neuroblastoma
    Hemophilia
Typically in preschool children
    Kawasaki disease
    Early onset pauciarticular JRA (mostly girls)
Typically in school-aged children and adolescents
    Acute rheumatic fever
    Henoch–Schonlein purpura
    Osteochondritis dissecans
    Posttrauma and other biomechanical problems
    Toxic synovitis
    Legg–Calve–Perthes
Typically in adolescents
    SLE, dermatomyositis, polyarteritis, scleroderma, other collagen vascular diseases
    Spondylarthritides, late-onset pauciarticular JRA (mostly boys), psoriatic arthritis, Reiter's
    Gonococcal arthritis
    Slipped capital femoral epiphysis
    Pigmented villondular synovitis

[a]This table gives general guidelines Exceptions can and do occur, see text

11.3.2. Age at Onset

Different kinds of arthritis affect different age groups (see Table 11.2). For example:

- **Traumatic arthritis** or arthritis resulting from biomechanical problems at the knees, like a torn meniscus or patellofemoral difficulties, uncommonly affects preadolescent children.
- **Pauciarticular JRA** (four of fewer joints) affects two particular age groups: preschoolers (usually girls) and early adolescents (usually boys).
- **Acute rheumatic fever** (ARF) is uncommon below the age of 5 and is rare below 2 years.
- **Pigmented villonodular synovitis** (PVNS), an unusual form of chronic knee or ankle arthritis associated with hemangiomatous lesions of the synovium, affects adolescents and young adults. It does occur in younger children but is rare.
- Conversely, **Kawasaki disease** is most often found affecting younger children with a mean age at onset of 1.5 years.
- **Henoch–Schönlein purpura** occurs most commonly in the 5 to 15 year age group and exhibits a distinct seasonal variation with most cases clustering in the winter months.

11.3.3. Pattern of Joint Involvement: Monarthritis

The pattern of joint involvement provides much information regarding etiology.

11.3.3.1. Bone and Joint Infection

Septic arthritis, for example, must always be considered in the child who presents acutely with a single, inflamed joint. **Osteomyelitis** may also be a consideration because with bacterial infection of the metaphysis there is often a sterile sympathetic effusion in the associated joint or both osteomyelitis and septic arthritis may be present. Bone scan, joint aspiration, and/or aspiration of the affected periosteum should be performed promptly.

Surgical anthrotomy for septic arthritis for drainage may be optional when knees or other joints are affected but should **always** be performed for septic arthritis of the hip if vascular compromise and necrosis of the femoral head is to be avoided (see Chapter 2).

Septic arthritis in children varies bacteriologically with age. Children under 5 years of age are more likely to have *Haemophilus influenzae* infection than older children though *Staphylococcus aureus* causes disease throughout childhood. Ten percent of children over 10 years of age with septic joints will have *Neisseria gonorrhoeae*. *Streptococcus pyogenes* also occasionally causes septic arthritis in children.

Predominant organisms causing osteomyelitis in children are *Staphylococcus aureus* and *Streptococcus pyogenes* (group A streptococcus). Unusual organisms occur in certain circumstances, however. *Pseudomonas aeruginosa*, for example, apparently likes living in the lining of tennis shoes and is associated with osteomyelitis resulting from a puncture wound through the sole of the shoe. Newborns with bony

infections often have the typical "newborn" organisms, including group B streptococcus and coliforms, and children with sickle-cell disease or an immunodeficiency
will have unusual organisms as well (see Fig. 11.2).

Monarthritis can also be caused by tuberculous infection or by fungi. Neither is
common and fungal infection of the joint is rare indeed, associated usually with children
who are immunocompromised or occasionally in the newborn period.

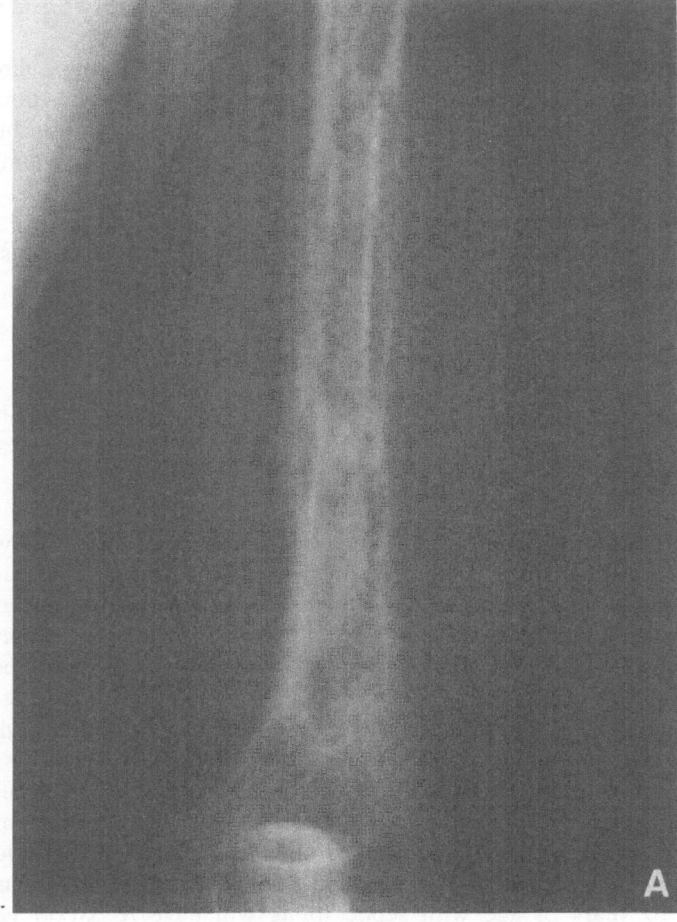

Figure 11.2. (A) Salmonella osteomyelitis of the left humerus in a 20-year-old woman with sickle-
cell disease. Note medullary destruction and periosteal new bone formation. Periosteal abscess may
be localized effectively for aspiration by ultrasound. (B) Technetium bone scan of same patient. The
dramatically increased radioisotope uptake in the left humerus is evident as is somewhat less
dramatically increased uptake in right humerus and ribs which may be related to infection or
infarction.

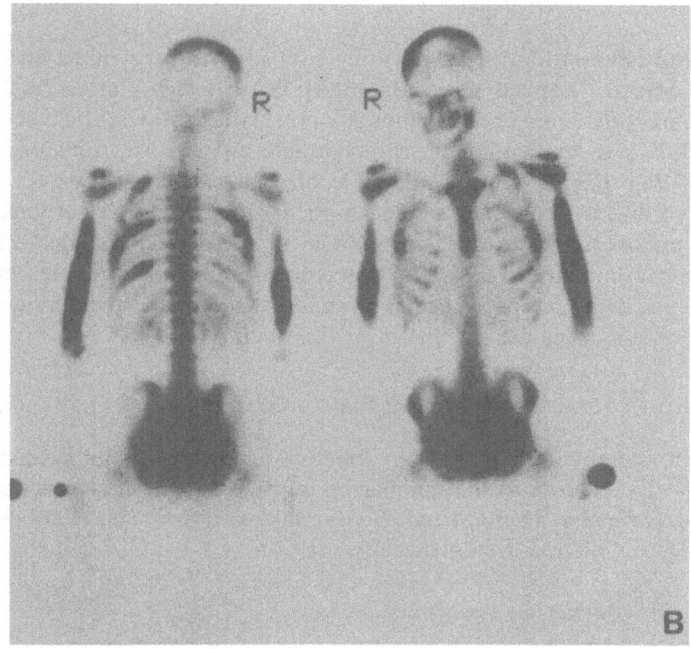

Figure 11.2. (*Continued*)

11 3 3 2 *Juvenile Rheumatoid Arthritis Presenting as Monarthritis*

Though **JRA** may present as arthritis in a single joint and in fact may persist as a monarticular arthritis, it has a specific predilection for certain joints Knees are affected in 75% of children with monarticular JRA with ankle or elbow next most common As mentioned above, monarthritis of the hip is an extremely uncommon way for JRA to present

11 3 3 3 *Traumatic Arthritis*

Traumatic arthritis with resulting hemarthrosis is most likely to be monarticular and accompanied by a history of trauma and external physical evidence of injury such as bruising or abrasion Coagulation studies for **hemophilia** or other coagulopathy should be performed when seeing a child with blood in any joint as well as consideration to a ligamentous tear or intraarticular fracture

Monarthritis can also be associated with a penetrating foreign body, often a thorn, which enters the joint and causes either a foreign body reaction or a low-grade indolent infection Often the penetrating injury happened months before the child presents and is not remembered

11.3.3.4. Other Causes for Monarthritis

Pigmented villonodular synovitis affects mostly knees or ankles and is usually a monarthritis. **Slipped capital femoral epiphysis or Legg–Calve–Perthes disease** (aseptic necrosis of the femoral head), though not truly arthritides, should be considered whenever a child presents with either demonstrable hip disease, limp, or medial thigh or knee pain. Pain referral from an irritable hip makes it important to consider hip disease in any child with obscure medial thigh, inguinal, buttock, or knee pain.

Though uncommon as a cause for monoarthritis, neoplasms should be included because of their importance to the health of the occasional child who presents with one. Included here are such rare malignancies as synovial sarcoma as well as more common ones like osteogenic sarcomas which are justaarticular.

11.3.4. Pattern of Joint Involvement: Pauciarticular

The most common type of JRA affects four or fewer joints and is termed *pauciarticular*. In addition to the number of joints, pauciarticular implies a specific pattern of joints affected. These include knees, ankles, wrists, and elbows with disease severity usually distributed asymmetrically.

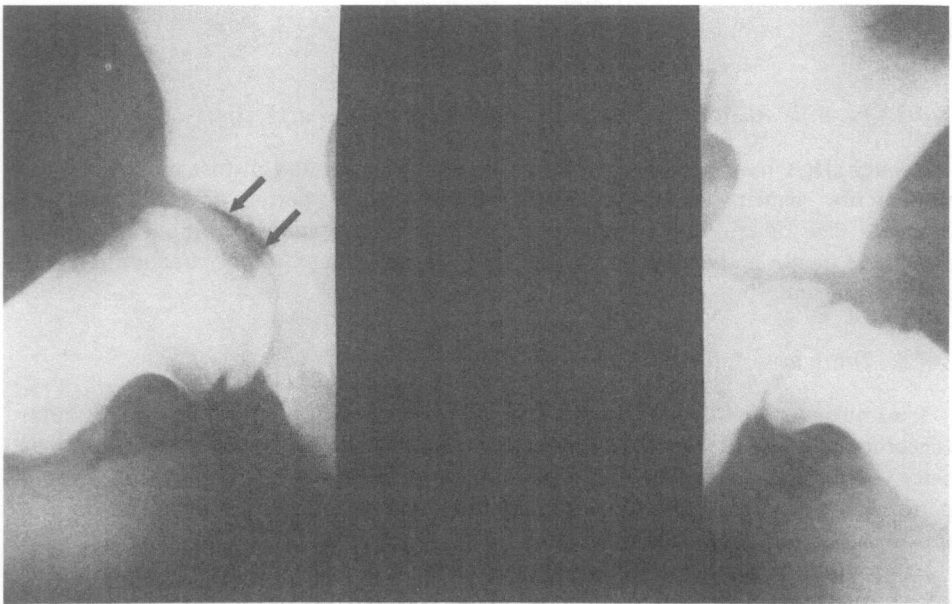

Figure 11.3. Legg–Calve–Perthes on the right is demonstrated on this frog-leg lateral film. Note widened head with reossification taking place. Vacuum arthrogram effect (arrows) reveals portion of cartilaginous head not yet reossified.

Table 11.3. Causes of Monarticular Arthritis in Children

Acute onset	Insidious onset or chronic course
Septic arthritis	JRA
Osteomyelitis with sympathetic effusion	Biomechanical—knee
Trauma	Patellofemoral syndrome
Hemophilia or other coagulopathy	Torn meniscus
Toxic synovitis of the hip	Osteochondritis dissecans
Slipped capital femoral epiphysis (acute)	Biomechanical—hip
	Legg–Calve–Perthes
	Slipped capital femoral epiphysis (chronic)
	Hemophilia or other coagulopathy
	Tuberculous or fungal arthritis
	Pigmented villonodular synovitis
	Foreign body (thorn) synovitis
	Psoriatic arthritis
	Chondrolysis of the hip
	Synovial tumors

11.3.5. Pattern of Joint Involvement: Low Back or Buttock Pain

The presence of low back or buttock pain, particularly if associated with demonstrable lumbar stiffness or sacroiliac joint disease, would lead one to consider spondylitis or inflammatory sacroiliitis as occurs with **juvenile ankylosing spondylitis** (JAS) or one of the spondylarthritides. Many of these exhibit peripheral large joint arthritis as well, usually asymmetrically affecting the lower extremities. Such biomechanical causes of low back pain and stiffness as spondylolisthesis, spondylolysis, intervertebral disc disease, and discitis would need to be ruled out as well.

Table 11.4. Arthritis in More Than One Joint

Acute onset	Slower onset (cont)
Acute rheumatic fever	Arthritis with
Systemic onset JRA	Leukemia
Henoch–Schonlein purpura	Neuroblastoma
Kawasaki disease	Sarcoidosis
Gonococcal arthritis	Immunodeficiency
Viral arthritis	Subacute bacterial endocarditis
Slower onset	Shunt infection
Other forms of JRA	Cystic fibrosis
Spondylarthritides, including	Pancreatitis
Juvenile ankylosing spondylitis	Acne
Reiter disease	Systemic lupus erythematosus[a]
Psoriatic arthritis	Other collagen vascular diseases, including
Arthritis with inflammatory bowel disease	Dermatomyositis
Reactive arthritis[a]	Scleroderma
Lyme disease	Polyarteritis nodosum[a]

[a]May also present acutely in some patients

Table 11.5. Juvenile Rheumatoid Arthritis Is:

1 Arthritis for more than 6 weeks, in
2 Children younger than 16 years of age, with
3 All other causes ruled out

11.3.6. Pattern of Joint Involvement: Migratory

Acute rheumatic fever (ARF) is a large-joint polyarthritis which generally affects the joints in the lower extremities in a migratory way. Each joint becomes involved for several days to a week before migrating to the next.

11.3.7. Preexisting or Coexisting Disease

Many diseases are associated with arthritis, including immune-mediated arthritis resulting from subacute bacterial endocarditis, infected ventriculoatrial shunts, severe cystic acne, and cystic fibrosis. Both reactive and true, hematogenously spread, septic arthritis have been described in children with such acute infections as bacterial meningitis.

Arthritis can also follow gastrointestinal or genitourinary infection. These "reactive" arthritides include not only **Reiter syndrome** (arthritis, conjunctivitis, and urethritis) but the arthritis which follows 1 to 2 weeks after acute shigella, yersinia, or salmonella infection.

Some children with evidence for a recent streptococcal infection and arthritis (**poststreptococcal reactive arthritis**) may not meet the revised Jones criteria for acute rheumatic fever. Their arthritis may not be migratory, may affect small joints as well as

Table 11.6. JRA May Be:

a Pauciarticular (four or fewer joints involved), with knees, ankles, wrists, and elbows most commonly involved
Pauciarticular JRA is further subdivided into
  • Early onset, affecting preschool children generally, mostly girls, and often associated with ANA positivity and chronic iritis, or
  • Late onset which most often affects teenage boys and is associated with HLA B-27 positivity and acute iritis
b Polyarticular (five or more joints involved), with symmetrical large- and small-joint disease affecting predominantly girls Some of the older girls with polyarticular disease will have rheumatoid factor positivity In either case, most of the invasive, destructive arthritis is in this polyarticular category
c Systemic onset which equally affects boys and girls and causes high fever, rash, lymphadenopathy, hepatosplenomegaly, and dramatic acute-phase reactants Occasionally, pericarditis, pleuritis, and hepatitis may also be part of the picture Most of these children transition to polyarticular or pauciarticular disease but some keep their systemic manifestations

large ones, and may persist for longer periods than expectable with ARF, often up to 6 months or more. Though lacking clinically apparent heart disease, some of these children will either demonstrate echocardiographic evidence of valvular abnormalities (Schaffer *et al.*, 1992) or will develop clinical valvular disease with subsequent streptococcal infection. Current thinking is that this poststreptococcal reactive arthritis is probably a clinical variant of acute rheumatic fever and that these children should receive long-term antibiotic prophylaxis.

Children with psoriasis or inflammatory bowel disease may develop arthritis. **Psoriatic arthritis** is most often pauciarticular and asymmetrical, with large joints involved, though it may include dactylitis. The arthritis associated with inflammatory bowel disease is most often peripheral in pattern though sacroiliitis or spondylitis may occur as well, presenting with low back or buttock pain.

Arthritis is a frequent and disabling complication of **hemophilia** because of the recurrent episodes of intraarticular bleeding. Blood in the joint space causes considerable inflammation and synovial hypertrophy which predisposes to future bleeding. As might be expected, joint disease most often affects children during their most active, ambulatory period and typically involves knee, elbow, ankle, shoulder, and hip (Cassidy and Petty, 1990).

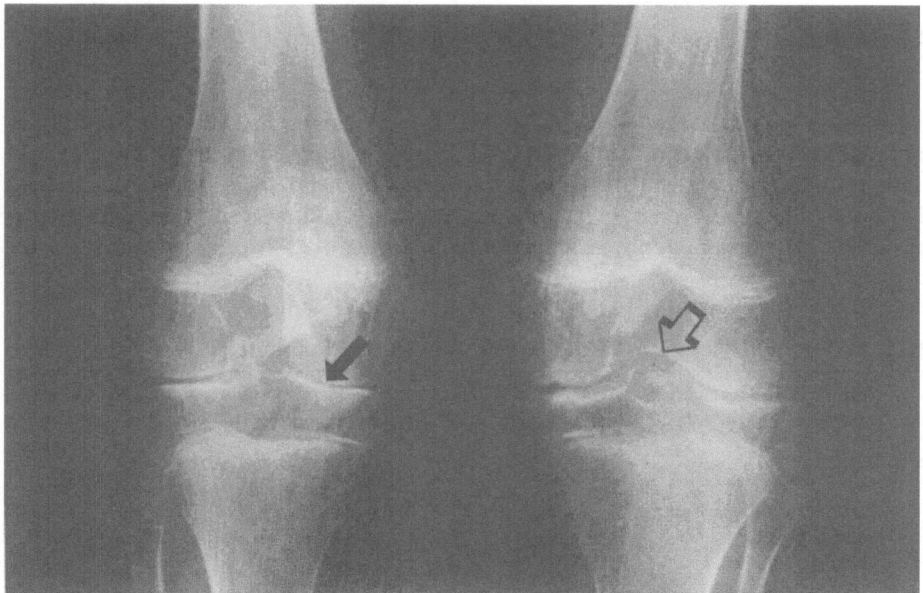

Figure 11.4. Residual of chronic arthritis caused by repeated hemarthroses in this 13-year-old male with hemophilia is evident on this anteroposterior film of both knees Note overgrowth of more seriously affected left knee, loss of articular cartilage with narrowing of joint space (closed arrow), widening and deepening of intercondylar notch (open arrow), and irregularity of subchondral surfaces These changes are typical of any chronic synovitis, a child with JRA might have the same picture

The dactylitis of **sickle-cell disease** may be difficult to tell from acute polyarthritis of the small joints of the hand or cellulitis of the soft tissues of the hand. Other joints may be affected as well, particularly the hips. Additionally, children with sickle-cell disease are particularly susceptible to infection with encapsulated organisms, including *Haemophilus influenzae*, *Streptococcus pneumoniae*, or salmonella, any of which can cause septic arthritis or osteomyelitis in these children (see Fig. 11.2).

11.3.8. Associated Symptoms

11.3.8.1. Systemic Onset Juvenile Rheumatoid Arthritis

In addition to such nonspecific symptoms as malaise, weight loss, and anorexia, many acute rheumatic syndromes cause fever and a variety of different kinds of rashes. Of these, the fever of **systemic onset JRA** (SOJRA) is the most dramatic. For months, such children will spike nightly or twice daily to 105°F (41°C). The fever, when it comes down, will often descend to below normal. The rash, malaise, and arthralgias are typically most pronounced when the temperature is at its peak. The rash of SOJRA is fleeting, macular, pink or salmon-colored, and is usually most prominent on the trunk or proximal extremities. Each lesion may range from several millimeters to several centimeters in diameter with larger lesions exhibiting some central clearing.

11.3.8.2. Kawasaki Disease

The rash of **Kawasaki disease** is also truncal but is variable from patient to patient and even with regard to one patient over time. It has been described as scarlatiniform, macular, papular, multiformis, and purpuric. It is, however, generally not vesicular or bullous. It can be accompanied by redness of the palms and soles, sometimes accompanied by edema of the dorsum of hands and feet. This is followed several weeks later by a characteristic desquamation which begins distally over the tips of fingers and toes and

---

Table 11.7. Revised Modified Jones Criteria for Acute Rheumatic Fever[a]

High probability of ARF if patient has evidence of recent streptococcal infection such as positive throat culture, or elevated ASO titer, plus either two major criteria or one major and two minor criteria:

Major criteria
  Carditis
  Polyarthritis (usually migratory, large joints)
  Sydenham's chorea
  Subcutaneous nodules
  Erythema marginatum
Minor criteria
  Fever (usually over 39°C)
  Arthralgia
  Prolonged PR interval on ECG
  Elevated erythrocyte sedimentation rate
  Elevated C-reactive protein

---

[a]Special Writing Group (1992).

works its way proximally. Other acute manifestations of Kawasaki disease include fever, lip erythema, strawberry tongue, nonpurulent bulbar conjunctivitis, and cervical lymphadenopathy, followed several weeks later by arthritis and thrombocytosis. Cardiac disease, specifically coronary artery aneurysm formation and thrombosis are the most serious complications. Initially high dose aspirin followed after the acute phase by low antiplatelet aspirin doses is recommended. Intravenous gamma globulin has been shown to be effective in reducing the serious complications of Kawasaki disease if begun during the first 10 or 12 days of the illness. It now has an established role in the treatment of these children.

11.3.8.3. Viral Infections Causing Arthritis

Viral infections are most often associated with arthralgias but can, on occasion, cause frank arthritis as well. Such virus-associated arthritis may result either from active viral infection of the synovium or from some immune-complex-mediated reactive process. This has been probably best demonstrated with rubella. Arthritis has also been described uncommonly as a transient complication of the rubella vaccine though more often in adult recipients than in children. The arthritis of the disease is both more common and more severe than that of the immunization. Other viruses which have been associated on occasion with arthritis include hepatitis B, adenovirus, Epstein–Barr virus, cytomegalovirus, varicella, herpes simplex, mumps, ECHO, Coxsackie B, and parvovirus B19, the viral agent which causes fifth disease or slapped cheek disease (erythema infectiosum). Though most viral arthritis is of short duration, usually of no more than 1 or 2 weeks, it is apparent now that parvovirus B19 can contribute to chronic arthritis in a small number of susceptible children.

11.3.8.4. Lyme Disease

Lyme disease, caused by the spirochete *Borrelia burgdorferi*, was first described in 1977 (Steere *et al.*, 1977) when a mother noticed that many other children in her neighborhood, in addition to her child, had "juvenile rheumatoid arthritis." The most common vector is the small "seed" tick *Ixodes dammini*. Lyme disease seems to occur in three phases. The first is associated with a rash which begins as a red spot and increases in size in a circular manner with central clearing (erythema chronicum migrans). Patients can sometimes remember being bitten by a tick at the location of this initial lesion. Nonspecific symptoms of malaise, arthralgia, and fever occur as well. Phase two occurs weeks to months later and is characterized by a variety of cardiac conduction abnormalities and neurologic manifestations, including aseptic meningitis, Bell's palsy, transverse myelitis, and chorea. Weeks to months later the arthritis of phase three develops, often involving the knee. Recurrent attacks tend to be more mild over time.

11.3.8.5. Other Collagen Vascular Diseases

Polyarthritis of a chronic nature is also associated with all of the other collagen vascular diseases of childhood, including **systemic lupus erythematosus** (SLE), **juve-**

nile dermatomyositis (JDM), and **systemic sclerosis** (SS). None are common and most provide some indication on physical or laboratory examination that one is dealing with a form of chronic arthritis other than JRA. SLE causes disease in a variety of body systems including nephritis, pericarditis, lymphopenia, thrombocytopenia or anemia, Raynaud phenomenon, mucosal ulcerations, photosensitivity, and rashes. JDM causes progressive symmetric proximal motor weakness with elevated muscle enzymes and EMG and biopsy evidence for myositis. Cutaneous manifestations of JDM include purplish discoloration of the eyelids (heliotrope rash) as well as red scaly patches over the extensor surfaces of the small joints of the hands, the elbows, and the knees (Gottron patches or papules). SS is even more rare in childhood than SLE or JDM and usually is associated more with arthralgia than arthritis. Other manifestations predominate and include Raynaud's phenomenon, contractures, tightening of the skin of the fingers, and dysphagia.

Case 1

PR is a 6-year-old boy with a 1-month history of pain and swelling in his knees Previously healthy, his mother first noticed a limp and subsequently knee swelling after a fall He was stiff in the morning There was no fever, weight loss, or rash There was no family history of rheumatologic disease Initial physical examination revealed tenderness of the right midfemoral region anteriorly There was a small effusion in the right knee which was sightly warm but without decreased range of motion The remainder of his examination was unrevealing He was begun on aspirin at 75 mg/kg daily with some relief

Initial laboratory evaluation revealed a WBC of 5200 with 82% polys, a mild normochromic and normocytic anemia, and a platelet count of 120,000 His ESR was 52 mm/hr and an ANA was negative Radiographs of both knees were normal Repeat CBC 1 week later showed worsening thrombocytopenia and abnormal cells in the peripheral smear Bone marrow aspirate revealed many lymphoblasts and he was begun shortly thereafter on therapy for his acute lymphocytic leukemia

Comment: We all live in fear of missing the child with neoplasia presenting as bone or joint disease It is not common but it is also not rare Acute lymphocytic leukemia is the most common cancer in children and about one-third will have bone pain at presentation Unlike many children with nonspecific lower extremity complaints, this patient consistently described discomfort in quite specific locations His ESR was inappropriately high for the mild nature of his arthritis and was not congruent with his low WBC and low platelet count

11.3.8.6. Henoch–Schönlein Disease and Other Vasculitides

Arthritis can also occur with any of the vasculitic syndromes of childhood, including **Henoch–Schönlein** (anaphylactoid) **purpura** (HSP), **serum sickness** (hypersensitivity angiitis), or **polyarteritis nodosa** (PAN). The large-joint arthritis of HSP is often overshadowed by the other manifestations of the disease, including palpable purpura over the lower extremities, cramping abdominal pain, and nephritis, with hematuria and proteinuria. Serum sickness is more likely nowadays to be caused by a drug reaction than by heterologous serum. The manifestations are the same, however, and reflect antigen–antibody complex-mediated disease 1 to 2 weeks after exposure. These include a rash, often urticarial or purpuric, with arthritis, edema, and fever. PAN is a severe but rare vasculitis which presents with weight loss, fever, abdominal pain, hypertension, and a petechial or vasculitic rash.

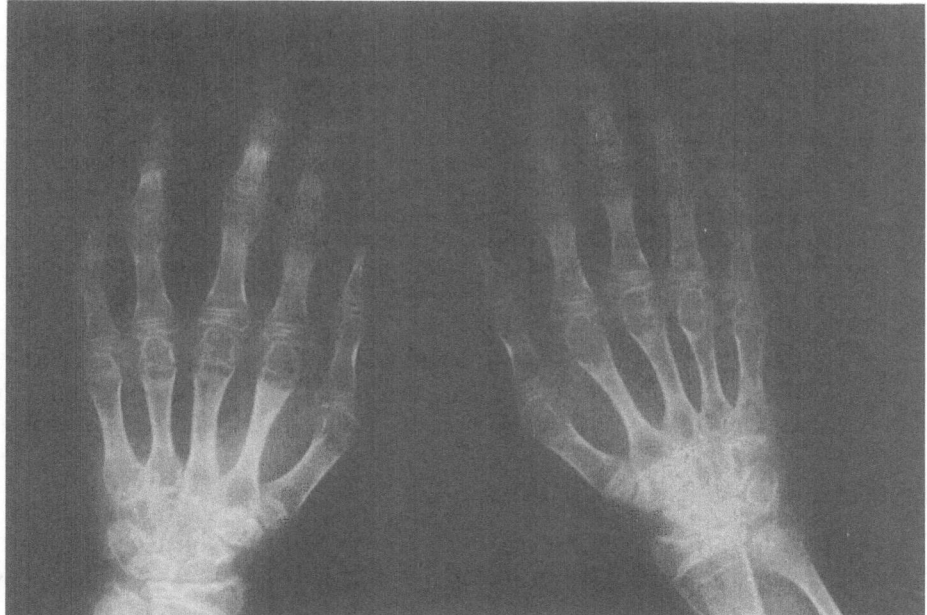

Figure 11.5. Hand films of a 13-year-old girl with long-standing polyarticular JRA and typical symmetrical large- and small-joint disease. The phalanges have become widened as a result of periosteal new bone growth. Note metaphyseal rarefaction of bone and metacarpal–phalangeal subluxation of both thumbs.

11.4. LABORATORY EVALUATION

11.4.1. Acute-Phase Reactants

Inflammatory or infectious conditions affecting the skeleton will often be associated with characteristic changes in several routine blood tests, the so-called acute-phase reactants. These include an **increase** in the WBC, platelet count (often over one million in SOJRA or Kawasaki disease), erythrocyte sedimentation rate, C-reactive protein (CRP), serum immunoglobulins, and ferritin and a **decrease** in serum albumin. Children with a chronic inflammatory process will also be anemic as a result of their disease. These are all nonspecific manifestations which don't distinguish one disease process from the other. The lack of acute-phase reactants, moreover, doesn't rule out the possibility of JRA since children with one or two affected joints may have normal blood counts and a normal erythrocyte sedimentation rate.

Case 2

S.H. is a 4-year-old white female with a 6-month history of swelling in the right knee. There is little pain but she limps and is stiff, particularly in the morning. There is a history of falling but her parents don't remember any specific serious traumatic episode before the onset of her knee difficulties. There are no other symptoms and her family history is negative.

Initial physical examination revealed bony enlargement, slight warmth, and soft-tissue swelling around the right knee, with a small amount of intra-articular fluid. She lacked full extension at the knee by about 5°. The remainder of her examination was normal.

Laboratory examination revealed a normal CBC with an ESR of 22 mm/hr An ANA was positive at a dilution of 1 to 160. She was begun on oral naproxen suspension at 12 mg/kg daily with improvement in her symptoms and also in the range of motion of her right knee. She has subsequently developed iritis controlled with topical steroid drops and arthritis of the proximal interphalangeal joint of the index finger of her left hand.

Comment: This little girl's story is a typical one for children with early onset pauciarticular JRA, with ANA positivity and iritis. The iritis is the source of most of the ultimate morbidity and the arthritis is usually easy to control. The small-joint disease of her right index finger is a little atypical and reminds us that, despite our well-thought-out categorizations, some children simply refuse to be pigeonholed.

The differential diagnosis of arthritis in childhood almost always includes JRA for which there are no pathognomonic lab tests. The laboratory evaluation in the child with arthritis is useful in order to rule out other causes of disease but not in ruling in JRA.

11.4.2. Antinuclear Antibodies (ANA)

Despite being highly associated with SLE, a positive ANA is often present in JRA and other collagen vascular diseases, though usually in lower titer. Overall, 40% of

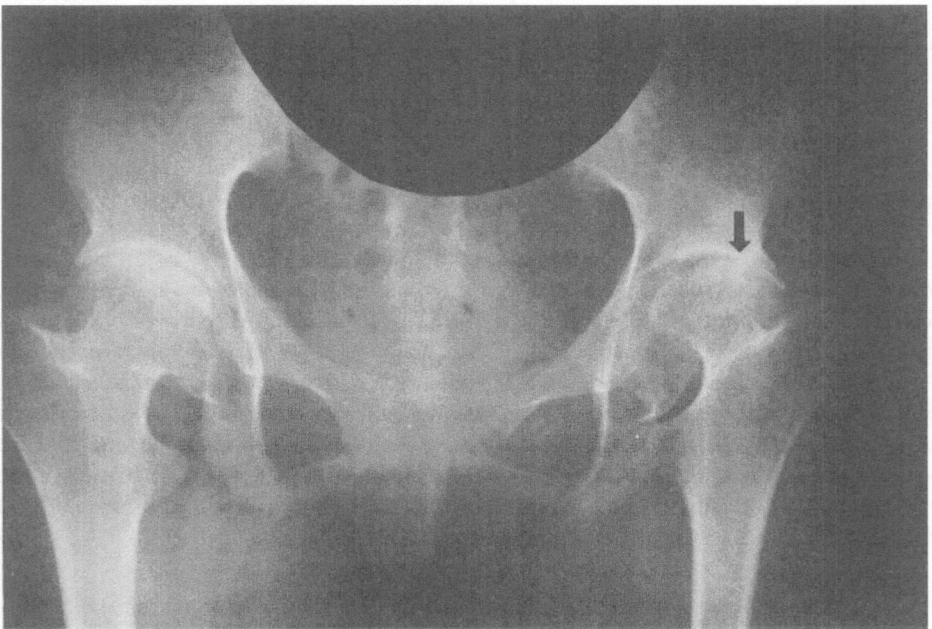

Figure 11.6. Hip films of same patient as in Fig. 11.5. The left hip in particular shows deformity with bony sclerosis and complete loss of articular surface (arrow).

children with JRA will have a positive ANA (Cassidy and Petty, 1990) with a higher likelihood of ANA positivity in preschool girls with pauciarticular disease (four or fewer joints). Most importantly, ANA positivity in JRA is highly associated with the development of ocular inflammation which is often asymptomatic. **Regular slit lamp examinations are therefore required in order to promptly diagnose and treat iritis early so that eye damage may be prevented.**

11.4.3. Rheumatoid Factor (RF)

RF positivity is unlikely in children with JRA except for teenage girls with symmetrical polyarticular disease who have "adult" rheumatoid disease. They are labeled as having JRA because they present when they are younger than 16 years of age.

11.4.4. Human Leukocyte Antigens (HLA)

HLA B-27 testing should be considered when a boy older than 7 years presents with pauciarticular chronic arthritis of the lower extremity with negative ANA and RF. All of the spondylarthritides, including Reiter's disease, reactive arthritis, juvenile ankylosing spondylitis, and some of the arthritis associated with psoriasis and inflammatory bowel disease, are associated with the presence of HLA B-27, a class I histocompatibility antigen. Ocular inflammation also occurs with this group and requires ophthalmologic consultation. Other HLA antigens are associated with pediatric rheumatologic disease including early onset pauciarticular JRA and RF-positive polyarticular JRA, though the associations have less clinical utility than research interest.

Case 3

A 13-year-old white male presents with a 2-month history of right hip and low back pain Fever as high as 39°C had been present intermittently and 400 mg of ibuprofen had not been helpful There had been no rash, GI symptoms, weight loss, or urethral discharge Sexual activity was denied The past medical history was significant for a 5-year history of mild psoriasis and allergy to penicillin There were two maternal uncles with psoriasis, though no family history of inflammatory bowel disease or spondylitis

Physical exam revealed a bed-bound male adolescent who was very uncomfortable when moved Significant atrophy of the right thigh was evident as was punch tenderness over the right sacroiliac joint and pain on pelvic compression Forward flexion at the lumbosacral spine was limited by his discomfort The FABER test (flexion, abduction, and external rotation) was positive on the right Hip range of motion was normal

Laboratory evaluation revealed a WBC of 12,500 with 78% polys, an ESR of 75 mm/hr, and blurring of the right SI joint on X-ray HLA B-27 was negative A technetium bone scan revealed increased uptake at the right SI joint Two blood cultures were negative as was culture of fluid obtained from direct aspiration of the SI joint on the right An MRI scan was interpreted as showing an abscess adjacent to the right SI joint

The patient was initially thought to have either an inflammatory or septic process involving the right SI joint and was begun on naproxen and intravenous clindamycin He was remarkably better after 1 week and was subsequently discharged on oral clindamycin and naproxen

Comment: In addition to MRI, the dramatic tenderness, asymmetry, markedly elevated ESR, and response to antibiotics all make a bacterial (probably staphylococcal) cause for his symptoms likely This case is a good example of why osteomyelitis/septic arthritis of the sacroiliac joint is a difficult diagnosis to make

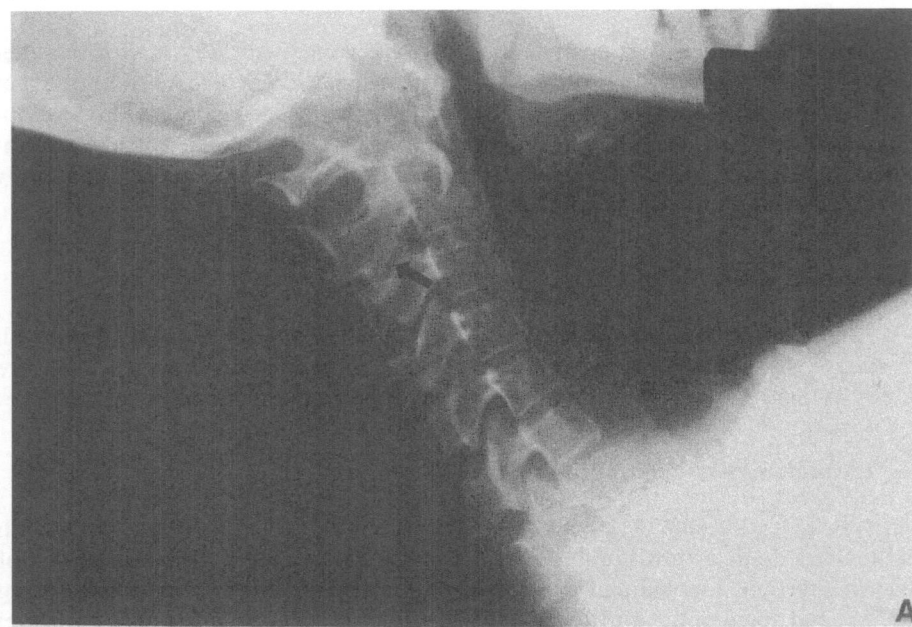

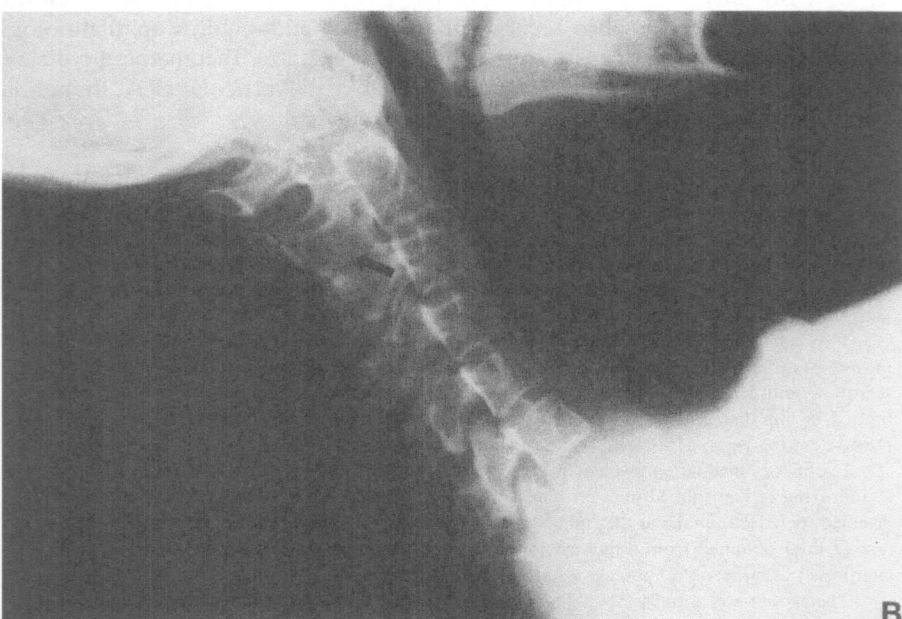

Figure 11.7. Almost all children with polyarticular JRA get cervical spine disease. The intervertebral joints aren't synovial joints and are therefore not involved in JRA. The facet joints are, however. (A) Facet joint narrowing between C-2 and C-3 (arrow). (B) Progression, 2 years later, to bony fusion of posterior elements (arrow). This is likely to progress to fusion of the entire cervical spine if disease activity continues, with resulting decreases in neck range of motion.

11.4.5. Antistreptolysin O (ASO) Titers

Certainly any child in whom ARF or poststreptococcal reactive arthritis is considered (and that includes many of the children who present with arthritis) should have an ASO titer and, if it is negative, antihyaluronidase, antistreptokinase, and antidesoxyribonuclease titers as well, if suspicion is high.

11.4.6. Radiography

Any child with persistent symptoms referable to a specific area should have radiographs done. Hip films (AP of the pelvis and frog-leg laterals) should be strongly considered when evaluating knee or medial thigh pain. This is particularly so in infants and toddlers who may have trouble cooperating with the examiner and with whom an adequate physical may not be possible.

11.4.7. Joint Aspiration

When septic arthritis is a consideration or when diagnosis is in doubt, joint fluid aspiration is indicated. Joint fluid is normally straw yellow and clear. As the degree of inflammation increases, so does the cloudiness. Mildly inflamed joints have fluid white cell counts below 5000 per cubic millimeter. Significantly inflamed rheumatoid joints might have fluid white cell counts between 15,000 and 80,000 (Morrissy, 1990). Septic joints frequently have white cell counts in excess of 100,000. The proportion of neutrophils also increases as the degree of inflammation increases with septic joints usually exhibiting at least 75% neutrophils. Joint fluid may clot after aspiration and should always be put in an anticoagulated tube. A Gram stain should always be performed if bacterial infection is a consideration as should an acid-fast stain if tuberculosis is a possibility. Appropriate cultures should be obtained. Synovial fluid glucose is reduced with bacterial joint infection and may prove useful. There is overlap in cell counts between severely inflamed joints and infected joints, but cell counts over 100,000 usually represent septic processes, particularly so if associated with a preponderance of neutrophils. However, a lower synovial fluid white cell count doesn't exclude a septic joint and neither does a sterile aspirate.

11.4.8. Other Tests

Other laboratory tests are indicated based on the child's clinical picture. These might include muscle enzymes or electromyography for dermatomyositis, technetium

Table 11.8. Basic Screening Laboratory[a] in Suspected Childhood Arthritis

White blood cell count	Antinuclear antibody
Platelet count	Antistreptolysin O
Erythrocyte sedimentation rate	Radiographs

[a]Other tests as indicated.

bone scanning for osteomyelitis, bone marrow aspirate for acute leukemia, or echocardiography for Kawasaki disease.

11.5. TREATMENT

A detailed description of the treatment of each of the above is beyond our scope here. Complicated problems will need to be referred to centers specialized in the care of pediatric rheumatologic or orthopedic conditions. There are some basic principles which are worth emphasizing, however.

11.5.1. Nonsteroidal Anti-inflammatory Drugs (NSAIDs)

Despite a dizzying proliferation of these medications for use in adult patients, there are a limited number of NSAIDs which are in common use in children. Four are worth being familiar with: ibuprofen, naproxen, tolmetin, and aspirin. Their primary care indications include symptomatic treatment of known, self-limited musculoskeletal pain and first-line treatment of mild to moderate chronic childhood arthritis. They should not be used as symptomatic treatment of undiagnosed musculoskeletal pain. All are antiprostaglandin drugs and all are renally excreted. All have similar toxicity which includes gastric irritation, renal side effects, and decreased platelet adhesion. Naproxen has also been associated with a blistering rash and with facial scarring (Wallace and Sherry, 1993). Though this is apparently rare, parents should be warned. Because of their gastric toxicity, all should be given with food.

Newer and more expensive NSAIDs should be used only with considerable discretion since they are generally not approved for use in pediatric patients. In general, using more than one NSAID at a time results in increased toxicity and should be avoided.

Many pediatric rheumatologists are using less aspirin and more of the other nonsteroidals. It is probably more irritating to the gastric lining than the other NSAIDs and also exhibits a specific effect on vitamin K-dependent coagulation in addition to its antiplatelet effects. A variety of other untoward effects have been described, including tinnitus, hepatitis, and bone marrow suppression. Aspirin has been associated with Reye syndrome and parents are therefore sometimes unenthusiastic. Education regarding

Table 11.9. Nonsteroidal Anti-inflammatory Drugs in Childhood

Drug	Dose (mg/kg/day)	Schedule	Cost[a]
Aspirin	75	qid	$18–54
Ibuprofen	35	qid	$5–7
Tolmetin	25	tid	$11–51
Naproxen	10	bid	$24–32

[a]Approximate monthly cost to the patient in 1992, assuming a 20-kg child; cost variation results from differing costs of proprietary versus generic brands as well as variation from store to store.

the need to discontinue the aspirin if the child develops symptoms of influenza or is exposed to chickenpox or shingles should be provided and influenza vaccination should be given to any child on aspirin. Aspirin may be more expensive than the other nonsteroidals (particularly ibuprofen and naproxen) when given at the usual dose of 75–90 mg/kg per day, divided into three or four doses with meals, though there is considerable overlap in prices. Parents should be advised to "shop around." When taken as the flavored chewable tablets, the child should rinse their mouth after each dose to reduce the likelihood of enamel etching.

The other three NSAIDs have equivalent potency and risk of toxicity. Naproxen is available as a liquid preparation with a concentration of 125 mg per 5 ml which makes its use in younger children easier. Its twice-daily dosing makes it particularly attractive. Ibuprofen is available also as a suspension, at 100 mg per 5 ml.

11.5.2. Steroids

Glucocorticoids are worth mentioning only to say that their use in childhood arthritis should be reserved to those working in specialty centers and only after a specific diagnosis is made. The indications for their use in pediatric musculoskeletal disease are relatively narrow. The inappropriate use of steroids will at least muddy the waters and often obscures the appropriate diagnosis, leading to delays or potentially dangerous mistreatment.

11.5.3. Antibiotics

The antibiotic treatment of bacterial joint infection depends on the organism involved and the age of the child. Empiric treatment initially will often be necessary while cultures are pending. Newborns with a septic joint will require antibiotic coverage for gram-positive organisms (*Staphylococcus aureus* and *group B streptococcus*) as well as gram-negative coliforms. Empiric coverage might be provided by methicillin and cefotaxime, a third-generation cephalosporin, though some might prefer methicillin plus an aminoglycoside. In the period from about 2 months to about 7 years, staphylococcal and other gram-positive coverage must be continued and *Haemophilus influenzae* coverage must also be provided. This might be accomplished empirically through the use of a second-generation cephalosporin like cefuroxime. Older children and adolescents are affected mainly by staphylococci and require methicillin or nafcillin, though *Neisseria gonorrhoeae* may also be responsible. Clindamycin or cefazolin, a first-generation cephalosporin, are alternatives for children allergic to penicillin if staphylococcal infection is thought responsible.

Empiric therapy for osteomyelitis before an organism is known is similar to that for septic arthritis. Ceftazidime, or other antipseudomonas medication, should be considered if pseudomonas osteomyelitis is being considered.

Bibliography

CHAPTER 1. SUGGESTED READING

Lourie, J , 1982, *Medical Eponyms Who Was Coude?* Pitman, London
Morrissy, R T (ed), 1990, *Lovell and Winter's Pediatric Orthopaedics*, 3rd ed , Lippincott, Philadelphia
Wenger, D R , and Rang, M , 1993, *The Art and Practice of Children's Orthopaedics*, Raven Press, New York

CHAPTER 2. REFERENCES

Cassidy, J T, and Petty, R E , 1990, *Textbook of Pediatric Rheumatology*, 2nd ed , Churchill Livingstone, Edinburgh
Crawford, A H , Kucharzyk, D W, Ruda, R , and Smitherman, H C , 1991, Diskitis in children, *Clinical Orthopaedics and Related Research* **266**:70
Dietz, F R , Mathews, K D, and Montgomery, W J , 1990, Reflex sympathetic dystrophy in children, *Clinical Orthopaedics and Related Research* **258**:225
Jackson, M A , and Nelson, J D , 1982, Etiology and management of acute suppurative bone and joint infections in pediatric patients, *Journal of Pediatric Orthopaedics* **2**:315
Morrissy, R T , 1990, Slipped capital femoral epiphysis, in *Lovell and Winter's Pediatric Orthopaedics*, 3rd ed (R T Morrissy, ed), Lippincott, Philadelphia, pp 885–904
Ostrov, B E , Goldsmith, D P, and Athreya, B H , 1993, Differentiation of systemic juvenile rheumatoid arthritis from acute leukemia near the onset of disease, *Journal of Pediatrics* **122**:595–598
Ozonoff, M B , 1992, *Pediatric Orthopedic Radiology*, 2nd ed , Saunders, Philadelphia
Shaw, B A , and Kasser, J R , 1990, Acute septic arthritis in infancy and childhood, *Clinical Orthopaedics and Related Research* **257**:212
Sherry, D D , and Weisman, R , 1988, Psychologic aspects of childhood reflex neurovascular dystrophy, *Pediatrics* **81**:572
Springfield, D S , 1990, Bone and soft tissue tumors, in *Lovell and Winter's Pediatric Orthopaedics*, 3rd ed (R T Morrissy, ed), Lippincott, Philadelphia, pp 325–364
Wallendal, M , Stork, L , and Hollister, J R , 1992, The discriminating value of serum LDH values in children with malignancy presenting as limb pain *56th Annual Scientific Meeting of the American College of Rheumatology* S56
Weinstein, S L , 1990, Legg–Calve–Perthes disease, in *Lovell and Winter's Pediatric Orthopaedics*, 3rd ed (R T Morrissy, ed), Lippincott, Philadelphia, pp 851–884
Wenger, D R, and Rang, M , 1993, *The Art and Practice of Children's Orthopaedics*, Raven Press, New York
Yunus, M B , and Masi, A T , 1985, Juvenile primary fibromyalgia syndrome A clinical study of thirty-three patients and matched controls, *Arthritis and Rheumatism* **28**:138

313

CHAPTER 3. REFERENCES

Ablin, D S , Greenspan, A , Reinhart, M , and Grix, A , 1990, Differentiation of child abuse from osteogenesis imperfecta, *American Journal of Roentgenology* **154:**1047–1048

Caffey, J , 1946, Multiple fractures in the long bones of infants suffering from chronic subdural hematoma *American Journal of Roentgenology* **56:**163–173

Caffey, J , and Silverman, F N , 1967, *Pediatric X-ray Diagnosis*, 5th ed , Year Book Medical Publishers, Chicago

Chapman, S , 1987, Child abuse or copper deficiency? A radiological view, *British Medial Journal* **294:**1370

Chapman, S , 1990, Radiological aspects of non-accidental injury, *Journal of the Royal Society of Medicine* **83:**67–71

Dalton, H J , Slovis, T , Helfer, R E , Comstock, J , Scheurer, S , and Riolo, S , 1990, Undiagnosed abuse in children younger than 3 years with femoral fracture, *American Journal of Diseases of Children* **144:** 875–878

Garcia, V F, Gotschall, C S , Eichelberger, M R , and Bowman, L M , 1990, Rib fractures in children A marker of severe trauma, *Journal of Trauma* **30:**695–700

Helfer, R E , Slovis, T L , and Black, M , 1977, Injuries resulting when small children fall out of bed, *Pediatrics* **60:**533–535

Kempe, C H , and Helfer, R E , 1987, *The Battered Child*, 4th ed , University of Chicago Press, Chicago

Kempe, C H , Silverman, F N , Steele, B F, Droegemueller, W , and Silver, H K , 1962, The battered child syndrome, *Journal of the American Medical Association* **181:**17–24

Kleinman, P K , 1990, Diagnostic imaging in infant abuse, *American Journal of Roentgenology* **155:**703–712

Kleinman, P K , and Zita, J L , 1984, Avulsion of the spinous processes caused by infant abuse, *Radiology* **151:**389

Kleinman, P K , Blackbourne, B D , Marks, S C , Karellas, A , and Belanger, P L , 1989, Radiologic contributions to the investigation and prosecution of cases of fetal infant abuse *New England Journal of Medicine* **320:**507–511

Kogutt, M S , Swischuk, L E , and Fagan, C J , 1974, Patterns of injury and significance of uncommon fractures in the battered child syndrome, *American Journal of Roentgenology* **121:**143

McClain, P W, Sacks, J J , Froehlke, R G , and Ewigman, B G , 1993, Estimates of fatal child abuse and neglect, United States, 1979 through 1988, *Pediatrics* **91:**338

Merten, D F, and Carpenter, B L , 1990, Radiologic imaging of inflicted injury in the child abuse syndrome, *Pediatric Clinics of North America* **37:**815–837

Merten, D F, Radkowski, M A , and Leonidas, J C , 1983, The abused child A radiological reappraisal, *Radiology* **146:**377

Ozonoff, M B , 1992, *Pediatric Orthopedic Radiology*, Saunders, Philadelphia

Robertson, D M , Barbor, P, and Hull, D , 1982, Unusual injury? Recent injury in normal children and children with suspected non-accidental injury, *British Medical Journal* **285:**1399–1401

Schmitt, B D , and Krugman, R D , 1992, Abuse and neglect of children, in *Nelson Textbook of Pediatrics* (R E Behrman, R M Kleigman, W E Nelson and V C Vaughan, eds), Saunders, Philadelphia

Silverman, F N , 1972, Unrecognized trauma in infants, the battered child syndrome, and the syndrome of Amboise Tardieu, *Radiology* **104:**337–353

Silverman, F N , 1980, Radiologic and special diagnostic procedures, in *The Battered Child*, 3rd ed (C H Kempe and R E Helfer, eds), University of Chicago Press, Chicago

Skinner, A E , and Castle, R L , 1969, *Battered Children A Retrospective Study*, National Society for the Prevention of Cruelty to Children, London

Tachdjian, M D , 1972, *Pediatric Orthopedics*, Saunders, Philadelphia

Taitz, L S , 1987, Child abuse and osteogenesis imperfecta, *British Medical Journal* **295:**1082–1083

Thomas, S A , Rosenfield, N S , Levental, J M , and Markowitz, R I , 1991, Long-bone fractures in young children Distinguishing accidental injuries from child abuse, *Pediatrics* **88:**471–476

Widom, C S , 1989, The cycle of violence, *Science* **244:**160–166

Worlock, P, Stower, M , and Barbor, P, 1986, Patterns of fractures in accidental and non-accidental injury in children A comparative study, *British Medical Journal* **293:**100–102

CHAPTER 4. REFERENCES

Edmonson, A S , and Crenshaw, A H , 1980, *Campbell's Operative Orthopedics*, 6th ed , Mosby, St Louis
Jacobs, J E , 1960, Metatarsus varus and hip dysplasia, *Clinical Orthopedics* **16**:203
Langenskiold, A , 1989, Tibia vara A critical review, *Clinical Orthopaedics and Related Research* **246**:195
Shopfner, C E , and Coin, C G , 1969, Genu varus and valgus in children, *Radiology* **92**:723
Smith, C F, 1982, Tibia vara (Blount's disease) Current concepts review, *Journal of Bone and Joint Surgery, American Volume* **64**:630
Staheli, L T , 1986, Torsional deformity, *Pediatric Clinics of North America* **33**(6):1373
Turek, S L , 1977, *Orthopaedics Principles and Their Application*, 3rd ed , Lippincott, Philadelphia
Wenger, D R , and Rang, M , 1993, *The Art and Practice of Children s Orthopaedics*, Raven Press, New York

CHAPTER 5. SUGGESTED READING

Bleck, E E , 1987, *Orthopaedic Management in Cerebral Palsy*, MacKeith Press, London
Farmer, T W (ed), 1983, *Pediatric Neurology*, Harper & Row, New York
Menkes, J H , 1985, *Textbook of Child Neurology*, 3rd ed , Lea & Febiger, Philadelphia
Wenger, D R , and Rang, M , 1993, *The Art and Practice of Children s Orthopaedics*, Raven Press, New York

CHAPTER 6. REFERENCES AND SUGGESTED READING

Aase, J M , 1990, *Diagnostic Dysmorphology*, Plenum Medical, New York
Beiser, G D , Epstein, S E , Stampfer, M , *et al* , 1972, Improvement of cardiac function in patients with pectus excavatum, with improvement after operative correction, *New England Journal of Medicine* **287**:267
Jones, K L (ed), 1988, *Smith's Recognizable Patterns of Human Malformation*, 4th ed , Saunders, Philadelphia
Morrissy, R T (ed), 1990, *Lovell and Winter's Pediatric Orthopaedics*, 3rd ed , Lippincott, Philadelphia
Ozonoff, M B , 1992, *Pediatric Orthopedic Radiology*, 2nd ed , Saunders, Philadelphia
Williams, P F, and Cole, W G (eds), 1991, *Orthopaedic Management in Childhood*, 2nd ed , Chapman & Hall Medical, London

CHAPTER 7. SUGGESTED READING

Beighton, P, 1988, *Inherited Disorders of the Skeleton*, 2nd ed , Churchill Livingstone, Edinburgh
Clark, C G D , 1991, *Clinical Paediatric Endocrinology*, 2nd ed , Blackwell Scientific, Oxford
Maroteaux, P, Faure, C , Fessard, C , and Rigault, P, translated by Kaufman, H , 1979, *Bone Diseases of Children*, Lippincott, Philadelphia
Wynne-Davies, R , Hall, C M , and Apley, A G , 1985, *Atlas of Skeletal Dysplasias*, Churchill Livingstone, Edinburgh

CHAPTER 8. REFERENCES AND SUGGESTED READING

DeHaven, K E , 1978, Athletic injuries in adolescents, *Pediatric Annals* **7**:704–714
Dupont, M , Beliveau, P, and Theriault, G , 1987, The efficacy of anti-inflammatory medication in the treatment of the acutely sprained ankle, *American Journal of Sports Medicine* **15**:41–45

Dyment, P G (ed), 1991, *Sports Medicine Health Care for Young Athletes*, 2nd ed , American Academy of Pediatrics, Elk Grove Village, Ill

Garrick, J G , and Requa, R K , 1978, Injuries in high school sports, *Pediatrics* **61**:465–469

Micheli, L J (ed), 1984, *Pediatric and Adolescent Sports Medicine*, Little, Brown, Boston

Sullivan, J A , and Grana, W A , 1990, *The Pediatric Athlete*, American Academy of Orthopaedic Surgeons, Park Ridge, Ill

Zaricznyj, B , Shattuck, L J , Mast, T A , Robertson, R V , and Delia, G , 1980, Sports related injuries in school-aged children, *American Journal of Sports Medicine* **8**:318–324

CHAPTER 9. REFERENCES AND SUGGESTED READING

Bradford, D S , and Hensinger, R M (eds), 1985, *The Pediatric Spine*, Thieme, Stuttgart

Crawford, A H , Kucharzyk, D W , Ruda, R , and Smitherman, H C , 1991, Diskitis in Children, *Clinical Orthopaedics and Related Research* **266**:70–79

Fredrickson, B E , Baker, D , McHolick, W J , Yuan, H A , and Lubicky, J P L , 1984, The natural history of spondylolysis and spondylolisthesis, *Journal of Bone and Joint Surgery* **66A**:699–707

Hensinger, R M , 1985, Back pain in children, in *The Pediatric Spine* (D S Bradford and R M Hensinger, eds), Thieme, Stuttgart, pp 41–60

Lonstein, J E , and Carlson, M J , 1981, Prognostication in idiopathic scoliosis, *Orthopaedic Transactions* **5**:22

Morrissy, R T (ed), 1990, *Lovell and Winter's Pediatric Orthopaedics*, 3rd ed , Lippincott, Philadelphia

Ozonoff, M B , 1992, *Pediatric Orthopedic Radiology*, Saunders, Philadelphia

CHAPTER 10. REFERENCES

Donn, S M , and Faix, R G , 1983, Long-term prognosis for the infant with severe birth trauma, *Clinics of Perinatology* **10**(2):507

Gobson, D A , and Carroll, N , 1970, Congenital pseudoarthrosis of the clavicle, *Journal of Bone and Joint Surgery* **52-B**:644

Gonik, B , Hollyer, V L , and Allen, R , 1991, Shoulder dystocia recognition Differences in neonatal risks for injury, *American Journal of Perinatology* **8**(1):31

Gresham, E L , 1975, Birth trauma, *Pediatric Clinics of North America* **22**(2):317

Jackson, T , Hoffer, M M , and Parrish, N , 1988, Brachial plexus palsy in the newborn, *Journal of Bone and Joint Surgery* **70-A**:1217

Nadas, S , and Reinberg, O , 1992, Obstetric fractures, *European Journal of Pediatric Surgery* **2**(3):165

Oppenheim, W L , Davis, A , Growden, W A , Dorey, F J , and Davlin, L B , 1990, Clavicle fractures in the newborn, *Clinical Orthopaedics and Related Research* **250**:176

Solonen, I S , and Uusitalo, R , 1990, Birth injuries Incidence and predisposing factors, *Zeitschrift fur Kinderchirurgie* **45**(3):133

CHAPTER 11. REFERENCES AND SUGGESTED READING

Cassidy, J T , and Petty, R E , 1990, *Textbook of Pediatric Rheumatology*, 2nd ed , Churchill Livingstone, Edinburgh

Jacobs, J C , 1982, *Pediatric Rheumatology for the Practitioner*, Springer-Verlag, Berlin

Morrissy, R T (ed), 1990, *Lovell and Winter's Pediatric Orthopaedics*, 3rd ed , Lippincott, Philadelphia

Schaffer, F M , Agarwal, R , Helm, J , Gingell, R L , Roland, J M A , and O'Neill, K M , 1992, Poststreptococcal reactive arthritis (PSA) The need for Doppler echocardiography and prophylactic antibiotic therapy, *56th Annual Scientific Meeting of the American College of Rheumatology* C137

Steere, A C , Malawista, S E , Snydman, D R , *et al* , 1977, Lyme arthritis An epidemic of oligoarticular arthritis in children and adults in three Connecticut communities, *Arthritis and Rheumatism* **20**:7

The Special Writing Group, 1992, Guidelines for the diagnosis of rheumatic fever Jones Criteria, 1992 update, *Journal of the American Medical Association* **268**:2069

Wallace, C A , and Sherry, D D , 1993, Facial scarring in children taking nonsteroidal anti-inflammatory drugs (NSAID), *57th Annual Scientific Meeting of the American College of Rheumatology* A151

Index

Figures are indicated by page numbers in italics and tables are indicated by page numbers in bold face.